Progress in Drug Research

Founded by Ernst Jucker

Progress in Drug Research

Advances in Targeted Cancer Therapy

Vol. 63

Edited by
Richard M. Schultz

Birkhäuser Verlag
Basel · Boston · Berlin

Editor

Dr. Richard M. Schultz
6551 Shelbyville Rd.
Indianapolis, IN 46237
USA

ISBN 10: 3-7643-7174-9 Birkhäuser Verlag, Basel – Boston – Berlin
ISBN 13: 978-3-7643-7174-6

Part of Springer Science+Business Media
Printed on acid-free paper produced from chlorine-free pulp. TCF ∞
Cover design and layout: Micha Lotrovsky, CH-4106 Therwil, Switzerland
Printed in Germany

ISBN 10: 3-7643-7174-9
ISBN 13: 978-3-7643-7174-6
e-ISBN: 3-7643-7414-4

9 8 7 6 5 4 3 2 1

www.birkhauser.ch

Contents

Foreword

Volume 63 of "Progress in Drug Research" is devoted to recent developments in targeted cancer therapy. Significant advances in the fields of molecular and tumor biology over the past decade have led to this exciting new era in cancer therapeutics with an intensive effort in rationally-designed cancer therapeutic strategies directed against selective molecular targets. These selective approaches may ultimately lead to tailoring treatments to individual patients where molecular biomarkers of sensitivity to therapy are identified, producing better tolerated therapies with less side effects than past experiences with cytotoxic cancer chemotherapy, and reducing cancer to a controlled, chronic state. This volume contains eleven chapters, including updated reviews on a range of targets, such as tumor angiogenesis, apoptosis/cell survival pathways, and various inhibitors of cyclin-dependent kinases, cyclooxygenase-2 (COX-2), epidermal growth factor receptor (EGFR), and histone deacetylases (HDAC). Additional topics, including target validation, polypharmacology and potential synergy of involving multiple targets, antisense approaches, animal models for preclinical development of targeted agents, and obstacles, including development of resistance are also presented. In addition, the particular challenges involved in translating preclinical data to clinical application are discussed. It gives me great pleasure to present this new volume. I would like to express my gratitude to the chapter authors, to Birkhauser Verlag and, in particular, to Dr. Beatrice Menz and Ms. Gabriele Poppen for their assistance in compiling and editing this volume.

April 2005 Richard M. Schultz

Progress in Drug Research, Vol. 63
(R. M. Schultz, Ed.)

Dawn of a new era in molecular cancer therapeutics

Richard M. Schultz

Division of Cancer Research
Lilly Research Laboratories
Lilly Corporate Center
Indianapolis, IN 46285, USA
<Rick_1252@msn.com>

1 Introduction to the new paradigm (molecular phenotype determines response)

The era of cancer chemotherapy began in the 1940s with the initial use of antifolate drugs and nitrogen mustards. The clinical use of these cytotoxic (cell-killing) chemotherapeutic agents against malignant tumors is successful in many cases, but suffers from major drawbacks: One being the lack of selectivity which leads to severe side effects and limited efficacy; the other being the emergence/selection of drug resistance. Traditional chemotherapy often debilitates patients with severe nausea, diarrhea and/or opportunistic infections. Moreover, cytotoxic chemotherapy is known to cause a range of long-term health problems to survivors, including hearing loss, heart damage, joint problems and memory impairment. Despite these limitations and the emergence of targeted agents with more tumor selectivity, many oncologists believe that these traditional agents will continue to be used for at least a decade due to the high unmet needs of the disease.

Cancer drug therapy is undergoing a major transition from the previous pregenomic cytotoxic era to the new postgenomic targeted era [1–6]. New cancer drugs that target tumor cells and leave normal healthy cells alone are just beginning to change the face of cancer treatment. The assessment of their efficacy will differ in terms of response however from that of traditional chemotherapy, since targeted treatments with cytostatic effect do not usually lead to reduction in tumor mass. Truly, the new knowledge of the regulation of cell growth and biochemical changes that lead to malignancy has created many new opportunities for targeted cancer drug discovery. Even if oncologists can't cure some tumors, they hope to use the new targeted therapies to turn them into chronic illnesses that are managed, for example, like diabetes.

One of the most frustrating aspects of traditional cancer treatment is the lack of knowledge why particular drug therapies help some patients yet fail to work in, or even significantly harm others. Researchers involved in the new field of individualized cancer care are seeking ways to predict in advance through genetic markers and molecular profiling whether a patient will respond to a given treatment. This should lead ultimately to a day when cancer care is commonly tailored or personalized to a particular patient's genetic make-up. For example, two teams of Boston (USA) scientists working separately at Massachusetts General Hospital and the Dana-Farber Cancer Institute recently announced they had found that lung cancer patients with specific genetic mutations were highly likely to respond to the new drug Iressa (gefitinib), while those without the mutations were not responsive [7–10]. This finding explains why the drug, which targets the cancer-fueling epidermal growth factor receptor (EGFR), only works in about 10 percent of these patients, those with abnormal EGFR genes. This discovery will help doctors determine whether to try Iressa versus another therapy in a particular patient.

Ultimately, oncologists should gain the ability to target the targeted therapies for optimizing patient outcomes.

Some examples of currently marketed, targeted drugs for cancer therapeutics are shown in Table 1. They represent several definitions (or subgroups) for the term *targeted therapy* [4, 11, 12]: 1) drugs requiring a diagnostic "eligibility" test, such as Trastuzumab in HER2/neu over-expressing metastatic breast cancer [13–15], Imatinib in bcr/abl-positive chronic myelogenous leukemia [10, 16, 17], and Cetuximab in EGFR over-expressing metastatic colorectal cancer [18–20]; 2) drugs targeting a specific pathway, such as Gefitinib targeting EGFR in lung cancer [7–9]; Bevacizumab targeting vascular endothelial growth factor (VEGF) in colorectal cancer [21–23], and Bortezomib targeting the proteasome in multiple myeloma [24, 25]; 3) antibody targeted therapies for hematologic malignancies guided by the immunophenotype, such as Rituximab (Rituxan, anti-CD20 antibody) in non-Hodgkin's lymphoma [26, 27], Gemtuzumab (Myelotarg, anti-CD33 antibody) in acute myelogenous leukemia [28], and Alemtuzumab (Campath, anti-CD52 antibody) in chronic lymphocytic leukemia [29]. Avastin (Bevacizumab), a monoclonal antibody therapeutic, is the first cancer drug to specifically target angiogenesis and does so by neutralizing VEGF.

A tremendous diversity of targets is available for potential cancer therapeutics. There are more than 100 distinct types of cancers and tumor subtypes, and tumorigenesis itself is a multistep process that involves a series of premalignant changes. The complex signaling pathways in tumor progression, the multiple stages in tumor growth, the dependence on the tumor microenvironment, the development of tumor cell invasion and metastasis formation, and the interaction of the tumor with complex cell types presents numerous targets for therapeutic intervention in cancer. Identification of the next generation of therapeutic targets for cancer drug development from among the products of the ~40000 genes in the human genome represents the paramount challenge for "post-genomics" drug discovery. The aim of this article is to give a brief introduction to the field of targeted cancer therapeutics.

Table 1.
Some examples of approved targeted drugs in cancer.

	Company	Mechanism	Indications	Toxicities
Trastuzumab (Herceptin) [13–15]	Genentech	Humanized monoclonal antibody against HER2	Metastatic breast cancer expressing HER2	Cardiotoxicity
Imatinib (Gleevec) [10, 16, 17]	Novartis	Small molecule inhibitor of Bcr-Abl and c-kit tyrosine kinases	Chronic myelogenous leukemia and gastro-intestinal stromal tumors	Nausea, diarrhea, myalgia, edema
Gefitinib (Iressa) [7–9]	AstraZeneca	Small molecule tyrosine kinase inhibitor of EGFR	Third-line treatment of non-small cell lung cancer	Diarrhea, nausea, rash, pulmonary toxicity
Cetuximab (Erbitux) [18–20]	Imclone/Bristol-Myers Squibb	Chimeric monoclonal antibody against EGFR	EGFR-positive, irinotecan-refractory metastatic colorectal carcinoma	Acneiform rash, folliculitis, hypersensitivity reactions
Bevacizumab (Avastin) [21–23]	Genentech	Humanized monoclonal antibody against vascular endothelial grow factor (VEGF)	First-line treatment for metastatic colorectal cancer	Hypertension, intestinal perforation (rare)
Bortezomib (Velcade) [24, 25]	Millennium co-developed with Johnson and Johnson	Small molecule protea-some inhibitor	Multiple myeloma relapsed after two prior treatments	Gastrointestinal symptoms, fatigue, thrombo-cytopenia, and sensory neuropathy
Rituximab (Rituxan) [26, 27]	IDEC Pharmaceuticals	Chimeric monoclonal antibody against CD20 antigen (expressed on mature B-cells)	Refractory low-grade and follicular B-cell non-Hodgkin's lymphoma	Infusion-related symptoms: fever, chills, nausea, urticaria

2 Identification of new molecular targets

Cancer is a stepwise process in which mutations in regulatory genes and epigenetic effects eventually progress to result in the loss of control of normal gene expression and, ultimately, cellular function [30]. Epidemiologic studies suggest that between seven and nine genetic or epigenetic changes must accumulate in a single cell to result in the acquisition of the spectrum of events required to become a clinically evident cancer. At the cellular level, the genetic and epigenetic changes must be "fixed" in the genome and inherited by daughter cells of the original clone. The corollary to this concept is that the spectrum of genetic changes that accumulate in a patient's tumor determines the aggressiveness of the tumor, which tumors will have high metastatic potential, which individuals will have a good or poor outcome, and which patients will respond to particular chemotherapy or molecular therapy approaches [31]. There is mounting evidence that each patient's cancer has a unique subset of molecular pathogenetic derangements, even for tumors that appear similar morphologically [32–34]. The identification of appropriate targets is based on a detailed understanding of the molecular changes underlying cancer.

In their paper entitled "The Hallmarks of Cancer" [35], Hanahan and Weinberg suggest that most or perhaps even all malignant cell types manifest six essential cellular alterations, referred to as acquired capabilities: self sufficiency to growth signals, insensitivity to growth-inhibitory signals (antigrowth), evasion of programmed cell death (apoptosis), limitless replicative potential, sustained angiogenesis, and tissue invasion and metastasis. The authors concluded "With holistic clarity of mechanism, cancer prognosis and treatment will become a rational science, unrecognizable by current practitioners". The oncology portfolio in most companies can be broken down across these six acquired capabilities of tumors [36].

Ross and colleagues identified seven features of the ideal anticancer target [11]: 1) crucial to the malignant phenotype; 2) not significantly expressed in vital organs and tissues; 3) a biologically relevant molecular feature; 4) expression reproducibly measurable in readily obtained clinical samples; 5) expression correlated with clinical outcome; 6) clinical response in a significant proportion of patients whose tumors express the target when target interrupted, interfered with, or inhibited; 7) minimal responses in patients whose tumors do not express the target.

High-throughput, global (genome-wide), unbiased technologies are rapidly developing a plethora of cellular events that correlate with patient outcomes [1, 37, 38]. Gene expression profiles from primary tumors are now being used to generate models that can be highly predictive of patient outcome [39, 40]. True cancer profiling is a complementary combination of genomics, transcriptional profiling, and proteomics [41]. These technologies include methods to globally assess changes at the DNA level (comparative genomic hybridization), loss of heterozygosity, DNA methylation (restriction landmark genomic scanning and methylation assays), RNA (transcriptional profiling and serial anaysis of gene expression), and protein level (2-dimensional gels, mass spectrometry, and protein and antibody arrays) [1, 42–52]. DNA microarrays have provided detailed molecular information, which is useful for target identification, prognostics and treatment options [42–46]. On the other hand, protein microarrays provide insights into cell signaling events that are evolving and adapting within a cell or a tumor [47–49]. A combination of laser capture microdissection (LCM) of tumors with multiplexed phosphoproteomic analysis using reverse phase protein microarray technology is being used to identify protein molecular signatures of individual tumors, including the *in vivo* state of multiple kinase-driven signaling pathways [37]. Currently, many efforts are concentrating on modulating cellular signaling pathways in cancer [53, 54]. Arrays that utilize LCM-procured cancer epithelial cells can assay the functional status of the pathways of interest and may be used to rapidly identify which target should undergo pharmacologic intervention, as well as assess how effective in mitigating changes in the deranged pathways a given therapy has become. These tools are illuminating the molecular derangements of individual tumors, even if these tumors have similar morphological characteristics, and assist in identifying new biomarkers for early detection/monitoring of the patient's tumor and new molecular targets for therapy.

3 Target validation

Initially core banked tumor tissue resources with annotated clinical follow-up are required to correlate expression or alteration of the candidate gene with clinical outcome. Those candidate targets with defined aberrant expression and/or genetic alteration, along with strong correlation with clinical prognosis, should be given the highest priority for development of new anti-cancer agents. The most commonly used strategy to validate a target once it has been shown to be aberrant or mutated in tumors is to alter its levels of expression or function, either in cell lines or in animal models, and to determine its effects on tumor development and growth. This can be accomplished by increasing or decreasing levels of expression or altering function by using chemical genetic approaches [55].

Target identification and validation can involve knocking down the target to see the desired biological effect in cells using approaches such as gene knockouts (even sophisticated "inducible knockouts" [56]) and RNA-based methods like small interfering RNA (siRNA) [57] or antisense RNA. The recent development of strategies to conditionally knock out the function of genes in a tissue specific manner has enabled investigators to engineer mice to demonstrate that the targeted inactivation of specific oncogenes can be effective in inducing sustained regression of tumors [56]. Genetic demonstration that loss of function is associated with a reduction in tumor formation or growth rate has been taken as support for the validity of a putative drug target. Expression of a potential target gene in a transgenic mouse can provide an *in vivo* model for evaluation of potential therapeutic strategies. However, these processes are time-consuming and fraught with technical and conceptual difficulties [31]. For example, if the levels of gene expression or activation assessed in the model systems do not match those present in tumors, the subsequent results may be noninformative. Similarly, multiple genetic aberrations may collaborate to generate the tumorigenic phenotype. Moreover, Higa [58] pointed out that the complexities involved in the pathways do not allow for a simple linear model (coupling cell surface message reception to nuclear gene expression) for signal transduction. Instead, a highly integrated circuit is comprised of numerous molecular components (some perhaps with overlapping, redundant, or compensating functions) that are harmoniously programmed to communicate a multitude of internal signals that control the cellular response.

Besides the validation of the target, the validation of the disease model creates a huge bottleneck in drug discovery. Studies of animal models are fraught with concerns that they may not reflect the pathophysiologic state of human tumors [59, 60]. This reinforces the requirement to validate the target in human clinical samples prior to investing the large time and monetary requirements for drug development. Validation of a model requires both a detailed understanding of the underlying scientific assumptions along with evidence of correspondence between the observed model disease phenotype and the human disease condition. Target validation is a process through which the proof of the causative role of the molecular target in a disease is discovered. However, the discovery of effective drugs requires a substantially different answer: Can the system, after perturbation by a small molecule or other therapeutic agent, return to a normal state, or counter the disease phenotype, to alleviate the symptoms [61]? Moreover, targets can only be considered fully validated when tested in patients in suitably designed clinical trials. Translating bench science to the clinic and feeding information from clinic back into discovery helps drive oncology research [62].

Pharmacodynamic evaluation of drug effects has become an integral feature of molecular targeted drug development. Gleevec targets specific kinases and has established a paradigm for the treatment of tumors whose growth is acutely dependent on specific kinase targets. Chronic myeloid leukemia is driven by the mutant kinase fusion protein Bcr-Abl, which displays constitutive activation of the Abl kinase, whereas gastrointestinal stromal tumors are caused by activating point mutations in the c-Kit and platelete derived growth factor (PDGF) receptor α-kinases. Gleevec effectively blocks the activity of all three kinases and produces dramatic clinical responses in all three situations in a manner that correlates precisely with the presence of these mutations in the tumor [5, 63]. The polypharmacology (inhibition of multiple mutant kinases) of Gleevec point to the requirement to fully understand target validation, since off-target effects may be responsible for antitumor activity in certain tumor models or individual patients. Gleevec has been extensively studied from the pharmacodynamic standpoint in preclinical models [64]. The Abl kinase is currently viewed as one of the best validated molecular targets in the new era of cancer drug discovery and development [17, 59, 65, 66]. Similarly, point mutations in the EGFR domain kinase domain are associated with clinical responses to Iressa in non-small cell lung cancer [7–9, 67] (thereby explaining the rather modest 10% response in all patients). These experiences clearly show that clinical responses to kinase inhibitors occur in tumors bearing specific activating mutations that drive tumor progression. The caveats/challenges for developing further therapies targeting mutant kinases have previously been reviewed [5, 68, 69]. Clinical studies with imatinib demonstrate the importance of identifying a molecular target that can be inhibited and that also provides a critical transforming signal for tumor cells. The requirement for accurate genetic diagnosis wherever possible is also emphasized (see next section).

4 Molecular diagnostics and patient selection for targeted therapies

The clinical development of targeted agents is particularly problematic because the current clinical trial paradigms were not developed for targeted therapeutics, which may be cytostatic rather than cytotoxic and also may not show toxicity at levels that effectively inhibit the target in the tumor tissue [70]. The question of whether patient enrollment should be restricted to patients whose tumor expresses the target of interest has been raised. For example, trastuzumab (Herceptin) only appears active in patients whose tumors over-express HER2 (30% of breast cancer patients). Had the trials been performed in all breast cancer patients, the effects would have been diluted with a large number of nonresponders. Indeed, modeling studies indicate that the effects of trastuzumab would not have been detected if all breast cancer patients had been included in the trials [31]. Dancey suggested that tumor imaging modalities for targeted agents may also play an important role in drug development [71]. Novel trial designs and approaches need to be implemented to fulfill the promise of individualized molecular medicine. Moreover, it is necessary to link targeted therapeutics to molecular diagnostics to identify individual patients most likely to respond to the targeted therapeutics under development. In this regard, accurate and reproducible assays must be developed to identify target patient populations, and these assays need to be validated in clinical trials, especially by analyzing the correlation of target expression (or over-expression) with clinical response to therapy. A strong commitment in clinical translational research is needed for parallel development of diagnostics/biomarkers along with investigational therapeutics. If the assay for a putative target does not identify a population that benefits, then therapy is not targeted [6, 68]. Similarly, if the target is known, but no reliable biomarker exists, therapy is not targeted. It is possible that more than one marker may be needed for testing, since the presence of the target might be necessary but not sufficient for antitumor activity. Moreover, if the treatment is effective but antitumor activity is not restricted to the population that expresses the target, therapy is again not targeted. Using molecular diagnostics to select the patient population most likely respond has important implications in statistical design and cost of clinical trials.

Hortobagyi [68] presented several important considerations for the future clinical development of targeted therapies: 1) select critical targets, i.e. those that drive the cancer cells' malignant behavior; 2) define molecular predictor(s) of response or resistance before clinical trials start, if possible; 3) develop relevant diagnostic test(s); 4) phase I studies should include proof of principle: *in vivo* inhibition of the target by the agent under investigation which requires, in most instances, tissue sampling at multiple times; 5) phase I studies should identify optimal (or effective) biological dose, rather than maximum tolerated dose; 6) evaluation of targeted therapies in unselected patient groups is wasteful; 7) phase II studies should not start until a targeted population can be confidently identified and an optimal biological dose has been identified (for some phase II studies, biological endpoints might lead to the most relevant assessment of activity); 8) endpoints of clinical trials need to be redefined (response rate does not necessarily predict patient benefit); and 9) for phase III studies, progression-free and overall survival should be optimal endpoints. It is critical that the clinical development of targeted therapy is concentrated in proof-of-principle trials to show that the drug reaches the tumor in sufficient concentrations to inhibit the target. Development of these newer therapeutic agents will require a cultural change in oncology, so that empirical trials are replaced by rational methods of drug development based on sound scientific principles.

5 Resistance to targeted agents

Although the development of molecular targeted antitumor agents is rapidly changing cancer therapeutics, drug resistance to these novel agents remains a real clinical concern [5, 69, 72–74]. For example, three broad mechanisms of resistance may inhibit the antitumor activity of imatinib in chronic myeloid leukemia [69]: 1) decreased intracellular levels of imatinib; 2) increased expression of the kinase; or 3) intrinsic changes in the kinase that affect its drug interaction or kinase activity. MDR1 overexpression causing drug efflux has been shown to cause imatinib resistance in Ph+ cell leukemia lines *in vitro* [75]. Increased levels of Bcr-Abl kinase, related to genomic amplification of the gene, or increased levels of expression have been observed [76, 77]. Moreover, exposure to low levels of imatinib *in vitro* promoted the development of genomic amplification, whereas effective drug levels did not [76]. Finally, mutations of Bcr-Abl may impair imatinib binding and appear to be the most common mechanism of resistance encountered in clinical practice [77–80]. In CML patients treated with imatinib, emergence of resistance due to mutations at amino positions 250–255, which form the adenosine triphosphate-binding loop (P-loop), produced an especially poor prognosis with 12 of 13 patients (92%) dying at a median of 18 weeks from the detection of the mutation [79]. It is possible that mutations conferring resistance are present in a small number of leukemic cells in CML prior to treatment and are positively selected by imatinib therapy [81]. Recent preclinical studies have identified second generation dual Src/Abl kinase inhibitors that retain activity against nearly all the imatinib-resistant mutants [82], raising the possibility that future therapy with dual inhibitors and/or cocktails of inhibitors may prevent the emergence of resistant subclones. It is also possible that the ongoing development of new targeted therapies may be useful in combating resistance from classical cytotoxic chemotherapy or radiation therapy [5, 83–85].

6 Concluding remarks

Exciting new research on the molecular pathways and mechanisms that control tumor cell growth and differentiation has resulted in a quantum leap in our understanding of the fundamental nature of cancer cells and has suggested valuable new approaches to cancer diagnosis and treatment. Indeed, the field of molecular therapeutics has clearly arrived, but patients and practitioners are yearning for this approach to have a broader impact. The successes of the past few years with Herceptin, Gleevec, and Iressa have exemplified the potential utility of innovative molecular therapeutics in the clinic. Developments in high throughput screening, structural biology, and microarray technology are increasing the speed of drug discovery. Drugs acting on a wide range of new genome–based molecular targets are now in preclinical and clinical development [53, 54, 68, 86–93]. We are progressing in the direction of customized cancer care for the individual patient due to the genetic make-up of their malignancy.

In a recent review, Seynaeve and Verweij [94] posed the following question in their title: "Targeted therapy: ready for prime time?" I believe that the answer is a resounding "yes" and look forward to the exciting developments of the future!

References

1 Desany B, Zemin Z (2004) Bioinformatics and cancer target discovery. *Drug Discovery Today* 9: 795–802

2 Workman P (2001) New drug targets for genomic cancer therapy: successes, limitations, opportunities and future challenges. *Curr Cancer Drug Targets* 1: 33–47

3 Guillemard V, Sargovi HU (2004) Novel approaches for targeted cancer therapy. *Curr Cancer Drug Targets* 4: 313–326

4 Segota E, Bukowski RM (2004) The promise of targeted therapy: Cancer drugs become more specific. *Cleveland Clinic J Med* 71: 551–560

5 Sawyers C (2004) Targeted cancer therapy. *Nature* 432: 294–297

6 Pegram M, Pietras R, Bajamonde A, Klein P, Fyfe G (2005) Targeted therapy: Wave of the future. *J Clin Oncol* 23: 1776–1781

7 Paez JG, Janne PA, Lee JC, Tracy S, Greulich H, Gabriel S, Herman P, Kaye FJ, Lindeman N, Boggon TJ et al (2004) EGFR mutations in lung cancer: Correlation with clinical response to gefitinib therapy. *Science* 304: 1497–1500

8 Lynch TJ, Bell DW, Sordella R (2004) Activating mutations in the epidermal growth factor receptor underlying responsiveness of non-small-cell lung cancer to gefitinib. *New Engl J Med* 350: 1–11

9 Golsteyn RM (2004) The story of gefitinib, an EGFR kinase that works in lung cancer. *Drug Discovery Today* 9: 587

10 Tibes R, Trent J, Kurzrock R (2005) Tyrosine kinase inhibitors and the dawn of molecular cancer therapeutics. *Annu Rev Pharmacol Toxicol* 45: 357–384

11 Ross JS, Schenkein DP, Pietrusko R, Rolfe M, Linette GP, Stec J, Stagliano NE, Ginsburg GS, Symmans WF, Pusztai L, Hortobagyi GN (2004) Targeted therapies for cancer 2004. *Am J Clin Pathol* 122: 598–609

12 Abou-Jawde R, Choueiri T, Alemany C, Mekhail T (2003) An overview of targeted treatments in cancer. *Cancer Therapeutics* 25: 2121–2129

13 Vogel CL, Cobleigh MA, Tripathy D, Gutheil JC, Harris LN, Fehrenbacher L, Slamon DJ, Murphy M, Novotny WF, Burchmore M et al (2001) First-line Herceptin monotherapy in metastatic breast cancer. *Oncology* 61 suppl 2: 37–42

14 Pegram MD, Konecny G, Slamon DJ (2000) The molecular and cell biology of HER2/neu gene amplification/overexpression and the clinical development of herceptin (trastuzumab) therapy for breast cancer. *Cancer Treatment and Res* 103: 57–75

15 Gianni L (2002) The future of targeted therapy: combining novel agents. *Oncology* 63 suppl 1: 47–56

16 Joensuu H, Dimitrijevic S (2001) Tyrosine kinase inhibitor imatinib (ST1571) as an anticancer agent for solid tumors. *Ann Med* 33: 451–455

17 Manley PW, Cowan-Jacob SW, Buchdunger E, Fabbro D, Fendrich G, Furet P, Meyer T, Zimmermann J (2002) Imatinib: a selective tyrosine kinase inhibitor. *Europ J Cancer* 38 suppl 5: S19–27

18 Cunningham D, Humblet Y, Siena S (2003) Cetuximab (C225) alone or in combination with irinotecan (CPT-11) in patients with epidermal growth factor receptor (EGFR)-positive, irinotecan-refractory metastatic colorectal cancer (MCRC). *Proc Am Soc Clin Oncol* 22: abstr 1012

19 O'dwyer PJ, Benson AB III (2002) Epidermal growth factor receptor-targeted therapy in colorectal cancer. *Semin Oncol* 29 suppl 14: 10–17

20 Waksal HW (1999) Role of an anti-epidermal growth factor receptor in treating cancer. *Cancer Metastasis Rev* 18: 427–436
21 Berlin JD (2002) Targeting vascular endothelial growth factor in colorectal cancer. *Oncology (Huntingt)*16 (8 suppl 7): 13–15
22 McCarthy M (2003) Antiangiogenesis drug promising for metastatic colorectal cancer. *Lancet* 361: 1959
23 Salgaller ML (2003) Technology evaluation: bevacizumab, Genentech/Roche. *Curr Opin Mol Ther* 5: 657–667
24 Richardson PG, Barlogie B, Berenson J (2003) A phase 2 study of bortezomib in relapsed, refractory myeloma. *N Engl J Med* 348: 2609–2617
25 Voorhees PM, Dees EC, O'Neil B, Orlowski RZ (2003) The proteasome as a target for cancer therapy. *Clin Cancer Res* 9: 6316–6325
26 McLaughlin P, Grillo-Lopez AJ, Link BK, Levy R, Czuczman MS, Williams ME, Heyman MR, Bence-Bruckler I, White CA, Cabanillas F et al (1998) Rituximab chimeric anti-CD20 monoclonal antibody therapy for relapsed indolent lymphoma: half of patients respond to a four-dose treatment program. *J Clin Oncol* 16: 2825–2833
27 Igarashi T, Itoh K, Kobayashi Y (2002) Phase II and pharmacokinetic study of rituximab with eight weekly infusions in relapsed aggressive B-cell non-Hodgkin's lymphoma (B-NHL). *Proc Am Soc Clin Oncol* 21: 286a
28 Sievers EL (2001) Efficacy and safety of gemtuzumab ozogamicin in patients with CD-33 positive acute myeloid leukemia in first relapse. *Expert Opin Biol Ther* 1: 893–901
29 Keating MJ, Flinn I, Jain V (2000) Therapeutic role of alemtuzumab (Campath-1H) in patients who have failed fludarabine: results of a large international study. *Blood* 99: 3554–3561
30 Mao JH, Wheldon TE (1995) A stochastic model for multistage tumorigenesis in developing and adult mice. *Math Biosci* 129: 95–110
31 Kohn EC, Lu Y, Wang H, Yu Q, Yu S, Hall H, Smith DL, Meric-Bernstam F, Hortobagyi GN, Mills GB (2004) Molecular therapeutics: promise and challenges. *Semin Oncol* 31 suppl 3: 39–53
32 Petricoin EF, Zoon KC, Kohn EC, Berrett JC, Liotta, LA (2002) Clinical proteomics: translating benchside promise into bedside reality. *Nat Rev Drug Discov* 9: 683–695
33 Liotta LA, Kohn EC (2001) The microenvironment of the tumour-host interface. *Nature* 6835: 375–379
34 Reed JC (1999) Dysregulation of apoptosis in cancer. *J Clin Oncol* 9: 2941–2953
35 Hanahan D, Weinberg R (2000) The hallmarks of cancer. *Cell* 100: 57–70
36 Hughes L (2004) Humanizing drug discovery. *Drug Discov Development* 7: 30–34
37 Espina V, Geho D, Mehta AI, Petricoin EF III, Liotta L, Rosenblatt KP (2005) Pathology of the future: molecular profiling for targeted therapy. *Cancer Investigation* 1: 36–46
38 Bichsel VE, Liotta LA, Petricoin EF III (2001) Cancer proteomics: from biomarker discovery to signal pathway profiling. *Cancer J* 7: 69–78
39 Van't Veer LJ, Dai H, van deVijer MJ, He YD, Hart AAM, Mao M, Peterse HL, van der Kooy K, Marton MJ, Witteveen AT (2002) Gene expression profiling predicts clinical outcome of breast cancer. *Nature* 415: 530–536
40 Yeoh EJ, Ross ME, Shertleff SA, Williams WK, Patel D, Mahfouz R, Behm FG, Raimondi SC, Relling MV, Patel A et al (2002) Classification, subtype discovery and prediction of outcome in pediatric acute lymphoblastic leukemia by gene expression profiling. *Cancer Cell* 1: 133–143

41 Ideker T, Thorsson V, Ranish JA, Christmas R, Buhler J, Eng JK, Bumgarner R, Goodlett DR, Aebersold R, Hood L (2001) Integrated genomic and proteomic analyses of a systematically perturbed metabolic network. *Science* 5518: 929–934

42 Miller LD, Long PM, Wong L, Mukherjee S, McShane LM, Liu ET (2002) Optimal gene expression analysis by microarrays. *Cancer Cell* 5: 353–361

43 Clarke PA, te Poele R, Wooster R, Workman P (2001) Gene expression microarray analysis in cancer biology, pharmacology, and drug development: Progress and potential. *Biochem Pharmacol* 62: 1311–1136

44 Ramaswamy S, Tamayo P, Rifkin R (2001) Multiclass cancer diagnosis using tumor gene expression signatures. *Proc Natl Acad Sci USA* 98: 15149–15143

45 Sorlie T, Perou CM, Tibshirani R, Aas T, Geisler S, Johnsen H, Hastie T, Eisen MB, van de Rijn M, Jeffrey SS et al (2001) Gene expression patters of breast carcinomas distinguish tumor subclasses with clinical implications. *Proc Natl Acad Sci USA* 98: 10869–10874

46 Beer DG, Kardia SL, Huang CC, Giordano TJ, Levin AM, Misek DE, Lin L, Chen G, Gharib TG, Thomas DG et al (2002) Gene-expression profiles predict survival of patients with lung adenocarcinoma. *Nat Med* 8: 816–824

47 Liotta L, Petricoin E (2000) Proteomic profiling of human cancer. *Nature Rev Genet* 1: 48–56

48 Liotta LA, Espina V, Mehta AI (2003) Protein microarrays: Meeting analytical challenges for clinical applications. *Cancer Cell* 3: 317–325

49 Liotta LA, Kohn EC, Petricoin EF (2001) Clinical proteomics: Personalized molecular medicine. *JAMA* 286: 2211–2214

50 Wei SH, Chen CM, Strathdee G, Harnsomburana J, Shyu CR, Rahmatpanah F, Shi H, Ng SW, Yan PS, Nephew KP et al (2002) Methylation microarry analysis of late-stage ovarian carcinoma distinguish progression-free survival in patients and identifies candidate epigenetic markers. *Clin Cancer Res* 8: 2246–2252

51 Rush LJ, Plass C (2002) Restriction landmark genomic scanning for DNA methylation in cancer: Past, present, and future applications. *Anal Biochem* 307: 191–201

52 Snijders AM, Nowak N, Segraves R, Blackwood S, Brown N, Conroy J, Hamilton G, Hindle AK, Huey B, Kimura K et al (2001) Assembly of microarrays for genome-wide measurement of DNA copy number. *Nat Genet* 29: 263–264

53 Kumar R and Hung M-C (2005) Signaling intricacies take center stage in cancer cells. *Cancer Res* 65: 2511–2515

54 Ravandi F, Talpaz M, Estrov Z (2003) Modulation of cellular signaling pathways: prospects for targeted therapy in hematological malignancies. *Clin Cancer Res* 9: 535–550

55 Shokat K, Velleca M (2002) Novel chemical genetic approaches to the discovery of signal transduction inhibitors. *Drug Discovery Today* 7: 872–879

56 Giuriato S, Rabin K, Fan AC, Shachaf CM, Felsher DW (2004) Conditional animal models: a strategy to define when ocogenes will be effective targets to treat cancer. *Semin Cancer Biol* 14: 3–11

57 Xie FY, Liu Y, Xu J, Tang QQ, Scaria PV, Zhou Q, Woodle MC, Lu PY (2004) Delivering siRNA to animal disease models for validation of novel drug targets in vivo. *Pharma Genomics* 4: 28–38

58 Higa GM (2004) Targeted therapies in oncology: in the crosshairs or at the crossroads? *Expert Rev Anticancer Ther* 4: 61–75

59 Kelland LR (2004) "Of mice and men": values and liabilities of the athymic nude mouse model in anticancer drug development. Europ J Cancer 40: 827–836
60 Roberts RB, Arteaga CL, Threadgill DW (2004) Modeling the cancer patient with genetically engineered mice: prediction of toxicity from molecular-targeted therapies. *Cancer Cell* 5: 115–120
61 Hopkins A (2004) Are drugs discovered in the clinic or in the laboratory. *Drug Discovery Today* 3: 173–175
62 Koppal T (2004) Humanizing drug discovery. *Drug Discovery and Development* 7: 30–34
63 Sawyers CL (2003) Opportunities and challenges in the development of kinase inhibitor therapy for cancer. Genes Dev 17: 2998–3010
64 le Coutre P, Mologni L, Cleris L, Marchesi E, Buchdunger E, Giardini R, Formelli F, Gambacorti-Passerini C (1999) In vivo eradication of human Bcr/Abl-positive leukemia cells with an Abl kinase inhibitor. *J Natl Cancer Inst* 91: 163–168
65 Buchdunger E, Zimmermann J, Mett H, Meyer T, Muller M, Druker BJ, Lydon NB (1996) Inhibition of the Abl protein-tyrosine kinase *in vitro* and *in vivo* by a 2-phenylaminopyrimidine derivative. *Cancer Res* 56: 100–104
66 Carroll M, Ohno-Jones S, Tamura S, Buchdunger E, Zimmermann J, Lydon NB, Gilliland DG, Druker BJ (1997) CGP 57148, a tyrosine kinase inhibitor, inhibits the growth of cells expressing Bcr-Abl, Tel-Abl, and Tel-PDGFR fusion proteins. *Blood* 90: 4947–4952
67 Khalil MY, Grandis JR, Shin DM (2003) Targeting epidermal growth factor receptor: novel therapeutics for the management of cancer. *Expert Rev Anticancer Ther* 3: 367–380
68 Hortobagyi GN (2004) Opportunities and challenges in the development of targeted therapies. *Semin Oncol* 31 suppl 3: 21–27
69 Ross DM, Hughes TP (2004) Cancer treatment with kinase inhibitors: what have we learnt from imatinib? *Br J Cancer* 90: 12–19
70 Schiller JH (2004) Clinical trial design issues in the era of targeted therapies. *Clin Cancer Res* 10: 4281s–4282s
71 Dancey JE (2003) Recent advances of molecular agents: opportunities for imaging. *Cancer Biol Ther* 2: 601–609
72 Vidal L, Attard G, Kaye S, DeBono J (2004) Reversing resistance to targeted therapy. *J Chemother* 16 suppl 4: 7–12
73 Akiyama S (2004) The mechanisms of the resistance to molecular targeted agents. *Nippon Rinsho* 62: 1297–1304
74 Kim R, Toge T (2004) Changes in therapy for solid tumors: potential for overcoming drug resistance in vivo for molecular targeted agents. *Surg Today* 34: 293–303
75 Mahon F-X, Belloc F, Legarde V, Chollet C, Moreau-Gaudry F, Reiffers J, Goldman JM, Melo JV (2003) MDR1 gene overexpression confers resistance to imatinib mesylate in leukemia cell line models. *Blood* 101: 2368–2373
76 Le Coutre, P, Tassi, E, Varella-Garcia M, Barni R, Mologna L, Cabrita G, Marchesi E, Supino R, Gamacorti-Passerini CB (2000) Inducion of resistance to the Abelson inhibitor ST1571 in human leukemia cells through gene amplification. *Blood* 95: 1758–1766.
77 Gorre ME, Mohammed M, Ellwood K, Hsu N, Paquette R, Rao PN, Sawyers CL (2001) Clinical resistance to STI-571 cancer therapy caused by Bcr-Abl gene mutation or amplification. *Science* 293: 876–880

78 Branford S, Rudzki Z, Walsh S, Grigg A, Arthur C, Taylor K, Herrmann R, Lynch KP, Hughes TP (2002) High frequency of point mutations clustered within the adenosine triphosphate-binding region of Bcr/Abl in patients with chronic myeloid leukemia or Ph-positive acute lymphoblastic leukemia who develop imatinib (STI571) resistance. *Blood* 99: 3472–3475
79 Branford S, Rudzki Z, Walsh S, Parkinson I, Grigg A, Szer J, Taylor K, Herrmann R, Seymour JF, Arthur C et al (2003) Detection of Bcr-Abl mutations in patients with CML treated with imatinib is virtually always accompanied by clinical resistance, and mutations in the ATP phosphate-binding loop (P-loop) are associated with a poor prognosis. *Blood* 102: 276–283
80 Hochhaus A, Kreil S, Corbin AS, La Rosee P, Muller MC, Lahaye T, Hanfstein B, Schoch C, Cross NCP, Berger U et al (2002) Molecular and chromosomal mechanisms of resistance to imatinib (STI571) therapy. *Leukemia* 16: 2190–2196
81 Roche-Lestienne C, Soenen-Cornu V, Grardel-Duflos N, Lai J-L, Philippe N, Falcon T, Fenaux P, Preudhomme C (2002) Several types of mutations of the Abl gene can be found in chronic myeloid leukemia patients resistant to STI571, and they can pre-exist to the onset of treatment. *Blood* 100: 1014–1018
82 Shah NP, Tran C, Lee FY, Chen P, Norris D, Sawyers CL (2004) Overriding imatinib resistance with a novel Abl kinase inhibitor. *Science* 305: 399–401
83 Tsurus T, Naito M, Tomida A, Fujita N, Mashima T, Sakamoto H, Haga N (2003) Molecular Targeting therapy of cancer: drug resistance, apoptosis and survival signal. *Cancer Sci* 94: 15–21
84 Tsuruo T (2003) Molecular cancer therapeutics: recent progress and targets in drug resistance. *Internal Med* 42: 237–243
85 Longley DB, Johnston PG (2005) Molecular mechanisms of drug resistance. *J Pathol* 205: 275–292
86 Yingling JM, Blanchard KL, Sawyers JS (2004) Development of TGF-beta signaling inhibitors for cancer therapy. *Nat Rev Drug Discov* 3: 1011–1022
87 Beeram M, Patnaik A (2002) Targeting intracellular signal transduction: a new paradigm for a brave new world of molecularly targeted therapeutics. *Hematol Oncol Clin N Am* 16: 1089–1100
88 Nam NH, Parang K (2003) Current targets for anticancer drug discovery. *Current Drug Targets* 4: 159–179
89 Zelent A, Petrie K, Chen Z, Lotan R, Lubbert M, Tallman MS, Ohno R, Degos L, Waxman S (2005) Molecular target-based treatment of human cancer: summary of the 10th international conference on differentiation therapy. *Cancer Res* 65: 1117–1123
90 Awada A, Mano M, Hendlisz A, Piccart M (2004) New anticancer agents and therapeutic strategies in development for solid cancers: a clinical perspective. *Expert Rev Anticancer Ther* 4: 53–60
91 Syed S, Rowisky E (2003) The new generation of targeted therapies for breast cancer. *Oncology (Huntington)* 17: 1339–1351
92 Liu MC, Marshall JL, Pestell RG (2004) Novel strategies in cancer therapeutics: targeting enzymes involved in cell cycle regulation and cellular proliferation. *Curr Cancer Drug Targets* 4: 403–424
93 El-Aneed A (2004) Current strategies in cancer gene therapy. *Eur J Pharmacol* 498: 1–8
94 Seynaeve C, Verweij J (2004) Targeted therapy: ready for prime time? *Cancer Treat Res* 120: 1–15

Progress in Drug Research, Vol. 63
(R. M. Schultz, Ed.)

Obstacles and opportunities in the clinical development of targeted therapeutics

Grace K. Dy[1] and
Alex A. Adjei[2]

[1]Department of Internal Medicine
Mayo Clinic College of Medicine
200 First St. SW, Rochester
MN 55905, USA

[2]Division of Medical Oncology
Mayo Clinic College of Medicine
200 First St. SW, Rochester,
MN 55905, USA
<adjei.alex@mayo.edu>

Glossary of abbreviations

DLTs, dose limiting toxicities; EGFR, epidermal growth factor receptor; FT, farnesyltransferase; GIST, gastrointestinal tumor; MTD, maximally tolerated doses; NSCLC, non-small cell lung cancer; PDGFR, platelet-derived growth factor receptor; VEGF, vascular endothelial growth factor.

1 Introduction

Cancer is a genetic disease arising from somatic mutations in cells that confer a survival advantage and invasive properties characteristic of the malignant phenotype [1]. The similarity between intracellular processes within malignant cells and those within normal host cells makes therapeutic approaches without substantial host toxicity challenging. Moreover, many of the mutations contributing to carcinogenesis affect gene products that are also important for normal cells. The inter- and intra-tumor heterogeneity as well as the inherent redundancy and overlap in biological response pathways, such as signal transduction and apoptosis, contribute to the complexity of selecting suitable drug targets. Nevertheless, increased knowledge of tumor biology has made the selection of drugs designed against specific molecules important in cancer pathogenesis possible. Research efforts exploiting distinctive 'molecular signatures' to improve tumor selectivity of cancer chemotherapy drugs has led to the emergence of new classes of drugs that have already revolutionized cancer therapy in recent years. Understanding key issues relevant to clinical application is thus vital to the continuing development of these and other novel targeted therapies.

2 Selection of valid targets

Genetic aberrations in cancer may be conceptualized as either 'gain-of-function', such as the activation of oncogenes, or 'loss-of-function', such as the inactivation of tumor suppressor genes and DNA methylation [2]. It has been proposed that neoplastic clones select out key oncogenic pathways and genomic stability that lead to the loss of multiple cross-checking signaling pathways present in normal cells. This 'oncogene addiction' [3] lends itself to therapeutic manipulation as cancer cells have reorganized aberrant oncogenic signaling networks, the deprivation or interruption of which will be lethal, but normal cells should be left unharmed as there is redundancy in the proto-oncogenic counterparts.

Ideally, the presence (or absence) of the purported target should be critical to the survival of cancer cells but be non-critical in the function of normal cells. Moreover, there should be unequivocal correlation of target modulation with clinical benefit. For successful target selection, it is essential to distinguish potential targets that are necessary for the maintenance of the malignant phenotype, from those that are simply correlative or implicated only in the early stages of tumorigenesis [4]. It can be generally stated that potentially useful targets include those that are mutated [e.g., K-ras, epidermal growth factor receptor (EGFR), c-kit] or amplify signals (e.g., Her-2/neu) along a proliferative pathway. Proteins that are at the site of convergence of aberrant upstream regulators (mTOR and PTEN, MEK and K-ras) or regulators of key malignant cell functions (e.g., ubiquitin, angiogenesis) are also relevant. On the other hand, oncogenic protein overexpression *per se* is insufficient to prove causality in initiating or maintaining the malignant phenotype. Indeed, as will be elaborated upon subsequently, target overexpression alone may not be as vital as initially perceived (e.g., EGFR, c-kit). Moreover, tissue-specific responses and multiple opposing effects of each individual pathway are context-dependent, such as the ras, NF-κB and TGF-β pathways [5–7], and thus introduce further elements of difficulty in the process of target selection.

Surface-expressed tumor-associated antigens are also appropriate anti-tumor targets for immunological strategies, such as vaccines and antibodies. However, it is important to recognize that many of the purported tumor-derived proteins are in fact tissue-specific differentiation antigens that are seen in normal tissues [8]. Targeting such a protein is thus confounded by the fact that the intervention affects both tumor and normal cells. Moreover, tumor cells are predisposed towards dedifferentiation, and thus may in fact express fewer receptors, such as the expression of CD20 in B cells [9]. An ideal antigenic target should be expressed differentially at reasonably higher levels, if not exclusively, in tumor cells. Its downregulation would be desired only if it is involved in pro-proliferative or anti-apoptotic signal transduction. Moreover, it preferably should not be shed or secreted into the circulation to avoid antibody-binding solely to the circulating soluble forms.

As has become evident over the last few years, the most rationally designed drug (antisense oligonucleotides, matrix metalloproteinase inhibitors) may fail because of the presence of redundant pathways, mutational changes downstream from the intended target or inability of the drug to reach its target. In the nascent stages of development of these new targeted therapeutics, many posit that such agents should be highly specific, mainly based on the concept of 'oncogene addiction'. Cumulative experience with several kinase inhibitors in fact demonstrate that the 'targeted' drugs with most clinical relevance (consider imatinib) are in fact pleiotropic in their activity, probably a function of the myriad interdependent and cross-talking cellular pathways. Another inherent weakness of drug design specific to a single target, regardless of approach or 'molecular promiscuity', is the emergence of resistance due to selection pressure.

3 Issues in clinical trials

3.1 Phase I trials

3.1.1 Determination of appropriate dose and schedule of administration

3.1.1.1 Classical dose-limiting toxicities

Systemic cancer therapy is conventionally administered at or near maximally tolerated doses (MTD) because of the long-held paradigm of a steep dose-response curve seen with standard cytotoxic chemotherapy. Standard approaches to phase I trial design assume that drug dose will be a significant determinant of toxicity, and dose-limiting toxicities (DLTs) are invariably defined. This may be true even for some novel agents, for example the nonspecific uptake of antibody molecules into the reticulo-endothelial system (i.e., liver, spleen and bone marrow) imposes dose restrictions in a traditional manner on the use of conjugated or radiolabeled monoclonal antibodies. Another similarity to conventional chemotherapy in the determination of schedule of drug administration is consideration of the drug effect on the physiological function of the purported target in normal tissues. The recovery period in normal tissues may in fact be a limiting factor to the duration of the intervals between cycles of therapy. This is exemplified by the limitations of prolonged inhibition of proteasome function. Traditional phase I designs are thus appropriate with novel agents that exhibit toxicity patterns leading to rapid occurrences of DLTs, as exemplified by proteasome inhibitors, mTOR inhibitors, farnesyltransferase (FT) inhibitors and other multi-kinase inhibitors.

3.1.1.2 Determination of appropriate dose in the absence of classical DLTs

A number of novel agents are generally well tolerated and classical DLTs are not observed, making the determination of MTD in the standard sense impossible. Examples include the antisense oligonucleotides and monoclonal antibodies. Technological and financial constraints in maintaining an adequate supply of the agent, albeit temporary obstacles, are practical issues that necessitate a more rational approach in dose determination. Similarly, physiological limitations in drug administration, such as volume of parenteral or enteral administration, introduce another aspect in the establishment of an optimum biologically effective dose of relatively non-toxic targeted therapies. Conversely, clinical activity may be observed several dose levels below the MTD, as demonstrated in the early trials of imatinib mesylate and gefitinib. In the phase I trial of imatinib, a small molecule that reversibly competes with ATP for binding to the kinase domain of the platelet-derived growth factor receptor (PDGFR), c-Kit and Abl tyrosine kinases, an MTD was never reached as clinical activity was demonstrated after a few dose escalations. The clinically active dose correlated well with Abl kinase inhibition [10]. In a similar vein, even though an MTD for gefitinib, an EGFR tyrosine kinase inhibitor, was achieved in early phase I testing from traditional toxicity endpoints, pharmacodynamic studies showed EGFR inactivation at doses well below the MTD [11]. Furthermore, large, randomized clinical studies demonstrated more adverse reactions at a higher dose without corresponding benefit to study outcomes [12, 13]. Lastly, efficacy of these novel agents as chemo-preventive agents in part rests upon minimal toxicity with chronic maintenance treatment.

Minimizing the number of patients enrolled to sub-therapeutic dose levels, while ensuring patient safety, is an inherent goal in phase I trials. With new targeted therapies that are relatively non-toxic, statistically-based alternative methods (to the traditional Fibonacci schema) allowing a reduction in the number of patients treated at sub-therapeutic doses as well as a more rapid completion of the trial are more feasible [14]. However, two elements remain crucial. Sufficient patients must be recruited to enable the study of inter-patient variability as well as dose-related pharmacokinetic and pharmacodynamic effects. Secondly, for all the reasons stated earlier, non-toxicity endpoints should be considered.

Table 1 summarizes the approaches other than MTD determination that may be employed as endpoints in the phase I evaluation of novel agents.

Table 1.
Approaches and limitations in selection of dose and schedule of administration of novel agents with minimal classic toxicity.

Dose and schedule selection approaches	Limitations
Pharmacokinetic parameters (AUC, steady state or trough concentrations, half-life)	Target levels defined from *in vitro* or animal xenograft studies that are not necessarily reflective of, or that can be directly extrapolated to, human patient populations (e.g., different schedules, metabolism, etc); inter-patient variability
Pharmacodynamic assays Biochemical *in vitro* assays Functional imaging Metabolomics	Cost, reproducibility of test, patient risk with invasive procedures, patient contraindications to imaging procedures, reliability of surrogate tissues (i.e., unsatisfactory correlation using surrogate tissues to reflect tumor tissue effect), validity of surrogate markers
Physiological and pharmaceutical limitations: e.g., maximal ingestable dose limited by oral absorption; volume of infusate; economical constraints on manufacturer (i.e., maximum affordable dose)	Empiric and not based on tumor biology

AUC, Area under the plasma concentration time curve.

Central to this paradigm shift is the concept of a minimal biologically effective dose alluded to previously. Pharmacokinetic parameters are useful in the early stages of clinical drug development, particularly in the absence of toxicity or efficacy endpoints. For example, if pharmacokinetic analyses demonstrate a saturable absorption or drug distribution beyond a certain dose or schedule, then there is no reason to administer higher or more frequent doses. Monoclonal antibodies can illustrate this model. The prolonged half-lives of monoclonal antibodies allow for intermittent administration on a weekly schedule or even longer intervals. A concentration-exposure profile can thus reasonably approximate interactions at the receptor level, allowing for antibody-based dosing approaches to be estimated using pharmacokinetic parameters.

Dose determination can be further refined by integrating pharmacodynamic endpoints. For example, the dose of bevacizumab currently utilized in the clinic is 5–10 mg/kg. It has been demonstrated, however, that as little as

0.3 mg/kg could remove all circulating free vascular endothelial growth factor (VEGF) from the blood [15]. Doses of >1 mg/kg produced serum levels of bevacizumab in the target range of ≥10 μg/ml, the trough plasma concentration necessary to achieve maximal tumor inhibition in preclinical models, for at least 14 days. On the other hand, there is suggestion of a dose response. In metastatic non-small cell lung cancer (NSCLC) and metastatic renal cell carcinoma, a direct dose-response relationship can be observed [16, 17]. In colorectal cancer, however, this is not apparent [18]. The context-dependent relationships can also be observed in the development of agents such as imatinib and other EGFR-directed therapies [10, 12, 13, 19]. The complexity in dose determination described here is due, at least in part, to the fact that circulating drug levels may differ significantly from concentrations achieved in the tumor.

3.1.2 Functional imaging

To ameliorate this problem, non-invasive imaging techniques are increasingly being incorporated into early phase clinical trials, not only to demonstrate biological activity, but also to aid in the pharmacodynamic determination of a biologically effective dose. Digital contrast-enhanced magnetic resonance imaging (DCE-MRI) can demonstrate alterations in tumor blood flow relevant to the development of anti-angiogenesis agents [20, 21]. Determining metabolic phenotypes of cancer cells may also be helpful in monitoring tumor growth and regression. PET scan can demonstrate rapid changes in tumor viability within a few hours of drug administration [22]. Features of high-throughput analysis and full automation enable a 'metabolomic' approach to be potentially feasible and practical [23]. Pattern-recognition models have been used to generate 'metabolic fingerprints' to analyze bioenergetic status and temporal changes in metabolites associated with numerous cell processes, such as lipid metabolism in apoptosis [24, 25]. Metabolic profiles may thus also serve as surrogate markers for the pharmacodynamic monitoring of tumor responses to therapy and in dose determination. Future research can help further characterize specific metabolic profiles that may be used not only to monitor response to therapy but also to predict response or resistance as well as understanding mechanisms of toxicity.

3.1.3 Biochemical assays in tumor or surrogate tissue

Although demonstrating target modulation in tumor tissue is the pharmacodynamic benchmark in dose determination, clinical settings with minimal tumor burden (e.g., adjuvant therapy, chemo-prevention), tumor tissue inaccessibility and other practical limitations to repeated tumor biopsies or imaging studies require the use of surrogate tissues. Peripheral blood mononuclear cells are easily obtained and are by far the most commonly utilized surrogate tissue for assays. Biochemical assays may measure the effect on the intended target directly, such as inhibition of FT by FT inhibitors, or indirectly through detection of expected changes downstream of the intended target, such as the accumulation of unfarnesylated proteins with FT inhibitors [26]. However, a surrogate marker rationally chosen to predict an intended effect may not consistently exhibit changes in response to therapy, and may be subject to inter-individual and inter-assay variability [27, 28]. More importantly, drug effects in surrogate tissues may have no relationship to effects in tumor tissue.

These difficulties highlight the uncertainties of using target modulation as an endpoint. Ideally, the targeted pharmacodynamic endpoint will have been shown to correlate with tumor response in animal models before its use for dose finding. However, primary drug targets are seldom known with certainty before phase I trials commence. For example, FT inhibitors were designed to inhibit the post-translational modification of ras, which they do, yet they exhibit activity against ras-independent tumors. Similarly, sorafenib was developed as a raf kinase inhibitor, but its antitumor activity in clinical testing seems more consistent with its activity as an inhibitor of VEGF receptor tyrosine kinase. It is, hence, important to point out that, whereas failure to observe an effect on the target or its downstream intended pathway most likely is an indication of drug ineffectiveness or inadequate dosage, the converse is not necessarily true – compounds with successful demonstration of target inhibition may not have any clinical activity despite satisfactory pharmacokinetic properties if the putative target is irrelevant to tumor response. Indeed, an inherent weakness of all surrogate endpoints is the assumption of a predictive relationship between the surrogate measure and the desired outcome. Two approaches can be recommended for dose selection in phase I trials of novel agents in the absence of traditional DLTs. First, while a number of novel agents may not yield traditional DLTs in cycle 1 of therapy, chronic toxicities precluding the administration of these agents chronically are invariably encountered. Incorporation of chronic toxicity determination into the definition of MTD will allow for a rational selection of phase II doses. In the exceptional cases where this approach is not feasible, the incorporation of functional imaging studies should be considered. This approach, when feasible, is valid since drug effects on tumor are measured *in situ*.

3.2 Phase II/III trials

3.2.1 Study designs and endpoints

Phase II studies in oncological practice serve to screen for agents that possess sufficient antitumor effect to warrant further investigation, thus minimizing the risk of conducting resource-consuming randomized phase III trials with ineffective therapies. Evaluation of cytotoxic anticancer drug efficacy in phase II trials has historically utilized tumor size reduction as an endpoint. Drugs are considered active when an equal or greater proportion of tumor shrinkage among patients is seen compared to currently available regimens.

The current thrust in the development of novel agents that can inhibit tumor growth, prevent metastasis or induce a state of tumor dormancy without effecting a measurable reduction in tumor volume has presented new problems in efficacy evaluation. Because of the difficulties encountered when assessing activity of a cytostatic compound in phase II trials, many pharmaceutical companies have moved directly from phase I to phase III testing. This is not prudent. As stated earlier, phase III trials have significant costs associated with them, both for patients and for sponsors. It comes as no surprise consequently, that there has been a spate of negative studies in recent years of many of these targeted therapies. It has long been recognized and recently reinforced that traditional phase II trial designs have to be modified to incorporate measures of antitumor effects that may indicate the potential for meaningful clinical benefit other than alterations in tumor size.

Several single-arm designs appropriate for the testing of novel agents have been described [29]. Enrollment of different tumor types in a single phase II study is a feasible variation from the traditional disease-specific paradigm [30]. Since the standard single-arm phase II studies are uncontrolled, one way of minimizing associated biases is the use of randomized designs. The candidate drug with the best observed outcome is selected for future testing among the group, regardless of the magnitude of the observed advantage over other treatments. This is determined by ranking and selection methods [31] in which formal statistical comparisons are not done and a standard treatment group is not required. As originally intended, this simple design provides a high probability of taking the superior treatment forward even when the observed superiority in efficacy occurred purely by chance. Sample sizes are kept small as the selection design makes no attempt to distinguish the false positive from the true positive. Hence, follow-up phase III studies where statistical error rates are properly controlled are mandatory. Unfortunately, randomized phase II selection designs are frequently misinterpreted and misused, leading to a lack of conclusive data from phase III trials that are delayed or omitted [32, 33]. This is particularly true when control arms and hypothesis testing are included, when in fact such settings give rise to an unacceptably high risk of false-positive results [32, 34]. Nevertheless, randomized phase II designs should be feasible as long as the results are interpreted in their proper context and the relevant phase III trials pursued.

Another approach that attempts to address the limitations of single-arm designs is the enrichment/re-randomization design, the first description of which is credited to Amery and Dony [35]. This type of design selects subjects for participation in a randomized comparison phase of a study on the basis of their prior response during a preliminary, often an open-labeled titration, phase of the same study. Many authors have proposed similar experimental designs under different names and with different goals. The randomized discontinuation approach is one such design relevant to cytostatic agents that has been employed [36]; in this, the investigational drug is given to all patients enrolled in the pre-randomization stage, but the random treatment assignments of discontinuing or continuing therapy are determined only for patients who tolerate treatment and exhibit stable disease. To facilitate patient compliance, resumption of therapy after placebo failure is allowed. Patients who experience a complete or partial response would not enter the randomization stage but would instead continue receiving therapy until toxicity or disease progression. This design claims the advantage of allowing every patient to be treated to the best possible response prior to randomization, and, among post-randomization patients, the ability to distinguish disease stability as being due either to the antitumor activity of the cytostatic agent under evaluation or to the natural history of the disease. The total sample size required, however, could be larger than that required in a standard design. Moreover, potential biases are seen in several aspects [37]. Treatment un-blinding may arise during the randomization phase when the active drug has a known side effect apart from its purported antitumor activity that the placebo drug does not exhibit, or when cross-over treatment to active agent must resume for placebo failures. A more serious flaw arises when treatment effects are underestimated due to a carryover treatment effect through the randomization stage from the first treatment stage.

Regardless of the statistical design chosen for phase II evaluation of novel targeted therapies that exhibit cytostatic activity, the key issue is defining the endpoint used in ascertaining drug efficacy. In these cases the standard benchmark of objective tumor size reduction may not be entirely relevant. Rate of early disease progression [38], time to disease progression or progression-free survival [39–41] have been suggested. However, the incorporation of stable disease as a measure of drug activity has often been criticized. This is highlighted by the fact that, unlike objective tumor responses that rarely occur in the absence of treatment, stable disease *per se* may be attributable to inherent tumor biology and does not necessarily imply drug activity. Incorporating quality-of-life or clinical-benefit endpoints in such circumstances may be useful. Moreover, the results from pivotal trials of novel therapies such as imatinib, erlotinib, cetuximab and bevacizumab still support the idea that tumor regression continues to be a valid predictor of ultimate survival outcomes. A number of purported failures of study design are indeed not valid. There has been a tendency for investigators to term ineffective agents "cytostatic" without any supporting data. In a number of cases, these agents lead to brisk tumor shrinkage in preclinical systems. It is fair to say that there are very few truly cytostatic agents in clinical development at the present time.

The demonstration of rapid achievement of tumor dormancy using FGD-PET imaging in gastrointestinal stromal tumors (GISTs) that antedate subsequent tumor size reduction with conventional imaging modalities such as CT scan and MRI [22] holds promise for functional imaging as a future tool that may be explored. Further refinements of such modalities to elicit drug-specific information on tumor activity, as well as validation of their use as surrogate measures of clinical outcome, are needed. Lastly, more opportunities should be provided for an expanded phase II trial of an agent that demonstrates promising activity, in which more patients are accrued to perform transcriptional profiling and validate biological assays for predicting drug sensitivity, as discussed in the next section.

3.2.2 Selection of target patient populations

The concept of targeted rationally based therapy is not new, and has been exploited in hormone-dependent malignancies. The availability of novel agents should be accompanied by more opportunities to precisely identify patient populations most likely to respond to the drug, adding another dimension to the meaning of targeted therapy. Acceptability of therapeutic risk vary in different cancer settings, which thus mandates more stringent criteria for adjuvant or chemo-preventive trials. While screening may limit enrollment, 'enrichment' in clinical trials of the target patient population would reduce the number of subjects required for clinical trials to demonstrate efficacy, and widen the benefit-risk ratio. This was certainly the case for trastuzumab, a humanized IgG1 monoclonal antibody against the HER2/neu receptor overexpressed in approximately 25% of invasive breast cancer [42]. The pivotal studies that led to its FDA approval showed striking improvement in survival and objective responses limited to HER2-overexpressing cancers [43, 44]. It is conceivable that such activity would be missed in an unselected group of patients. This readily represents the current dilemma of other novel agents in that treatment effects may be diluted in an unselected population if only a small subgroup of patients is likely to respond.

A major challenge in administering new target-specific drugs is the ability to predict the outcome of therapy, which encompasses tumor response, clinical toxicity and resistance. Despite intensive research, validated biological markers predictive of response to targeted therapies are multifactorial and not always apparent. Emerging evidence from various studies show that the paradigm of target overexpression in tumor samples as criteria for patient selection may be erroneous. A distinction early on should be made between predictive markers of treatment response and prognostic markers of clinical outcomes. Although therapeutic approaches designed against poor prognostic markers intuitively should correlate with improved outcomes, such a relationship is not consistently observed due to a variety of tumor-, drug- and host-related factors. Increased EGFR expression is common in lung cancers, but neither EGFR expression levels nor phosphorylation state correlate with response to EGFR-directed therapies. In contrast, the chimeric neutralizing

EGFR antibody cetuximab is beneficial only in EGFR-expressing colon cancer. Imatinib mesylate shows remarkable activity in c-kit-positive GISTs, yet are not effective in small cell lung cancers that overexpress c-kit.

Some of the discernible differences in drug response may be attributable to pharmacogenetic variability independent of the tumor phenotype. Illustrative of this statement is the experience with rituximab, a chimeric monoclonal anti-CD20 IgG1 used in the treatment of B lymphoproliferative malignancies. Cytotoxic effector cells such as natural killer cells and macrophages bear receptors for the Fc portion of the IgG (FcγR), linking IgG-sensitized tumor cells to inflict antibody-dependent cell-mediated cytotoxicity (ADCC), an important mechanism in the eradication of tumor cells by rituximab [45]. A single nucleotide polymorphism at position 158 of FcγRIIIa (FCGR3A) molecule seem to affect activity of anti-CD20 monoclonal antibody. Human IgG1 binds more strongly to the homozygous FcγRIIIa -158V (valine) natural killer cells than to homozygous FcγRIIIa -158F (phenylalanine) or heterozygous natural killer cells [46]. The genotype homozygous for FcγRIIIa -158V (VV) is associated with higher clinical and molecular response to rituximab [47].

More commonly, the determinants of response to therapy are not only tumor-dependent, but are also defined by the inherent characteristics and limitations of the individual agents. For example, truncated receptor variants may preclude the use of monoclonal antibody approaches. Nevertheless, a recurring theme is the correlation of the presence of activating mutations in the oncogenic protein, which ultimately reflects oncogenic dependence by various malignancies, with response to kinase inhibitors. Clinical activity of imatinib in GISTs is highest in tumor with activating mutations at exons 9 and 11 of the Kit gene [48]. In about a third of GISTs expressing wild-type Kit, imatinib's efficacy can be explained by the presence of intragenic mutations in the PDGFRA gene that yields a constitutively active PDGFR [49]. Activating mutations that involve the ATP-binding pocket of receptor tyrosine kinases may confer hyperresponsiveness to cognate ligands, explaining the ~10-fold increased sensitivity of tumors with EGFR kinase domain mutations to gefitinib [50, 51]. Although it is tempting based on these data to select patients with tumor harboring such mutations, our current information is incomplete as responses were also seen in tumor samples that do not harbor mutations. As it is, we cannot definitely exclude the possibility of therapeutic benefit to patients without kinase mutations.

3.2.3 Combination of novel agents with standard chemotherapy agents

Cellular damage induced by cytotoxic chemotherapy activates survival pathways for cancer cells to escape death. Moreover, emergence of resistance clones to single-agent therapy, whose main mechanism of action is directed against one specific target in a tumor, is likely to occur due to selection pressure, regardless of the drug's molecular promiscuity. It has been hypothesized that combination of novel agents with cytotoxic chemotherapy will result in enhanced antitumor effects.

Four phase III well-designed and adequately powered trials, with over 4000 NSCLC patients combined, comparing the combination of the EGFR tyrosine kinase inhibitors and standard chemotherapy to standard chemotherapy alone did not meet either the primary endpoint of survival or the secondary endpoints of time to disease progression or response rates, thus indicating that concomitant administration of these agents does not add clinical benefit to conventional chemotherapy in NSCLC [52–55].

These results were unexpected as preclinical data supported such combinations [56, 57], and both gefitinib and erlotinib demonstrate single-agent activity in NSCLC [12, 13, 58]. The reasons for these surprising results are unclear, but several explanations have been offered. Schedule-dependent antagonism could have occurred. Both novel agents possess anti-proliferative effects and cause G_1 cell cycle arrest [59, 60]. It may be that continuous kinase inhibition could render tumor cells less sensitive to cytotoxic agents. Indeed, intermittent gefitinib administration is significantly superior to continuous dosing in combination with paclitaxel in preclinical studies [61].

On the other hand, interim results from a multicenter phase III combination chemotherapy trial of gemcitabine and erlotinib or placebo in locally advanced or pancreatic cancer met its primary endpoint, demonstrating statistically significant improvements in overall survival with the combination [62]. In irinotecan-refractory EGFR-expressing metastatic colorectal cancer, clinical benefit is also shown upon combination of cetuximab with irinotecan [63].

Echoing similar discrepancies and context-dependent clinical activity is the combination of anti-angiogenic agents with cytotoxic chemotherapy. Whereas bevacizumab improves overall survival in combination with chemotherapy in colorectal cancer, this endpoint is not met in the phase III trial of combination chemotherapy in metastatic breast cancer in spite of improved objective tumor responses [64]. Of note, the colorectal cancer study was in front-line advanced disease, whereas the breast cancer study was in the third-line setting. Another unresolved issue is the optimal sequence of combination therapy.

As discussed above, the desired clinical endpoints are not consistently met despite preclinical proof. In some instances, the schedule of drug treatment utilized in clinical trials does not reliably re-produce the preclinical schedules. For example, the preclinical studies of gefitinib and paclitaxel utilized pulse dosing of gefitinib [61], whereas in clinical studies, gefitinib was administered continuously [53]. Another contributing factor to these results relates to the inherent limitations of the preclinical models used to validate therapeutic rationale. An almost obligatory component in the progress to clinical development of new anticancer agents is the initial screening using panels of disease-oriented human tumor cell lines grown *in vitro* or xenografted *in vivo* with the assumption that such cell lines might possess tissue-specific targets not exhibited in murine-based tumor models, and thus would more adequately reflect the behavior of human cancer. Although there are data to suggest that the human tumor xenograft model is a good predictor of clinical activity of cytotoxic anticancer drugs [65], the appropriateness of this paradigm is subject to question in the evaluation of contemporary targeted agents that focuses heavily on various signaling and gene expression pathways, the responses to which are highly dependent on microenvironmental conditions. The fidelity of human tumor cell lines to the original tumor phenotype is likely confounded by variability over successive passages, time and nature of selection pressures. For example, xenografts derived from cell lines generally demonstrate a more homogeneous, undifferentiated histology and, on occasion, loss of the target receptors/proteins. It has been demonstrated that cell lines demonstrate a significant shift towards higher growth rate and reduced drug response, such as to EGFR signal transduction inhibitors, in comparison to primary cultures of surgical tumor specimens [66]. This is consistent with the variation seen in specific gene expression pathways that may account for drug resistance and increased proliferation in cell lines, despite overall gene expression patterns that correlated with their histological origins [67].

On the other hand, although xenografts derived directly from patient tumor specimens appear to better retain the morphological and molecular properties, the chief disadvantage in their use is the technical difficulty in establishing such xenografts. Alternatives to these transplantation models are animals that naturally develop cancers with features relevant to the human disease, such as companion animals. Recent advances have made possible the creation of genetically engineered mice that develop cancers with an order of progression that mimic their human counterparts in a wide variety of organs. The limited use of genetically engineered mice in preclinical drug development may in part relate to the spontaneous, asynchronous and mostly protracted nature of tumor development. Nonetheless, as chronic treatment may be foreseen with the new targeted agents, the use of genetically engineered mice may help predict side effects that may not be uncovered with the relatively brief treatment duration in early clinical trials. Full phenotypic expression, however, may take years to manifest. An example is seen with anti-EGFR strategies. Cardiac valvular abnormalities and ventricular hypertrophy took over 60 years to surface in EGFR mutant mice [68]. Moreover, species-specific and drug-dependent variations in metabolism and organ toxicity in preclinical animal models compared to humans is a well-established fact. In addition, there are instances where animal models are likely inappropriate for evaluating clinical outcomes with certain therapeutic interventions, such as anti-angiogenic strategies when the vasculature is of murine origin. Despite these issues, spontaneous cancer models are feasible [69, 70] and hopefully will play a major role in bridging the gap between previous *in vivo* models and human clinical trials.

3 Conclusion

In this genomic era, new discoveries rapidly inundate and overwhelm our ability to test and rank individual cancer gene products according to their hierarchical importance. Appropriate target selection and drug selection using more stringent criteria serve as a crucial initial step in the success of new drug development. Full characterization of the cellular function of a frequently dysregulated or abnormal protein and its pathway is imperative to validate the therapeutic value of a potential target. Ideally, such a target should be differentially expressed in tumor tissue compared to normal cells. There should be more effort invested in improving and conducting more comprehensive preclinical evaluation, particularly in the identification of pharmacodynamic markers of drug efficacy in preclinical animal models, which may subsequently be applied in the clinic. Development of assays to test target inhibition in tumor tissue is essential, as many of these drugs are relatively non-toxic and the conventional phase I design of MTD in determining dose may not be as relevant, or needed. However, because of the existence of redundancy in cellular pathways, drugs with pleiotropic targets will prove to be more versatile and clinically effective. Mechanism-based combination therapy with other novel agents likewise is warranted. Results from preclinical models, although certainly valuable, do not reliably reproduce treatment effects seen in human cancer and should be interpreted carefully.

New paradigms in clinical trial design and endpoints are needed. As in preclinical evaluation, documentation of target inhibition should be incorporated in early clinical trials. The incorporation of functional imaging studies is gaining acceptance and efforts should continue in further refining these tests. As investigators strive to improve the efficiency of phase I clinical trials, provisions for adequate pharmacokinetic studies should be maintained, not only to aid dose escalation, but also to clarify important pharmacological details that may otherwise not be studied in later phases of drug development.

The large number of negative phase III studies suggest that phase II testing remains relevant in determining an agent's clinical efficacy before deciding on further development. Consequently, novel phase II designs and modification of efficacy endpoints should be adopted and reassessed to avoid such high-profile 'failures'.

On the other hand, early stopping rules should be routinely incorporated in phase III designs to avoid committing large numbers of patients to trials unlikely to yield positive results. With genomic and proteomic technology becoming increasingly available, it is imperative that molecular signatures of prognosis [71], prediction of response [72] and toxicity [73, 74] be established to aid in the selection of the most suitable target patient populations for specific agents. Ultimately, the final determinant of success remains a clinically significant impact on survival, the "*ne plus ultra*" of all measured outcomes.

References

1 Vogelstein B, Kinzler KW (2004) Cancer genes and the pathways they control. *Nat Med* 10: 789–799

2 De Vita V, Hellman S, Rosenberg S (eds) (2001) *Cancer principles and practice of oncology, 6th edition*. Lippincott Williams and Wilkins, Philadelphia

3 Weinstein IB (2002) Cancer. Addiction to oncogenes: the Achilles heal of cancer. *Science* 297: 63–64

4 Nowak MA, Iwasa Y, Michor F (2004) Dynamics of cancer progression. *Nat Rev Cancer* 4: 197–205

5 Skinner J, Bounacer A, Bond JA, Haughton MF, deMicco C, Synford-Thomas D (2004) Opposing effects of mutant ras oncoprotein on human fibroblast and epithelial cell proliferation: implications for models of human tumorigenesis. *Oncogene* 23: 5994–5999

6 Aggarwal BB (2004) Nuclear factor-κB. The enemy within. *Cancer Cell* 6: 203–208

7 Byfield SD, Roberts AB (2004) Lateral signaling enhances TGF-beta response complexity. *Trends Cell Biol* 14: 107–111

8 Overwijk WW, Restifo NP (2000) Autoimmunity and the immunotherapy of cancer: targeting the 'self' to destroy the 'other'. *Crit Rev Immunol* 20: 433–450

9 Rossman ED, Lundin J, Lenkei R, Mellstedt H, Osterborg A (2001) Variability in B-cell antigen expression: implications for the treatment of B-cell lymphomas and leukemias with monoclonal antibodies. *Hematol J* 2: 300–306

10 Druker BJ, Talpaz M, Resta DJ, Peng B, Buchdunger E, Ford JM, Lydon NB, Kantarjian H, Capdeville R, Ohno-Jones S, Sawyers CL (2001) Efficacy and safety of a specific inhibitor of the BCR-ABL tyrosine kinase in chronic myeloid leukemia. *N Engl J Med* 344: 1031–1037

11 Albanell J, Rojo F, Averbuch S, Feyereislova A, Mascaro JM, Herbst R, LoRuss P, Rischin D, Sauleda S, Gee J et al (2002) Pharmacodynamic studies of the epidermal growth factor receptor inhibitor ZD1839 in skin from cancer patients: histopathologic and molecular consequences of receptor inhibition. *J Clin Oncol* 20: 110–124

12 Fukuoka M, Yano S, Giaccone G, Tamura T, Nakagawa K, Douillard JY, Ishiwaki Y, Vansteenkiste J, Kudoh S, Rschin D et al (2003) A multi-institutional randomized phase II trial of genfitini for previously treated patients with advanced non-small cell lung cancer (THE IDEAL 1 Trial). *J Clin Oncol* 21: 2237–2246

13 Kris MG, Natale RB, Herbst RS, Lynch TJ Jr, Prager D, Belani CP, Schiller JH, Kelly K, Spiridonidis H, Sandler A et al (2003) Efficacy of gefitinib, an inhibitor of the epidermal growth factor receptor tyrosine kinase, in symptomatic patients with non-small cell lung cancer: A randomized trial. *JAMA* 290: 2149–2158

14 Eisenhauer EA, O'Dwyer PJ, Christian M, Humphrey JS (2000) Phase I clinical trial design in cancer drug development. *J Clin Oncol* 18: 684–692

15 Gordon MS, Margolin K, Talpaz M, Sledge GW Jr, Holmgren E, Benjamin R, Stalter S, Shak S, Adelman DC (2001) Phase I safety and pharmacokinetic study of recombinant human anti-vascular endothelial growth factor in patients with advanced cancer. *J Clin Oncol* 19: 843–850

16 Johnson DH, Fehrenbacher L, Novotny WF, Herbst RS, Nemunaitis JJ, Jablons DM, Langer CJ, DeVore RF 3rd, Gaudreault J, Damico LA et al (2004) Randomized phase II trial comparing bevacizumab plus carboplatin and paclitaxel with carboplatin and paclitaxel alone in previously untreated locally advanced or metastatic non-small-cell lung cancer. *J Clin Oncol* 22: 2184–2191

17 Yang JC, Haworth L, Sherry RM, Hwu P, Schwartzentruber DJ, Topalian SL, Steinberg SM, Chen HX, Rosenberg SA (2003). A randomized trial of bevacizumab, an anti-vascular endothelial growth factor antibody, for metastatic renal cancer. *N Engl J Med* 349: 427–434

18 Kabbinavar F, Hurwitz H, Fehrenbacher L, Meropol NJ, Novotny WF, Lieberman G, Griffing S, Bergsland E (2003) Phase II, randomized trial comparing bevacizumab

plus fluorouracil (FU)/leucovorin (LV) with FU/LV alone in patients with metastatic colorectal cancer. *J Clin Oncol* 21: 60–65
19 Fischer PM (2004) The design of drug candidate molecules as selective inhibitors of therapeutically relevant protein kinases. *Curr Med Chem* 11: 1563–1583
20 Xiong HQ, Herbst R, Faria SC, Scholz C, Davis D, Jackson EF, Madden T, McConkey D, Hicks M, Hess K et al (2004) A phase I surrogate endpoint study of SU6668 in patients with solid tumors. *Invest New Drugs* 22: 459–466
21 Morgan B, Thomas AL, Drevs J, Hennig J, Buchert M, Jivan A, Horsfield MA, Mross K, Ball HA, Lee L et al (2003) Dynamic contrast-enhanced magnetic resonance imaging as a biomarker for the pharmacological response of PTK787/ZK 222584, an inhibitor of the vascular endothelial growth factor receptor tyrosine kinases, in patients with advanced colorectal cancer and liver metastases: results from two phase I studies. *J Clin Oncol* 21: 3955–3964
22 Gayed I, Vu T, Iyer R, Johnson M, Macapinlac H, Swanston N, Podoloff D (2004) The role of 18F-FDG PET in staging and early prediction of response to therapy of recurrent gastrointestinal stromal tumors. *J Nucl Med* 45: 17–21
23 Griffin JL, Shockcor JP (2004) Metabolic profiles of cancer cells. *Nat Rev Cancer* 4: 551–561
24 Hakumaki JM, Poptani H, Puumalainen AM, Loimas S, Paljarvi LA, Yla-Herttuala S, Kauppinen RA (1998) Quantitative ^{1}H NMR diffusion spectroscopy of pf BT4C rat glioma during thymidine kinase-mediated gene therapy *in vivo*: identification of apoptotic response. *Cancer Res* 58: 3791–3799
25 Chung YL, Troy H, Banerji U, Jackson LE, Walton MI, Stubbs M, Griffiths JR, Judson IR, Leach MO, Workman P et al (2003) Magnetic resonance spectroscopic pharmacodynamic markers of HSP90 inhibitor, 17-allylamino-17-demethoxygeldanamycin, in human colon cancer models. *J Natl Cancer Inst* 95: 1624–1633
26 Adjei AA, Davis JN, Erlichman C, Svingen PA, Kaufmann SH (2000) Comparison of potential markers of farnesyltransferase inhibition. *Clin Cancer Res* 6: 2318–2325
27 Drevs J (2003) Soluble markers for the detection of hypoxia under antiangiogenic treatment. *Anticancer Res* 23: 1159–1161
28 Davis DW, McConkey DJ, Abbruzzese JL, Herbst RS (2003) Surrogate markers in antiangiogenesis clinical trials. *Br J Cancer* 89: 8–14
29 Korn EL, Arbuck SG, Pluda JM, Simon R, Kaplan RS, Christian MC (2000) Clinical trial designs for cytostatic agents: are new approaches needed? *J Clin Oncol* 19: 265–272
30 Rinehart J, Adjei AA, LoRusso PM, Waterhouse D, Hecht JR, Natale RB, Hamid O, Varterasian M, Asbury P, Kaldjian EP et al (2004) Multicenter Phase II study of the oral MEK inhibitor, CI-1040 in patients with advanced non-small cell lung, breast, colon and pancreatic cancer. *J Clin Oncol* 22: 4456–4462
31 Simon R, Wittes RE, Ellenberg SS (1985) Randomized phase II clinical trials. *Cancer Treat Rep* 69: 1375–1381
32 Liu PY, LeBlanc M, Desai M (1999) False positive rates of randomized phase II designs. *Control Clin Trials* 20: 343–352
33 Perrone F, Di Maio M, De Maio E, Maione P, Ottaiano A, Pensabene M, De Lorenzo G, Lombardi AV, Signoriello G, Gallo C (2003) Statistical design in phase II clinical trials and its application in breast cancer. *Lancet Oncol* 4: 305–311
34 Sylvester RJ (1988) A bayesian approach to the design of phase II clinical trials. *Biometrics* 44: 823–836

35 Amery W, Dony J (1975) A clinical trial design avoiding undue placebo treatment. *J Clin Pharmacol* 15: 674–679
36 Rosner GL, Stadler W, Ratain MJ (2002) Randomized discontinuation design: application to cytostatic antineoplastic agents. *J Clin Oncol* 20: 4478–4484
37 Leber PD, Davis CS (1998) Threats to the validity of clinical trials employing enrichment strategies for sample selection. *Control Clin Trials* 19: 178–187
38 Zee B, Melnychuk D, Dancey J, Eisenhauer E (1999) Multinomial phase II cancer trials in incorporating response and early progression. *J Biopharm Stat* 99: 351–363
39 Mick R, Crowley JJ, Carroll RJ (2000) Phase II clinical trial design for nocytotoxic anticancer agents for which time to disease progression is the primary endpoint. *Control Clin Trials* 21: 343–359
40 Liu PY, Dahlberg S, Crowley J (1993) Selection designs for pilot studies based on survival. *Biometrics* 49: 391–398
41 Schaid DJ, Ingle JN, Wieand S, Ahman DL (1988) A design for phase II testing of anticancer agents within a phase III clinical trial. *Control Clin Trials* 9: 107–118.
42 Slamon DJ, Godolphin W, Jones LA, Holt JA, Wong SG, Ketih E, Levin WJ, Stuart SG, Udove J, Ullrich A et al (1989) Studies of the HER-2/neu proto-oncogene in human breast and ovarian cancer. *Science* 244: 707–712
43 Vogel CL, Cobleigh MA, Tripathy D, Gutheil JC, Harris LN, Fehrenbacher L, Slamon DJ, Murphy M, Novotny WF, Burchmore M et al (2002) Efficacy and safety of trastuzumab as a single agent in first-line treatment of HER2-overexpressing metastatic breast cancer. *J Clin Oncol* 20: 719–726
44 Slamon DJ, Leyland-Lones B, Shak S, Fuchs H, Paton V, Bajamonde A, Fleming T, Eiermann w, Wolter J, Pegram M et al (2001) Use of chemotherapy plus a monoclonal antibody against HER2 for metastatic breast cancer that overexpressed HER2. *N Engl J Med* 344: 783–792
45 Shan D, Ledbetter JA, Press OW (1998) Apoptosis of malignant human B cells by ligation of CD20 with monoclonal antibodies. *Blood* 91: 1644–1652
46 Koene HR, Kleijer M, Algra J, Roos D, von dem Borne AE, de Haas M (1997) FcγRIIIa-158V/F polymorphism influences the binding of IgG by natural killer cell FcγRIIIa, independently of the FcγRIIIa-48L/R/H phenotype. *Blood* 90: 1109–1114
47 Cartron G, Dacheux L, Salles G, Solal-Celigny P, Bardos P, Colombat P, Watier H (2002) Therapeutic activity of humanized anti-CD20 monoclonal antibody and polymorphism in IgG Fc receptor FcγRIIIa gene. *Blood* 99: 754–758
48 Heinrich MC, Corless CL, Demetri GD, Blanke CD, von Mehren M, Joensuu H, McGreevey LS, Chen C-J, Van Den Abbeele AD, Druker BJ et al (2003) Kinase mutations and imatinib response in patients with metastatic gastrointestinal stromal tumor. *J Clin Oncol* 21: 4342–4349
49 Heinrich MC, Corless CL, Duensing A, McGreevey L, Chen C-J, Joseph N, Singer S, Griffith DJ, Haley A, Town A et al (2003) PDGFRA activating mutations in gastrointestinal stromal tumors. *Science* 299: 708–710
50 Lynch TJ, Bell DW, Sordella R, Gurubhagavatula S, Okimoto RA, Brannigan BW, Harris PL, Haserlat SM, Supko JG, Haluska FG et al (2004) Activating mutations in the epidermal growth factor receptor underlying responsiveness of non-small cell lung cancer to gefitinib. *N Engl J Med* 350: 2129–2139

51 Paez JG, Janne PA, Lee JC, Tracy S, Greulich H, Gabriel S, Herman P, Kaye FJ, Lindeman N, Boggon TJ et al (2004) EGFR mutations in lung cancer: Correlation with clinical response to gefitinib therapy. *Science* 304: 1497–1500

52 Giaccone G, Herbst RS, Manegold C, Scagliotti G, Rosell R, Miller V, Natale RB, Schiller JH, von Pawel J, Pluzanska A et al (2004) Gefitinib in combination with gemcitabine and cisplatin in advanced non–small-cell lung cancer: A phase III trial – INTACT 1. *J Clin Oncol* 22: 777–784

53 Herbst RS, Giaccone G, Schiller J, Natale RB, Miller V, Manegold C, Scagliotti G, Rosell R, Oliff I, Reeves JA et al (2004) Gefitinib in combination with paclitaxel and carboplatin in advanced non-small-cell lung cancer: a Phase III trial – INTACT 2. *J Clin Oncol* 22: 785–794

54 Gatzemeier U, Pluzanska A, Szczesna A, Kaukel E, Roubec J, Brennscheidt U, De Rosa F, Mueller B, Von Pawel J (2004) Results of a phase III trial of erlotinib (OSI-774) combined with cisplatin and gemcitabine (GC) chemotherapy in advanced non-small cell lung cancer (NSCLC). *J Clin Oncol* 22(14S): 7010

55 Herbst RS, Prager D, Hermann R, Miller V, Fehrenbacher L, Hoffman P, Johnson B, Sandler AB, Mass R, Johnson DH (2004) TRIBUTE - A phase III trial of erlotinib HCl (OSI-774) combined with carboplatin and paclitaxel (CP) chemotherapy in advanced non-small cell lung cancer (NSCLC). *J Clin Oncol* 22(14S): 7011

56 Sirotnak FM, Zakowsky MF, Miller VA, Scher HI, Kris MG (2000) Efficacy of cytotoxic agents against human tumor xenographs is markedly enhanced by coadministration of ZD1839 (Iressa) an inhibitor of tyrosine kinase. *Clin Cancer Res* 6: 4885–4892

57 Ciardiello F, Caputo R, Bianco R, Damiano V, Pomatico G, De Placido S, Bianco AR, Tortora G (2000) Antitumor effect and potentiation of cytotoxic drugs activity in human cancer cells by ZD-1839 (Iressa), an epidermal growth factor receptor-selective tyrosine kinase inhibitor. *Clin Cancer Res* 6: 2053–2063

58 Shepherd FA, Pereira J, Ciuleanu TE, Tan EH, Hirsh V, Thongprasert S, Bezjak A, Tu D, Santabarbara P, Seymour L (2004) A randomized placebo-controlled trial of erlotinib in patients with advanced non-small cell lung cancer (NSCLC) following failure of 1st line or 2nd line chemotherapy. A National Cancer Institute of Canada Clinical Trials Group (NCIC CTG) trial. *J Clin Oncol* 22(14S): 7022

59 Di Gennaro E, Barbarino M, Bruzzese F, de Lorenzo S, Caraglia M, Abbruzzese A, Avallone A, Comella P, Caponigro F, Pepe S et al (2003) Critical role of both p27KIP1 and p21CIP1/WAF1 in the antiproliferative effect of ZD1839 ('Iressa'), an epidermal growth factor receptor tyrosine kinase inhibitor, in head and neck squamous carcinoma cells. *J Cell Physiol* 195: 139–150

60 Moyer JD, Barbacci EG, Iwata KK, Arnold L, Boman B, Cunningham A, DiOrio C, Doty J, Morin MJ, Moyer MP et al (1997) Induction of apoptosis and cell cycle arrest by CP-358,774, an inhibitor of epidermal growth factor receptor tyrosine kinase. *Cancer Res* 56: 3666–3669

61 Solit DB, She Y, Moasser M, Hudis C, Kris M, Scher H, Rosen N, Sirotnak FM (2003) Pulsatile administration of the EGF receptor inhibitor (Iressa, ZD1839) is significantly more effective that continuously dosing for sensitizing tumors to Taxol. *Clin Cancer Res*. 19(16S): 70, abstract A83

62 Genentech press release September 20, 2004: *http://www.gene.com/gene/news/press-releases/display/.do?method=detail&id=7747&categoryid=3* (Accessed May 2005)

63 Cunningham D, Humblet Y, Siena S, Khayat D, Bleiberg H, Santoro A, Bets D, Mueser M, Harstrick A, Verslype C et al (2004) Cetuximab monotherapy and cetuximab plus irinotecan in irinotecan-refractory metastatic colorectal cancer. *N Engl J Med* 351: 337–345
64 Miller KD, Rugo HS, Cobleigh MA, Marcom PK, Chap LI, Holmes FA, Fehrenbacher L, Overmoyer BA, Reimann JD, Vassel AV et al (2002) Phase III trial of capecitabine (Xeloda) plus bevacizumab (Avastin) versus capecitabine alone in women with metastatic breast cancer previously treated with an anthracycline and a taxane. *Breast Cancer Res Treat* 76: S37, abstract 36
65 Johnson JI, Decker S, Zaharevitz D, Rubinstein LV, Venditti JM, Schepartz S, Kalyandrug S, Christian M, Arbuck S, Hollingshead M, Sausville EA (2001) Relationships between drug activity in NCI preclinical *in vitro* and *in vivo* models and early clinical trials. *Br J Cancer* 84: 1424–1431
66 Baguley BC, Marshall ES (2004) *In vitro* modeling of human tumour behaviour in drug discovery programmes. *Eur J Cancer* 40: 794–801
67 Ross DT, Scherf U, Eisen MB, Perou CM, Rees C, Spellman P, Iyer V, Jeffrey SS, van de Rijn M, Waltham M et al (2000) Systematic variation in gene expression patterns in human cancer cell lines. *Nat Genet* 24: 227–235
68 Roberts RB, Arteaga CL, Threadgill DW (2004) Modeling the cancer patient with genetically engineered mice: Prediction of toxicity from molecule-targeted therapies. *Cancer Cell* 5: 115–120
69 Frijhoff AFW, Conti CJ, Senderowicz AM (2004) Advances in molecular carcinogenesis: current and future use of mouse models to screen and validate molecularly targeted anticancer drugs. *Mol Carcinog* 39: 183–194
70 Hansen K, Khanna C (2004) Spontaneous and genetically engineered animal models: use in preclinical cancer drug development. *Eur J Cancer* 40: 858–880
71 van de Vijver MJ, He YD, van't Veer LJ, Dai H, Hart AAM, Voskuil DW, Schreiber GJ, Peterse JL, Roberts C, Marton MJ et al (2002) A gene-expression signature as a predictor of survival in breast cancer. *N Engl J Med* 347: 1999–2009
72 Ayers M, Symmans WF, Stec J, Damokosh AI, Clark E, Hess K, Lecocke M, Metivier J, Booser D, Ibrahim N et al (2004) Gene expression profiles predict complete pathologic response to neoadjuvant paclitaxel and fluorouracil, doxorubicin, and cyclophosphamide chemotherapy in breast cancer. *J Clin Oncol* 22: 2284–2293
73 Pennie WD, Woodyatt NJ, Aldridge TC, Orphanides G (2001) Application of genomics to the difinition of the molecular bass for toxicity. *Toxicol Lett* 120: 353–358
74 Kennedy S (2002) The role of proteomics in toxicology: identification of biomarkers of toxicity by protein expression analysis. *Biomarkers* 7: 1–22

Progress in Drug Research, Vol. 63
(R. M. Schultz, Ed.)

Tumor models for preclinical development of targeted agents

Beverly A. Teicher

Genzyme Corporation
1 Mountain Road, Framingham
MA 01701, USA
<Beverly.Teicher@Genzyme.com>

1 Introduction

The *in vivo* efficacy testing of potential new anticancer therapies is one of the most important, most misunderstood and most maligned phases of drug development in oncology [1, 2]. The criticism that currently used tumor models are not representative of human disease of the same histological type is frequently heard; however, those in the field are well aware of the significant impact of results from such studies on whether a new agent moves forward or not, and on the selection of diseases where new agents are anticipated to have activity. For many years both syngeneic tumor models and human tumor xenograft models were 'black boxes' that the investigator, without direct knowledge, hoped were generic representations of broad swatches of human malignant disease. Single tumor lines were often taken to represent all breast cancers, all lung cancers or all prostate cancers. As molecular biology techniques have been refined and targeted therapeutics have come to the fore, analysis of both syngeneic and human xenograft tumor tissues have allowed some light into the 'black boxes'. It is now possible to select tumor cell lines that are known to express the anticipated molecular target of the test agents. The Developmental Therapeutics program NCI/NIH (http://dtp.nci.nih.gov/mtargets/mt_index.html) has measured thousands of molecular targets in the NCI panel of 60 human tumor cell lines. The measurements include protein levels, RNA measurements, mutation status and enzyme activity levels.

2 HER-2/neu and Herceptin™

Among the first signal transduction inhibitors proven to be therapeutically useful in the treatment of human cancer is the humanized mouse monoclonal antibody to HER-2 designated trastuzumab (Herceptin™), which neutralizes the activity of the p185HER2 growth factor receptor [3]. Several human tumor cell lines were shown to have high endogenous expression of the HER-2/Neu receptor, including SKOV-3 ovarian carcinoma, and SKBR3 breast carcinoma and other human tumor cell lines such as MCF-7 human breast carcinoma were engineered to overexpress the target [4, 5]. Preclinical studies, strengthened by the knowledge of the HER-2/neu expression status of the tumor models, have been invaluable in elucidating the therapeutic value of trastuzumab. The binding of trastuzumab stabilizes HER-2 homodimer formation, and prevents the receptor from interacting with other HER co-receptors. Trastuzumab binding induces phosphorylation of specific C-terminal resides on the receptor that recruit chaperon proteins and lead to receptor ubiquitination and degradation [6]. Binding of trastuzumab to the HER-2 receptor ultimately results in decreased levels of cyclin D1 and increased steady-state levels of the cyclin-dependent kinase inhibitor p27, leading to cell cycle arrest [7]. A consequence of these events is reduced expression and secretion of critical angiogenic factors by the cancer cells [8]. Another antitumor mechanism triggered by binding of trastuzumab to tumor cells may be recruitment of Fc receptor-expressing immune effector cells leading to antibody-dependent cell-mediated cytotoxicity (ADCC) [9].

HER-2 is amplified and overexpressed in 25–30% of human breast cancers [10–13]. In NIH-3T3 cells and immortalized human breast cells, overexpression of the HER-2 gene produces a neoplastic transformation [13–17]. Pegram et al. [18] found that transfecting human breast and ovarian cancer cell lines with HER-2/neu did not significantly alter their response to a variety of chemotherapeutic agents in cell culture, or when grown as xenograft tumors. However, when human breast and ovarian cell lines that overexpress HER-2 were grown as xenografts in nude mice, their growth was inhibited by administration of a recombinant humanzied monoclonal antibody to HER-2 [19, 20]. Tumor growth was decreased in a manner that was dependent upon the dose of the antibody. Tumor growth resumed when the antibody therapy was stopped, indicating a primarily cytostatic effect of the antibody. The antibody was an effective addition to treatment regimens in combination with cisplatin or doxorubicin. Thus, there was an anti-proliferative effect of the humanized recombinant antibody to HER-2 when tumors expressed the HER-2 receptor, and there was a therapeutic advantage to administration of the anti-HER-2 receptor antibody in combination with anticancer chemotherapy. *In vivo* experiments with chemotherapy with or without the humanized recombinant antibody to HER-2 were conducted with HER-2/neu-transfected human MCF7 breast cancer xenografts in nude mice [21]. Combination regimens with the humanized recombinant antibody to HER-2 and cyclophosphamide, doxorubicin, paclitaxel, methotrexate, etoposide and vinblastine resulted in additive to greater-than-additive tumor response, while combination regimens with 5-fluorouracil resulted in sub-additive tumor response.

Using several ovarian cancer cell lines including SKOV-3 cells that overexpressed HER-2 (10^5 receptors/cell), Xu et al. [22] found that antibodies to

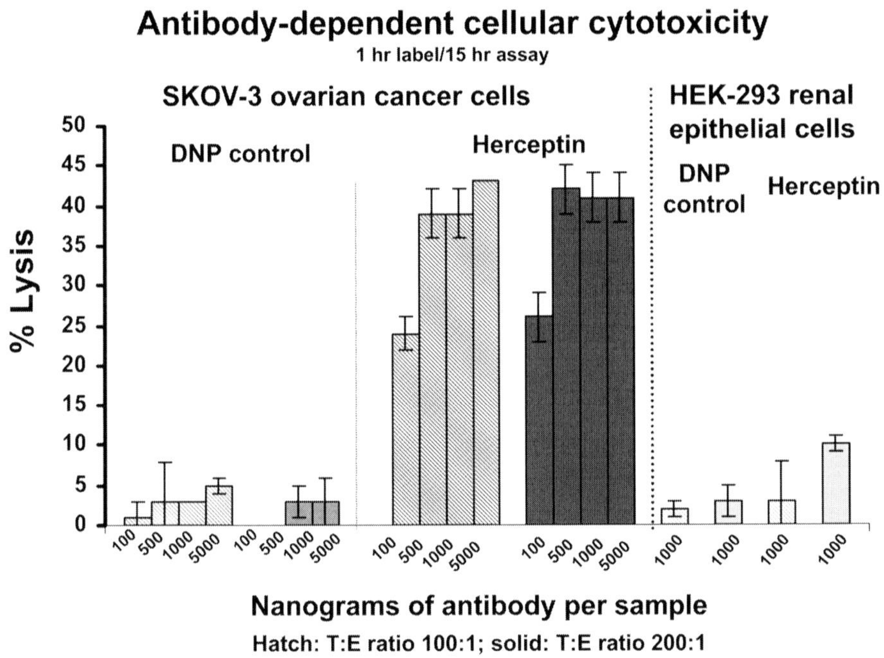

Figure 1.
Antibody-dependent cellular cytotoxicity (ADCC) mediated by Herceptin. Human SKOV-3 ovarian cancer cells, which express HER-2/neu in co-culture with human PBMC (100:1 or 200:1), were exposed to various concentrations of the isotype control antibody DNP or to Herceptin, and SKOV-3 cell lysis as determined by release of ^{51}Cr was measured. Human HEK293 renal epithelial cells, which do not express HER-2/neu, were treated in the same way. Two independent experiments were performed; bars represent SEM.

HER-2 inhibited the growth of transfectants with high levels of HER-2 expression independent of HER-3 and HER-4 expression, and that agonistic antibodies that bind to HER-2 alone inhibit anchorage-independent growth of the cells. ADCC has been described as a potentially important mode of action for antibody therapeutics *in vivo*. Human SKOV-3 ovarian carcinoma cells express very high levels of Her2/neu. These cells were used as target-expressing cells, and HEK 293 cells were used as cells not expressing the target, allowing the use of Herceptin as an antibody in an ADCC assay (Fig. 1). The isotype control antibody was anti-dinitro-phenol (DNP). SKOV-3 cells or relevant target cells were labeled overnight with ^{51}Cr, and then washed in DMEM to remove unincorporated ^{51}Cr. The Cr-labeled SKOV-3 cells (7×10^4)

were mixed with 300 ng–5 μg Herceptin in 1.4 ml DMEM. The reaction mixture was divided into 12 wells of a 96-well plate (5×10^3 cells/well in 100 μl DMEM). Human peripheral blood mononuclear cells (PBMC) or monocyte effector cells were added to the wells at an effector: target cell (E:T) ratio of 200:1 and 100:1 in 100 μl DMEM bringing the total volume per well to 200 μl (final antibody concentrations: 0.012–0.18 μg/well). The plate was centrifuged at 900 rpm for 3 min and then incubated at 37°C for 5 h or overnight (20 h). The ^{51}Cr released was measured using a beta counter. All samples were assayed in triplicate with two E:T ratios. Percent specific lysis was calculated as: % target cell lysis = 100 × (experimental cpm – spontaneous cpm)/(total cpm – spontaneous cpm). As is evident from Figure 1, exposing SKOV-3 cells and PBMC to various concentrations of Herceptin resulted in the lysis of about 40% of the SKOV-3 cells, while exposing the same cultures to DNP resulted in lysis of only about 5% of the SKOV-3 cells. On the other hand, exposure to Herceptin was much less lethal when non-HER-2/neu expressing HEK 293 cells and PBMC were treated with the antibody. Recently, Konecny et al. [23] found a significant positive association between HER-2/neu and vascular endothelial growth factor (VEGF) expression by ELISA in primary breast tumor tissue lysates from 611 unselected patients with a median clinical follow-up of 50 months. The positive association between HER-2/neu and VEGF expression implicates VEGF in the aggressive phenotype exhibited by HER-2/neu overexpression.

3 Epidermal growth factor receptor (EGFR) and EGFR inhibitors

As the understanding of cancer has increased, the complexity of the molecular events that comprise malignant disease has become evident [24–28]. Interactions involved in intertwining signaling networks, including membrane receptors, enzymes along with activators, deactivators and regulators, protein-protein interactions, protein-nucleic acid interactions and small molecule effectors in multiple cell types, are all recognized targets for therapeutic attack. Agents are targeted to specific abnormalities in the sequence and expression of genes/proteins that operate in a stepwise, combinatorial manner to permit the malignant disease to progress [29]. Cell growth, motility, differentiation and death are regulated by signals received from the environment in either an autocrine or paracrine manner [30]. Signals may come from interactions with other cells or components of the extracellular matrix, or from binding of soluble signaling molecules to specific receptors at the cell membrane, thereby initiating different signaling pathways inside of the cell. Cancer may be visualized as a critical perturbation of signaling pathways [31–43]. Receptor tyrosine kinases (RTKs) are key mediators of many normal cellular processes and of human malignant disease processes. Several signaling pathways controlled by tyrosine kinases have been selected as important targets for anticancer therapeutic intervention [45–48]. Kinase inhibitors can be antiangiogenic through activity in the malignant cells and other cells that secrete angiogenic factors and by blocking intracellular signal transduction in cells that respond to angiogenic factors (Fig. 2).

The EGFR is targeted by both monoclonal antibodies to prevent ligand binding, and small molecule inhibitors of the tyrosine kinase enzymatic activity to inhibit auto-phosphorylation and downstream intracellular signaling by the receptor [49–57]. The inhibitors of EGFR are grouped amongst the 'targeted' cancer therapeutics, even though EGFR is widely expressed in normal tissues. EGFR mRNA is found at fairly low levels in a variety of breast,

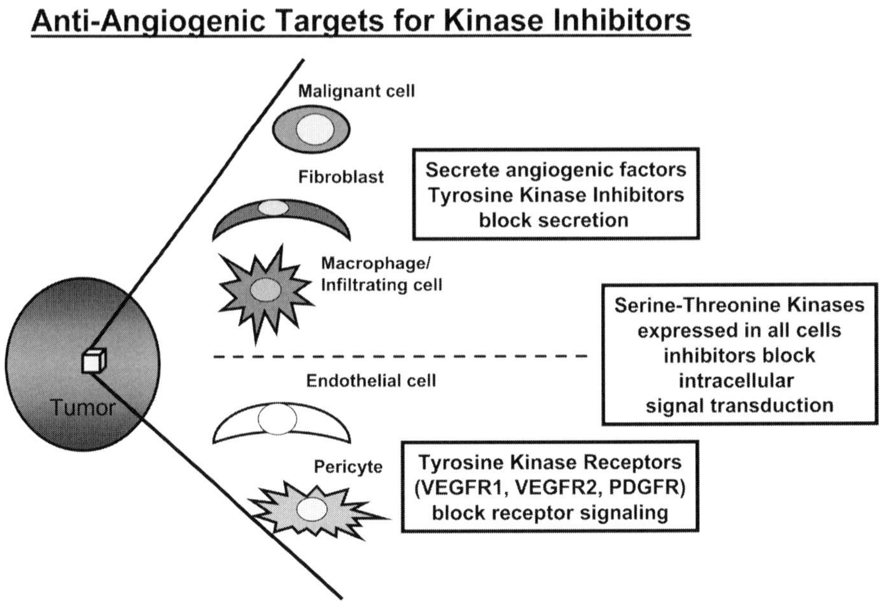

Figure 2.
Schematic of antiangiogenic kinase targets in a variety of cell-types involved in malignant disease.

lung, prostate and other cancer cell lines, and is found at higher levels in some breast (MD-MBA-468) and ovarian (OVT1) cancer cell lines. The murine MAb 225 antibody, a mouse monoclonal antibody to EGFR, was shown to have antitumor activity against human A431 epidermoid carcinoma and human MDA-MB-468 breast carcinoma grown as xenografts in combination with doxorubicin or cisplatin [58–61]. The humanized MAb 225 antibody C225 has been studied alone and in combination with gemcitabine, topotecan, paclitaxel and radiation therapy in several human tumor xenograft models [62–65]. In the fast growing GEO human colon carcinoma, C225 (10 mg/kg, i.p., 2× weekly for 5 weeks) produced a tumor growth delay of 24 days; topotecan (2 mg/kg, i.p., 2× weekly for 5 weeks), a camptothecin analog, produced a tumor growth delay of 14 days and the combination regimen produced a tumor growth delay of 86 days (Fig. 3) [62]. At least part of the activity of C225 can be attributed to antiangiogenic activity [66–68]. Bruns et al. [63] implanted L3.6pl human pancreatic carcinoma cells into the pancreas of nude mice, and, beginning on day 7 post tumor cell implantation, treatment was initiated with C225 (40 mg/kg, i.p., 2× weekly for 4 weeks), gemcitabine (250 mg/kg, i.p., 2× weekly for 4 weeks) or the combination. The animals were sacrificed on day 32 at completion of the treatment regimen; therefore, no definitive endpoints could be assessed. Gemcitabine appeared to be most effective against the liver and lymph node metastasis, and C225 appeared to be most effective against the primary disease. The combination regimen appeared to be more effective than either treatment alone. Combination treatment regimens including C225 with radiation therapy appeared to produce at least additive tumor growth delay in two head and neck squamous carcinoma xenograft models [52, 55, 65]. C225 has undergone three consecutive phase I clinical trials, a phase Ib clinical trial, several single agent and combination phase II and phase III clinical trials, and has received FDA approval as Erbitux [42, 59, 67–69].

Among the several small-molecule ATP-binding site competitive inhibitors of EGFR kinase activity, ZD1839 (gefitinib, Iressa) has reached clinical approval [70–73]. ZD1839 has been studied in combination with cisplatin, carboplatin, oxaliplatin, paclitaxel, docetaxel, doxorubicin, etoposide, raltitrexed and radiation therapy in human tumor xenograft models [67–69, 74–77]. The contribution of ZD1839 to the anticancer activity of combination treatment regimens is due, at least in part, to activity as an antiangiogenic agent [69, 78]. When nude mice bearing the fast growing human GEO

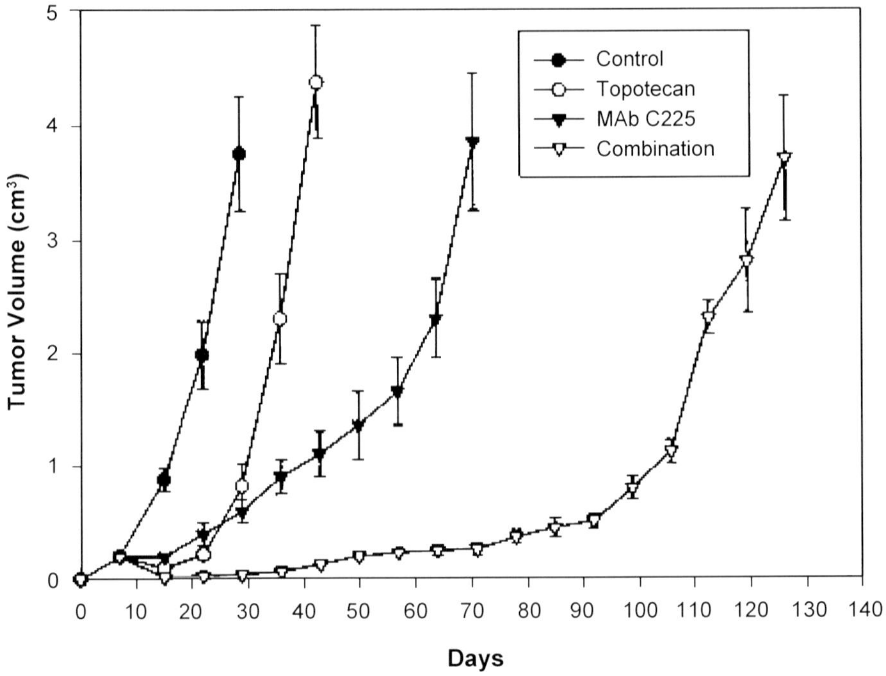

Figure 3.
Antitumor activity of topotecan and MAb C225 on established GEO human colon carcinoma xenografts. Mice were injected s.c. in the dorsal flank with 10^7 human GEO colon carcinoma cells. After 7 days (average tumor size, 0.2 cm^3), mice were treated i.p. with topotecan alone (2 mg/kg/dose, twice weekly on days 1 and 2 of each week for 2 weeks) or with MAb C225 alone (0.25 mg/dose, twice weekly on days 3 and 6 of each week for 5 weeks), or with both drugs with the same sequential schedule. Each group consisted of ten mice. The experiment was repeated three times. Data represent the average of 30 mice for each group; bars represent SD. Student's *t*-test was used to compare tumor sizes among different treatment groups at day 29 after tumor cell implantation. MAb C225 *vs* control ($P < 0.001$); topotecan *vs* control ($P < 0.001$); topotecan followed by MAb C225 *vs* control ($P < 0.001$); topotecan followed by MAb C225 *vs* MAb C225 ($P < 0.001$); topotecan followed by MAb C225 *vs* topotecan ($P < 0.001$).

colon carcinoma were treated with ZD1839 daily for 5 days per week for 4 weeks at doses of 50, 100 or 200 mg/kg i.p., tumor growth delays of 4, 6 and 18 days, respectively, resulted [67, 68]. The 100 mg/kg dose of ZD1839 was selected for combination studies. Using the GEO colon xenograft tumor model, Ciardiello et al. [67, 68] found that ZD1839 administered daily i.p. for 5 days per week for 4 weeks produced a 6- to 10-day tumor growth delay, while standard regimens for paclitaxel (20 mg/kg), topotecan (2 mg/kg) and tomudex (12.5 mg/kg) resulted in 9, 7 and 10 days of tumor growth delay, respectively. The combination treatment regimens of ZD1839 with each cytotoxic agent resulted in 33, 27 and 25 days of tumor growth delay, respectively. Sirotnak et al. [74] administered ZD1839 (150 mg/kg) p.o. daily for 5 days for 2 weeks to nude mice bearing A431 human vulvar epidermoid carcinoma, A549, SK-LC-16 or LX-1 human non-small cell lung carcinomas or PC-3 or TSU-PR1 human prostate carcinomas, as a single agent or along with cisplatin, carboplatin, paclitaxel, docetaxel, doxorubicin, edatexate, gemcitabine or vinorelbine. ZD1839 was a positive addition to all of the treatment combinations except gemcitabine, where it did not alter the antitumor activity compared with gemcitabine alone, and vinorelbine where the combination regimen was toxic. For example, in the LX-1 non-small cell lung carcinoma xenograft, ZD1839 (150 mg/kg, p.o.) produced a tumor growth delay of 8 days, paclitaxel (25 mg/kg, i.p.) produced a tumor growth delay of 16 days and the combination treatment regimens resulted in a tumor growth delay of 26 days. Working in the human GEO colon carcinoma, Ciardiello et al. [69] found that ZD1839 (150 mg/kg, i.p., daily for 5 days per week for 3 weeks; total dose 2250 mg/kg) was a more powerful antiangiogenic therapy than paclitaxel (20 mg/kg, i.p., once per week for 3 weeks; total dose 60 mg/kg) and that the combination treatment regimen was most effective. Expanding upon these studies, Tortora et al. [79] examined combinations of an antisense oligonucleotide targeting protein kinase A, a taxane and ZD1839 in the fast growing human GEO colon carcinoma xenograft. The tumor growth delays were 8 days with the taxane IDN5109 (60 mg/kg, p.o.), 20 days with ZD1839 (150 mg/kg, p.o.), 23 days with the antisense AS-PKAI (10 mg/kg, p.o.), and 61 days with the three agent combination treatment regimen. Naruse et al. [80] found that a subline of human K562 leukemia made resistant to the phorbol ester TPA and designated K562/TPA was more sensitive to ZD1839 administered i.v. or s.c. to nude mice bearing s.c. implanted tumors than was the parental K562 line. Given these results, it is unlikely that ZD1839 would be a highly effective single agent in the clinic, but it could be a useful component in combination treatment regimens.

ZD1839 was evaluated in five phase I clinical trials including 254 patients, and it appeared that response to ZD1839 did not correspond to tumor EGFR expression [81]. A phase I study of 26 colorectal cancer patients showed that ZD1839 could be combined safely with 5-fluorouracil and leucovorin [73, 82]. Two large multicenter phase III clinical trials of ZD1839

(250 or 500 mg daily) in combination with carboplatin/paclitaxel or cisplatin/gemcitabine as first-line treatment in non-operable stage III and stage IV non-small cell lung cancer patients were conducted [81, 83, 84].

Like ZD1839, OSI-774 (erlotinib, Tarceva) is a small molecule ATP-competitive inhibitor of EGFR kinase function of the 4-phenylamino-quazoline class [71]. The antitumor activity of OSI-774 was explored in two human tumor cell lines known to overexpress the EGFR and known to be sensitive to antibodies to EGFR, the LICR-LON-HN5 head and neck carcinoma (HN5; [85–87]) and A431 epidermoid carcinoma [60, 88]. For administration of OSI-774 to animals either by i.p. injection or by oral gavage (p.o.), the compound was formulated in a vehicle containing 10% DMSO by volume [89]. By either route, OSI-774 produced a significant dose-related inhibition of EGFR tyrosine phosphorylation in HN5 tumors collected 1 h after administration of the compound. Orally administered OSI-774 was tested in nude mice bearing s.c. implanted HN5 tumors. When the compound was given daily beginning on day 4 post tumor cell implant and continued until day 24, doses of OSI-774 between 1.6 and 6.2 mg/kg produced tumor growth delays of 2–10 days, while doses of the compound between 12.5 and 100 mg/kg produced tumor growth delays of 32–38 days (Fig. 4) [89]. OSI-774 was then evaluated in the HN5 tumor beginning treatment when the tumors were well established, on about day 18 post s.c. tumor implantation and continuing daily until about day 38. Doses of the compound between 2.9 and 5.7 mg/kg produced tumor growth delays of 0–8 days and doses between 11 and 92 mg/kg result in a tumor growth delay of about 30 days (Fig. 4). Finally, nude mice bearing a human A431 epidermoid carcinoma s.c. xenograft were treated orally, beginning day 4 post tumor cell implantation, with OSI-774 daily until day 24. While treatment was on-going, the tumor growth delays produced by doses of the compound between 3.1 and 12.5 mg/kg were 0-7 days and at doses between 25 and 100 mg/kg were =14 days (Fig. 4). OSI-774 was tested in two phase I clinical trials using daily or weekly oral dosing [90]. The dose-limiting toxicities were rash and diarrhea, and the final recommended dose was 150 mg/day. Three phase II clinical trials explored the efficacy of OSI-774 (150 mg/day) in non-small cell lung cancer, ovarian cancer and head and neck cancers. The single agent activity of OSI-774 was modest. Subsequently, a number of phase III clinical trials were initiated in non-small cell lung cancer in combination with cisplatin and gemcitabine (TALENT), with carboplatin and paclitaxel (TRBUTE), in second-

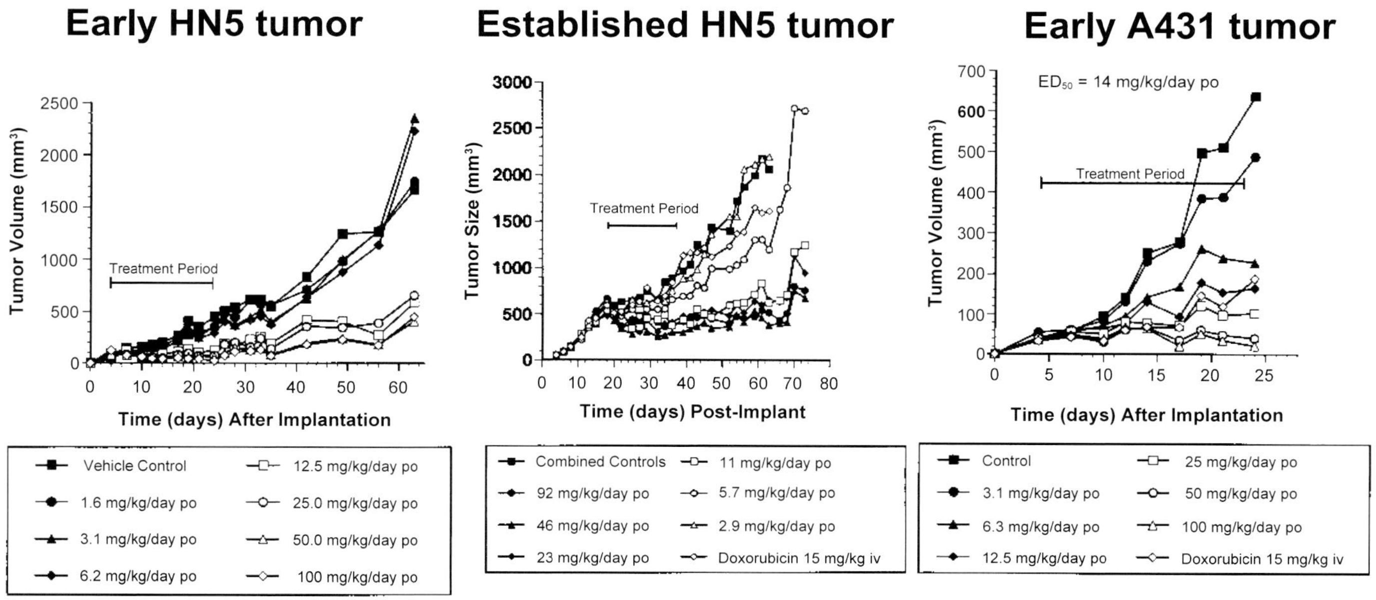

Figure 4.
Antitumor activity of OSI-774 administered orally to athymic mice bearing s.c. implanted human tumor xenografts. In each experiment, OSI-774 was administered once daily for 20 consecutive days in a vehicle consisting of sterile, pyrogen-free 10% DMSO, 0.85% sodium chloride and 0.1% Pluronic P105. Doxorubicin was administered as a single dose by i.v. injection into a tail vein. The data are representative of two independent experiments (adapted from [89]).

line therapy with docetaxel and as second/third-line monotherapy [90–92]. OSI-774 was successful in meeting the clinical goals in the TRIBUTE phase II trial.

The deregulated tyrosine kinase activity of the BCR-ABL fusion protein has been established as a causative molecular event in chronic myelogenous leukemia (CML). The BCR-ABL fusion protein has proven to be an ideal tyrosine receptor kinase target for pharmacological inhibition. STI571 (Gleevec; Glivec; CGP57148B) is a potent inhibitor of the Abl tyrosine kinase that is present on the malignant cells in 95% of patients with CML. The STI571 selectively kills v-Abl- and Bcr-Abl-expressing cells and has antitumor activity as a single agent in animal models at well-tolerated doses [71, 93–101]. Unlike many other tyrosine kinase inhibitors that are cytostatic, STI571 is cytotoxic toward CML-derived cell lines as demonstrated in colony formation assays using the surviving fraction endpoint [102]. In cell culture STI571 adds to the cytotoxicity of other cytotoxic agents, such as etoposide, in the cells that express the BCR-ABL mutation [102–104]. In cell culture studies modeling combinations that may be used for bone marrow pre-transplantation conditioning regimens, using the BV173 and EM-3 BCR-ABL-positive cell lines with an MTT growth inhibition endpoint, Topaly et al. [105] found that STI571 produced greater-than-additive growth inhibition in combination with radiation therapy and produced additive to less-than-additive growth inhibition with busulfan and treosulfan by the combination index method. Mice reconstituted with P210 (BCR/ABL)-transduced bone marrow cells succumb to a rapidly fatal leukemia [106]. When these animals were treated with STI571, survival time was increased. In contrast to the polyclonal leukemia in control mice, STI571-treated mice develop a CML-like leukemia that is generally oligoclonal, suggesting that STI571 eliminated or severely suppressed certain leukemic clones. None of the STI571-treated mice were cured of the CML-like myeloproliferative disorder, and STI571-treated murine CML transplanted with high efficiency to fresh recipient animals.

Progression of CML to acute leukemia (blast crisis) in humans has been associated with acquisition of secondary chromosomal translocations frequently resulting in the NUP98/HOXA9 fusion protein. Dash et al. [107] developed a murine model expressing BCR/ABL and NUP98/HOXA9 to cause blast crisis. The phenotype depends upon expression of both mutant proteins, and the tumor retains sensitivity to STI571. Despite the success of STI571, resistance can develop to this agent in the clinic [108–111].

STI571 is not a specific inhibitor of BCR/ABL and is, indeed, also a potent inhibitor of other tyrosine kinases including the receptor tyrosine kinase KIT and the platelet-derived growth factor receptor (PDGFR). About 90% of malignant gastrointestinal stromal tumors (GISTs) have a mutation in c-kit, leading to KIT receptor autophosphorylation and ligand-independent activation. Initial clinical studies have found that about 50% of GISTs respond to STI571 [112–117]. PDGFR is expressed in several human cancers and is also expressed by tumor endothelial cells, thus, enabling STI571 to be used as an antiangiogenic agent.

4 Genetically engineered mouse models

The wide-spread use of genetically engineered murine cancer models for testing potential therapeutics has had a difficult beginning for several reasons. The first is that of maintenance in producing large breeding colonies with sufficient animals to perform efficacy testing. Second is that the tumor nodules arising in these mice generally occur at 'old-age' so that large numbers of animals must be housed for long periods before they can be used in experiments. Third is that many of the models develop tumor nodules originating from a single gene alteration and are overly responsive to therapy. The hypothesis is that the transformation of a normal cell to a malignant tumor cell occurs as a result of a relatively small number of critical genetic changes [118]. Transgenic models of mammary, pancreas, prostate, stomach and lung adenocarcinoma have been developed by genetically engineering mice that express polyoma middle T (MMTV) alone or along with activated neu or Wnt1, c-myc (WAP) alone or along with TGF-α, elastase-T antigen (ET), or prostate steroid binding protein alone or along with T antigen [119]. Several approaches have been applied to genetically engineered models of brain tumors; these include embryonic stem cell-mediated transgenesis, injection of cells producing an oncogene by infection with a retroviral victor, and targeted gene disruption [120].

The more recently developed approaches allow the use of latent, conditional and inducible alleles to better mimic appropriate expression of human genes in engineered mice [121]. Chromosome translocations, latent alleles and tissue-specific and temporally regulated mutations provide a better model of human disease [122]. Multiple mutations are often introduced into animals by interbreeding. The Cancer Genome Anatomy Project (http://cgap.nci.nih.gov) established by the National Cancer Institute in 1997 is cataloging all cancer-related changes in both human and mouse tumors using EST and SAGE cDNA sequencing methods to examine large proportions of the genome for aberrant expression and sequence alterations. While most current transgenic oncomouse models fail to produce malignant disease, as defined by ability to metastasize, future generations of genetically engineered animal models will likely be moving closer to true disease models [123].

The main focus of cancer research and tumor model development has been on the alteration in cells that enable enhanced growth properties, evasion of apoptotic signals, immortality, and invasive and metastatic properties to become malignant. The roles of the microenvironment, that is stromal cells including stromal fibroblasts and inflammatory cells that support/promote tumor growth, are also an area of active investigation [124]. It is evident that early and persistent inflammatory responses observed in or around many solid tumors have an important role in establishing a molecular environment supportive of neoplastic progression by providing growth factors, cytokines, chemokines and other factors that alter tissue homeostasis [124]. The phenomenon designated as epithelial to mesenchymal transition (EMT), which refers to the breakdown of epithelial cell homeostasis leading to aggressive cancer progression, can be promoted and potentially driven by molecules secreted by stromal cells [125]. An example of the power of stroma on tumor growth is the prostate carcinoma and bone-stroma interaction [126]. In a cell-based three-dimensional co-culture assay system established with prostate cancer cells and bone cells, both genotypical and phenotypical responses were observed; responses that were demonstrated when tumor epithelial cells were co-cultured with bone stroma.

5 Conclusions

The cancer research community realizes that human cancer in its limitless forms is a very difficult disease to model and very difficult to treat. The notion of 'targeted' therapeutics that would selectively block molecular processes required for tumor growth, but that are not expressed by or needed by normal tissues, has generally not had the successes hoped for. There have been, however, subgroups of patients whose malignant disease has responded very well to specific 'targeted' therapeutics, and in a few cases a molecular alteration or expression of the target can account for those responses. Examples of these cases may be expression of specifically mutated EGFR and responses to erlotinib or gifitinib, and expression of HER-2/neu and responses to Herceptin. These findings have encouraged the development of diagnostic tests that can be applied to select patients with the best chance of responding to a specific targeted agent. Clinical colleagues again turn to preclinical models with questions to be answered before an appropriate clinical trial design can be defined for a particular agent [127]. Question such as: (1) Can any serious toxicity be predicted based upon preclinical data?; (2) Can single agent activity including tumor regression be predicted from preclinical efficacy data?; (3) Is there a clear molecular target?; (4) Does inhibition or neutralization of the target molecule correlate with tumor response in the preclinical efficacy models?; (5) Can inhibition or neutralization of the target be detected in tumor materials or in surrogate tissues in preclinical models?; (6) Are there surrogate measurements that can be correlated with target inhibition? The answers to these types of questions test the value of preclinical models, but also influence the selection of targets and therapeutic agents to address those targets.

References

1 Teicher BA (ed) (2001) *Tumor models in cancer research.* Humana Press, Totowa

2 Schuh JCL (2004) Trials, tribulations and trends in tumor modeling in mice. *Toxicol Pathol* 32 (Suppl 1): 53–66

3 Coussens L, Yang-Feng TC, Liao YC, Chen E, Gray A, McGrath J, Seeburg PH, Lieberman TA, Schlessinger J, Francke U et al (1985) Tyrosine kinase receptor with extensive homology to EGF receptor shares chrmosomal location with neu oncogene. *Science* 230: 1132–1139

4 Pirollo KF, Hao Z, Rait A (1997) Evidence supporting a signal transduction pathway leading to the radiation-resistant phenotype in human tumor cells. *Biochem Biophys Res Commun* 230: 196–201

5 Pietras RJ, Poen JC, Gallardo D, Wongvipat PN, Lee HJ, Slamon DJ (1999) Monoclonal antibody to HER-2/neu receptor modulates repair of radiation-induced DNA damage and enhances radiosensitivity of human breast cancer cells overexpressing this oncogene. *Cancer Res* 59: 1347–1355

6 Klapper LN, Waterman H, Sela M, Yarden Y (2000) Tumor-inhibitory antibodies to HER-2/ErbB-2 may act by recruiting c-CBL and enhancing ubiquitination of HER-2. *Cancer Res* 60: 3384–3388

7 Sliwkowski MX, Lofgren JA, Lewis GD, Hotaling TE, Fendly BM, Fox JA (1999) Nonclinical studies addressing the mechanism of action of Trastuzumab (Herceptin). *Semin Oncol* 26 (Suppl 12): 60–70

8 Petit AM, Rak J, Hung MC, Rockwell P, Goldstein N, Fendly B, Kerbel RS (1997) Neutralizing antibodies against epidermal growth factor and ErbB-2/neu receptor tyrosine kinases downregulate vascular endothelial growth factor production by tumor cells *in vitro* and *in vivo*. *Am J Pathol* 151: 1523–1530

9 Clynes RA, Towers TL, Presta LG, Ravetch JV (2000) Inhibitory Fc receptors modulate *in vivo* cytotoxicity against tumor targets. *Nat Med* 6: 443–446

10 Slamon DJ, Clark GM, Wong SG, Levin W, Ullrich A, McGuire WL (1987) Human breast cancer: correlation of relapse and survival with amplification of the HER-2/neu oncogene. *Science* 235: 177–182

11 Slamon DJ, Godolphin W, Jones L, Holt J, Wong S, Keith D, Levin W, Stuart S, Udove J, Ullrich A et al (1989) Studies of the HER-2/neu proto-oncogene in human breast cancer and ovarian cancer. *Science* 244: 707–712

12 Slamon D, Press M, Godolphin W, Ramos L, Haran P, Shek L, Stuart S, Ullrich A (1989) Studies of the HER-2/neu oncogene in human breast cancer. *Cancer Cells* 7: 371–379

13 Reese D, Slamon D (1997) HER-2/neu signal transduction in human breast and ovarian cancer. *Stem Cells* 15: 1–8

14 DiFiore PP, Pierce JH, Kraus MH, Segatto O, King CR, Aaronson SA (1987) erbB2 is a potent oncogene when expressed in NIH-3T3 cells. *Science* 237: 178–181

15 Hudziak RM, Schlessinger J, Ullrich A (1987) Increased expression of the putative growth factor receptor p185HER-2 causes transformation and tumorigenesis of NIH-3T3 cells. *Proc Natl Acad Sci USA* 84: 7159–7163

16 Chazin V, Kaleko M, Miller A, Slamon DJ (1992) Transformation mediated by the human HER-2 gene independent of the epidermal growth factor receptor. *Oncogene* 7: 1859–1865

17 Pierce J, Arnstein P, Dimarco E, Artrip J, Kraus M, Lonardo F, Di Fiore P, Aaronson S (1991) Oncogenic potential of erbB-2 in human mammary epithelial cells. *Oncogene* 6: 1189–1194

18 Pegram MD, Finn RS, Arzoo K, Beryt M, Pietras RJ, Slamon DJ (1997) The effect of HER-2/neu overexpression on chemotherapeutic drug sensitivity in human breast and ovarian cancer cells. *Oncogene* 15: 537–547

19 Pietras RJ, Pegram MD, Finn RS, Maneval DA, Slamon DJ (1998) Remission of human breast cancer xenografts on therapy with humanized monoclonal antibody to HER-2 receptor and DNA-reactive drugs. *Oncogene* 17: 2235–2249

20 Pegram MD, Pauletti G, Slamon DJ (1998) HER-2/neu as a predictive marker of response to breast cancer therapy. *Breast Cancer Res Treat* 52: 65–77

21 Pegram M, Hsu S, Lewis G, Pietras R, Beryt M, Sliwkowski M, Coombs D, Baly D, Kabbinavar F, Slamon D (1999) Inhibitory effects of combinations of HER-2/neu antibody and chemotherapeutic agents used for treatment of human breast cancers. *Oncogene* 18: 2241–2251

22 Xu F, Yu Y, Le X-F, Boyer C, Mills GB, Bast RC (1999) The outcome of heregulin-induced activation of ovarian cancer cells depends on the relative levels of HER-2 and HER-3 expression. *Clin Cancer Res* 5: 3653–3660

23 Konecny GE, Meng YG, Untch M, Wang H-J, Bauerfeind I, Epstein M, Stieber P, Vernes J-M, Gutierrez J, Hong K et al (2004) Association between HER-2/neu and vascular endothelial growth factor expression predicts clinical outcome in primary breast cancer patients. *Clin Cancer Res* 10: 1706–1716

24 Kohn EC, Lu Y, Wang H, Yu Q, Yu S, Hall H, Smith DL, Meric-Bernstam F, Hortobagyi GN, Mills GB (2004) Molecular therapeutics: promise and challenges. *Semin Oncol* 31: 39–53
25 Chakravarthy B, Pietenpol JA (2003) Combined modality management of breast cancer: development of predictive markers through proteomics. *Semin Oncol* 30: 23–36
26 Petricoin EF, Liotta LA (2003) Clinical applications of proteomics. *J Nutr* 133: 2476S–2484S
27 Frank R, Hargreaves R (2003) Clinical biomarkers in drug discovery and development. *Nat Rev Drug Discov* 2: 566–580
28 Hamid O (2004) Emerging treatments in oncology: focus on tyrosine kinase (erbB) receptor inhibitors. *J Am Pharm Assoc* 44: 52–58
29 Workman P (2001) Scoring a bull's-eye against cancer genome targets. *Curr Opin Pharmacol* 1: 342–352
30 Heldin CH (2001). Signal transduction: multiple pathways, multiple options for therapy. *Stem Cells* 19: 295–303
31 Elsayed YA, Sausville EA (2001) Selected novel anticancer treatments targeting cell signaling proteins. *Oncologists* 6: 517–537
32 Hondermarck H, Vercoutter-Edouart AS, Revillion F, Lemoine J, er-Yazidi-Belkoura I, Nurcombe V, Peyrat JP (2001) Proteomics of breast cancer for marker discovery and signal pathway profiling. *Proteomics* 1: 1216–1232
33 Arteaga CL, Khuri F, Krystal G, Sebti S (2002) Overview of rationale and clinical trials with signal transduction inhibitors in lung cancer. *Semin Oncol* 29 (1 suppl 4): 15–26
34 Fodde R, Smits R, Clevers H (2001) APC, signal transduction and genetic instability in colorectal cancer. *Nat Rev Cancer* 1: 55–67
35 Graff JR (2002) Emerging targets in the AKT pathway for treatment of androgen-independent prostatic adenocarcinoma. *Exp Opin Ther Targets* 6: 103–113
36 Lango MN, Shin DM, Grandis JR (2001) Targeting growth factor receptors: integration of novel therapeutics in the management of head and neck cancer. *Curr Opin Oncol* 13: 168–175
37 Bode AM, Dong Z (2000) Signal transduction pathways: targets for chemoprevention of skin cancer. *Lancet Oncol* 1: 181–188
38 Heymach JV (2001) Angiogenesis and antiangiogenic approaches to sarcomas. *Curr Opin Oncology* 13: 261–269
39 Reddy SA (2001) Signaling pathways in pancreatic cancer. *Cancer J* 7: 274–286
40 Lieberman SM, Horig H, Kaufman HL (2001) Innovative treatments for pancreatic cancer. *Surg Clin N Am* 81: 715–739
41 Folkman J (1971) Tumor angiogenesis: therapeutic implications. *N Engl J Med* 285: 1182–1186
42 Ciardiello F, Bianco R, Caputo R, Caputo R, Damiano V, Triani T, Melisi D, De Vita F, De Placido S, Bianco AR et al (2004) Antitumor activity of ZD6474, a vascular endothelial growth factor receptor tyrosine kinase inhibitor, in human cancer cells with acquired resistance to antiepidermal growth factor receptor therapy. *Clin Cancer Res* 10: 784–793
43 El-Rayes BF, LoRusso PM (2004) Targeting the epidermal growth factor receptor. *Br J Cancer* 91: 418–424

44 Herbst RS (2004) Review of epidermal growth factor receptor biology. *Int J Radiat Oncol Biol Phys* 59 (2 suppl): 21–26

45 Teicher BA (1996) Systems approach to cancer therapy (antiangiogenics + standard cytotoxics – mechanism(s) of interaction). *Cancer Metastasis Rev* 15: 247–272

46 Teicher BA (ed) (1999) *Antiangiogenic agents in cancer therapy.* Humana Press, Totowa

47 Zwick E, Bange J, Ullrich A (2001) Receptor tyrosine signaling as a target for cancer intervention strategies. *Endocr Relat Cancer* 8: 161–173

48 Ciardiello F, Tortora G (2001) A novel approach in the treatment of cancer: targeting the epidermal growth factor receptor. *Clin Cancer Res* 7: 2958–2970

49 Sedlacek HH (2000) Kinase inhibitors in cancer therapy. A look ahead. *Drugs* 59: 435–476

50 Moscatello DK, Holgado-Madruga M, Emlet DR, Montgomery RB, Wong AJ (1998) Constitutive activation of phosphatidylinositol 3-kinase by a naturally occurring mutant epidermal growth factor receptor. *J Biol Chem* 273: 200–206

51 Kari C, Chan TO, de Quadros MR, Roderick U (2003) Targeting the epidermal growth factor receptor in cancer: apoptosis takes center stage. *Cancer Res* 63: 1–5

52 Huang S, Armstrong EA, Benavente S, Chinnaiyan P, Harari PM (2004) Dual-agent molecular targeting of the epidermal growth factor receptor (EGFR): combining anti-EGFR antibody with tyrosine kinase inhibitor. *Cancer Res* 64: 5355–5362

53 Kim DW, Choy H (2004) Potential role for epidermal growth factor receptor inhibitors in combined-modality therapy for non-small cell ling cancer. *Int J Radiat Oncol Biol Phys* 59 (2 suppl): 11–20

54 Thomas SM, Grandis JR (2004) Pharmacokinetic and pharmacodynamic properties of EGFR inhibitors in combined-modality therapy for non-small cell lung cancer. *Int J Radiat Oncol Biol Phys* 59 (2 suppl): 11–20

55 Harari PM, Huang SM (2004) Combining EGFR inhibitors with radiation or chemotherapy: will preclinical studies predict clinical results? *Int J Radiat Oncol Biol Phys* 58: 976–983

56 Li B, Chang CM, Yuan M, McKenna WG, Shu HK (2003) Resistance to small molecule inhibitors of epidermal growth factor receptor in malignant gliomas. *Cancer Res* 63: 7443–7450

57 Arteaga CL (2003) EGF receptor as a therapeutic target: patient selection and mechanisms of resistance to receptor-targeted drugs. *J Clin Oncol* 21 (23 suppl): 289s–291s

58 Mendelsohn J (2000) Blockade of receptors for growth factors: an anticancer therapy. *Clin Cancer Res* 6: 747–753

59 Mendelsohn J (1997) Epidermal growth factor receptor inhibition by a monoclonal antibody as anticancer therapy. *Clin Cancer Res* 3: 2703–2707

60 Fan Z, Baselga J, Masui H, Mendelsohn J (1993) Antitumor effect of anti-epidermal growth factor receptor monoclonal antibodies plus cis-diamminedichloroplatinum on well established A431 cell xenografts. *Cancer Res* 53: 4637–4642

61 Baselga J, Norton L, Masui H, Pandiella A, Coplan K, Miller WH, Mendelsohn J (1993) Antitumor effects of doxorubicin in combination with anti-epidermal growth factor receptor monoclonal antibodies. *J Natl Cancer Inst* 85: 1327–1333

62 Ciardiello F, Bianco R, Damiano V, De Lorenzo S, Pepe S, De Placido S, Fan Z, Mendelsohn J, Bianco AR, Tortora G (1999) Antitumor activity of sequential treatment with topotecan and anti-epidermal growth factor receptor monoclonal antibody C225. *Clin Cancer Res* 5: 909–916

63 Bruns CJ, Harbison MT, Davis DW, Portera CA, Tsan R, McConkey DJ, Evans DB, Abbruzzese JL, Hicklin DJ, Radinsky R (2000) Epidermal growth factor receptor blockade with C225 plus gemcitabine results in regression of human pancreatic carcinoma growing orthotopically in nude mice by antiangiogenic mechanisms. *Clin Cancer Res* 6: 1936–1948
64 Inoue K, Slaton JW, Perrotte P, Davis DW, Bruns CJ, Hicklin DJ, McConkey DJ, Sweeney P, Radinsky R, Dinney CP (2000) Paclitaxel enhances the effects of the anti-epidermal growth factor receptor monoclonal antibody ImClone C225 in mice with metastatic human bladder transitional cell carcinoma. *Clin Cancer Res* 6: 4874–4884
65 Huang S-M, Harari P (2000) Modulation of radiation response after epidermal growth factor receptor blockade in squamous cell carcinomas: inhibition of damage repair, cell cycle kinetics and tumor angiogenesis. *Clin Cancer Res* 6: 2166–2174
66 Perrotte P, Matsumoto T, Inoue K, Kuniyasu H, Eve BY, Hicklin DJ, Radinsky R, Dinney CP (1999) Anti-epidermal growth factor receptor antibody C225 inhibits angiogenesis in human transitional cell carcinoma growing orthotopically in nude mice. *Clin Cancer Res* 5: 257–265
67 Ciardiello F, Bianco R, Damiano V, Fontanini G, Caputo R, Pomatico G, De Placido S, Damiano V, De Lorenzo S, Pepe S et al (2000) Antiangiogenic and antitumor activity of anti-epidermal growth factor receptor C225 monoclonal antibody in combination with vascular endothelial growth factor antisense oligonucleotide in human GEO colon cancer cells. *Clin Cancer Res* 6: 3739–3747
68 Ciardiello F, Caputo R, Bianco R, Damiananco V, Pomatico G, De Placido S, Bianco AR, Tortora G (2000) Antitumor effect and potentiation of cytotoxic drug activity in human cancer cells by ZD-1839 (Iressa), an epidermal growth factor receptor-sensitive tyrosine kinase inhibitor. *Clin Cancer Res* 6: 2053–2063
69 Ciardiello F, Caputo R, Bianco R, Damiano V, Fontanini G, Cuccato S, De Placido S, Bianco AR, Tortora G (2001) Inhibition of growth factor production and angiogenesis in human cancer cells by ZD1839 (Iressa), a selective epidermal growth factor receptor tyrosine kinase inhibitor. *Clin Cancer Res* 7: 1459–1465
70 Woodburn JR, Kendrew J, Fennell M, Wakeling AE (2000) ZD1839 ('Iressa') a selective epidermal growth factor receptor tyrosine kinase inhibitor (EGFR-TKI): inhibition of c-fos mRNA, an intermediate marker of EGFR activation, correlates with tumor growth inhibition. *Proc Am Assoc Cancer Res* 41: 402
71 Traxler P (2003) Tyrosine kinases as targets in cancer therapy – successes and failures. *Expert Opin Ther Targets* 7: 215–234
72 Traxler P, Bold G, Buchdunger E, Caravatti G, Furet P, Manley P, O'Reilly T, Wood J, Zimmermann J (2001) Tyrosine kinase inhibitors: from rational design to clinical trials. *Med Res Rev* 21: 499–512
73 Douglass EC (2003) Development of ZD1839 in colorectal cancer. *Semin Oncol* 30: 17–22
74 Sirotnak FM, Zakowsky MF, Miller VA, Scher HI, Kris MG (2000) Efficacy of cytotoxic agents against human tumor xenografts is markedly enhanced by coadministration of ZD1839 (Iressa) an inhibitor of EGFR tyrosine kinase. *Clin Cancer Res* 6: 4885–4892
75 Ohmori T, Ao Y, Nishio K, Saijo N, Arteaga CL, Kurki T (2000) Low dose cisplatin can modulate the sensitivity of human non-small cell lung carcinoma cells to EGFR tyrosine kinase inhibitor (ZD1839; Iressa) *in vivo*. *Proc Am Assoc Cancer Res* 41: 482

76 Williams K, Telfer BA, Stratford IJ, Wedge SR (2000) An evaluation of the EGFR tyrosine kinase inhibitor ZD1839 (Iressa) in combination with ionizing radiation. *11th NCI-EORTC-AACR Symposium on New Drugs in Cancer Therapy:* Amsterdam, November 7–10. Abstract LB3

77 Harari PM, Huang SM (2001) Radiation response modification following molecular inhibition of epidermal growth factor receptor signaling. *Semin Radiat Oncol* 11: 281–289

78 Hirata A, Ogawa S-I, Kometani T, Kuwano T, Naito S, Kuwano M, Ono M (2002) ZD1839 (Iressa) induces antiangiogenic effects through inhibition of epidermal growth factor receptor tyrosine kinase. *Cancer Res* 62: 2554–2560

79 Tortora G, Caputo R, Damiano V, Fontanini G, Melisi D, Veneziani BM, Zunino F, Bianco AR, Ciardiello F (2001) Oral administration of a novel taxane, an antisense oligonucelotide targeting protein kinase A, and the epidermal growth factor receptor inhibitor Iressa causes cooperative antitumor and antiangiogenic activity. *Clin Cancer Res* 7: 4156–4163

80 Naruse I, Ohmori T, Ao Y, Fukumoto H, Kuroki T, Mori M, Saijo N, Nishio K (2002) Antitumor activity of the selective epidermal growth factor receptor-tyrosine kinase inhibitor (EGFR-TKI) Iressa (ZD1839) in an EGFR-expressing multidrug-resistant cell line *in vitro* and *in vivo*. *Int J Cancer* 98: 310–315

81 Drucker BJ, Schwartz L, Marion S, Motzer R (2002) Phase II trial of ZD1839 (Iressa), an EGF receptor inhibitor, in patients with advanced reanl cell carcinoma. *Proc Am Soc Clin Oncol* 2002: abstract 720

82 Cho CD, Fisher GA, Halsey JZ, Advani RH, Yuen AR, Sikic BI (2002) A phase I study ZD1839 (Iressa) in combination with oxaliplatin, 5-fluororuacil (5-FU) and leucovorin (LV) in advanced solid malignancies. *Proc Am Soc Clin Oncol.* 2002: abstract 38

83 Albanell J, Rojo F, Baselga J (2001) Pharmacodynamic studies with the epidermal growth factor receptor tyrosine kinase inhibitor ZD1839. *Semin Oncol* 28 (5 suppl 16): 56–66

84 Dancey J (2004) Epidermal growth factor receptor inhibitors in clinical development. *Int J Radiat Oncol Biol Phys* 58: 1003–1007

85 Modjtahedi H, Eccles S, Box G, Styles J, Dean C (1993) Immunotherapy of human tumour xenografts overexpressing the EGF receptor with rat antibodies that block growth factor-receptor interaction. *Br J Cancer* 67: 254–261

86 Modjtahedi H, Styles J, Box G, Eccles S, Gusterson B, Dean C (1993) Antitumour activity of rat Mabs to the human receptor for EGF. In: AA Epenetos, NR Lemonie (eds): *Mutant oncogenes: targets for therapy?* Chapman and Hall, London, 35–47

87 Modjtahedi H, Styles J, Dean C (1993) The growth response of human tumour cell lines expressing the EGF receptor to treatment with EGF and/or Mabs that block ligand binding. *Int J Oncol* 3: 237–243

88 Fan Z, Baselga J, Masui H, Mendelsohn J (1992) Antitumor effect of anti-epidermal growth factor receptor monoclonal antibodies plus cis-diamminedichloroplatinum on well established A431 cell xenografts. *Cancer Res* 53: 4637–4642

89 Pollack VA, Savage DM, Baker DA,Tsparikos KE, Sloan DE, Moyer JD, Barbacci EG, Pustilnik LR, Smolarek TA, Davis JA et al (1999) Inhibition of epidermal growth factor receptor-associated tyrosine phosphorylation in human carcinomas with CP-358,774: dynamics of receptor inhibition in situ and antitumor effects in athymic mice. *J Pharmacol Exp Ther* 291: 739–748

90 Grunwald V, Hidalgo M (2003) Development of the epidermal growth factor receptor inhibitor OSI-774. *Semin Oncol* 30: 23–31
91 Miller VA (2004) Long survival of never smoking non-small cell lung cancer (NSCLC) patients (pts) treated with relotinib HCl (OSI-774) and chemotherapy: subgroup analysis of TRIBUTE. *Proc Am Soc Clin Oncol* 2004: abstract 7061
92 Tran HT (2004) Pharmacokinetic study of the phase III randomized, double-blind, multicenter trial of paclitaxel (Pac) and carboplatin (C) combined with erlotinib (E) or placebo in patients with advanced non-small cell lung cancer. *Proc Am Soc Clin Oncol* 2004: abstract 2050
93 Mauro MJ, Druker BJ (2001) STI571: targeting BCR-ABL as therapy for CML. *Oncologist* 6: 233–238
94 Mauro MJ, Druker BJ (2001) STI571: a gene product-targeted therapy for leukemia. *Curr Oncol Reports* 3: 223–227
95 Mauro MJ, O'Dwyer M, Heinrich MC, Druker BJ (2002) STI571: a paradigm of new agents for cancer therapies. *J Clin Oncol* 20: 325–334
96 Griffin J (2001) The biology of signal transduction inhibition: basic science to novel therapies. *Semin Oncol* 28 (5 suppl 17): 3–8
97 Thambi P, Sausville EA (2002) STI571 (imatinib mesylate): the tale of a targeted therapy. *Anti-Cancer Drugs* 13: 111–114
98 Olavarria E, Craddock C, Dazzi F, Marin D, Marktel S, Apperley JF, Goldman JM (2002) Imatinib mesylate (STI571) in the treatment of relapse of chronic myeloid leukemia after allogenic stem cell transplantation. *Blood* 99: 3861–3862
99 Gorre ME, Sawyer CL (2002) Molecular mechanisms of resistance to STI571 in chronic myeloid leukemia. *Curr Opin Hematol* 9: 303–307
100 O'Dwyer ME, Mauro MJ, Druker BJ (2002) Recent advances in the treatment of chronic myelogenous leukemia. *Annu Rev Med* 53: 369–381
101 La Rose P, O'Dwyer ME, Druker BJ (2002) Insights from pre-clinical studies for new combination treatment regimens with the Bcr-Abl kinase inhibitor imatinib mesylate (Gleevec/Glivec) in chronic myelogenous leukemia: a translational perspective. *Leukemia* 16: 1213–1219
102 Liu WM, Stimson LA, Joel SP (2002) The *in vitro* activity of the tyrosine kinase inhibitor STI571 in BCR-ABL positive chronic myeloid leukemia cells: Synergistic interactions with anti-leukemic agents. *Br J Cancer* 86: 1472–1478
103 Marley SB, Davidson RJ, Goldman JM, Gordon MY (2002) Effects of combinations of therapeutic agents on the proliferation of progenitor cells in chronic myeloid leukemia. *Br J Hematol* 116: 162–165
104 Avramis IA, Laug WE, Sausville EA, Avramis VI (2003) Determination of drug synergism between the tyrosine kinase inhibitors NSC680410 (adaphostin) and/or STI571 (imatinib mesylaste, Gleevec) with cytotoxic drugs against human leukemia cell lines. *Cancer Chemother Pharmacol* 52: 307–318
105 Topaly J, Fruehauf S, Ho AD, Zeller WJ (2002) Rationale for combination therapy of chronic myelogenous leukemia with imatinib and irradiation or alkylating agents: implications for pretransplant conditioning. *Br J Cancer* 86: 1487–1493
106 Wolff NC, Ilaria RL (2001) Establishment of a murine model for therapy-treated chronic myelogenous leukemia using the tyrosine kinase inhibitor STI571. *Blood* 98: 2808–2816
107 Dash AB, Williams IR, Kutok JL, Tomasson MH, Anastasiadou E, Lindahl K, Li S, Van Etten RA, Borrow J, Housman D et al (2002) A murine model of CML blast crisis

induced by cooperation between BCR/ABL and NUP98/HOXA9. *Proc Natl Acad Sci USA* 99: 7622–7627

108 Krystal GW (2001) Mechanisms of resistance to imatinib (STI571) and prospects for combination with conventional chemotherapeutic agents. *Drug Resist Updat* 4: 16–21

109 Krystal GW, Honsawek S, Kiewlich D, Liang C, Vasile S, Sun L, McMahon G, Lipson KE (2001) Indoline tyrosine kinase inhibitors block kit activation and growth of small cell lung cancer cells. *Cancer Res* 61: 3660–3668

110 Weisberg E, Griffin JD (2001) Mechanisms of resistance imatinib (STI571) in preclinical models and in leukemia patients. *Drug Resist Updat* 4: 22–28

111 Donato NJ, Wu JY, Stapley J, Lin H, Arlinghaus R, Aggarwal BB, Shisshodia S, Albitar M, Hayes K, Kantarjian H, Talpaz M (2004) Imatinib mesylate resistance through BCR-ABL independence in chronic myelogenous leukemia. *Cancer Res* 64: 672–677

112 Demetri GD (2004) SU11248, a multi-targeted tyrosine kinase inhibitor, can overcome imatinib (IM) resitance caused by diverse genomic mechanisms in patients (pts) with metastatic gastrointestinal stromal tumor (GIST). *Proc Am Soc Clin Oncol* 2004: abstract 3001

113 Demetri GD (2001) Targeting c-kit mutations in solid tumors: scientific rationale and novel therapeutic options. *Semin Oncol* 28 (5 suppl 17): 19–26

114 Joensuu H, Dimitrijevic S (2001) Tyrosine kinase inhibitor imatinib (STI571) as an anticancer agent for solid tumors. *Ann Med* 33: 451–455

115 Joensuu H, Krause A, Demetri GD, Blanke C, von Mehren M, Heinrich MC, Eisenberg B, Roberts PJ, Silberman S, Dimitrijevic S et al (2002) Gastrointestinal stromal tumor (GIST) patients who respond to imatinib (STI571, Gleevec) show marked decline of circulating levels of VEGF, KIT, and bFGF in serum, but not stem cell factor (SCF) levels. *Proc Am Soc Clin Oncol* 2002: abstract 552

116 Heinrich MC, Blanke CD, Druker BJ, Corlees CL (2002) Inhibition of KIT tyrosine kinase activity: a novel molecular approach to the treatment of KIT-positive malignancies. *J Clin Oncol* 20: 1692–1703

117 Sawaki A, Yamao K (2004) Imatinib mesylate acts in metastatic or unresectable gastrointestinal stromal tumor by targeting KIT receptors: a review. *Cancer Chemotherap Pharmacol* 54 (suppl 1): S44–S49

118 Herzig M, Christofori G (2002) Recent advances in cancer research: mouse models of tumorigenesis. *Biochim Biophys Acta* 1602: 97–113

119 Gendler SJ, Mukherjee P (2001) Spontaneous adenocarcinoma mouse models for immunotherapy. *Trends Mol Med* 7: 471–475

120 Lampson LA (2001) New animal models to probe brain tumor biology, therapy, and immunotherapy: advantages and remaining concerns. *J Neurooncol* 53: 275–287

121 Tuveson DA, Jacks T (2002) Technologically advanced cancer modeling in mice. *Curr Opin Genet Dev* 12: 105–110

122 Jackson-Grusby L (2002) Modeling cancer in mice. *Oncogene* 21: 5504–5514

123 Kerbel RS (2003) Human tumor xenografts as predictive preclinical models for anticancer drug activity in humans. *Cancer Biol Ther* 2 (4 suppl 1): S134–S139

124 van Kempen LCLT, Ruiter DJ, van Muijen GNP, Coussens LM (2003) The tumor microenvironment: a critical determinant of neoplastic evolution. *Eur J Cell Biol* 82: 539–548

125 Gotzmann J, Mikula M, Eger A, Schulte-Hermann R, Foisner R, Beug H, Mikulits W (2003) Molecular aspects of epithelial cell plasticity: implications for local tumor invasion and metastasis. *Mutat Res* 566: 9–20
126 Chung LWK (2003) Prostate carcinoma bone-stroma interaction and its biologic and therapeutic implications. *Cancer* 97 (3 suppl): 772–778
127 Hoekstra R, Verweij J, Eskens FALM (2003) Clinical trial design for target specific anticancer agents. *Invest New Drugs* 21: 243–250

Progress in Drug Research, Vol. 63
(R. M. Schultz, Ed.)

Angiogenesis inhibitors: what is the clinical future?

Henk M. W. Verheul[1]
and Herbert M. Pinedo[2]

[1]Department of Medical Oncology
Johns Hopkins University
1650 Orleans Street CRB 162
Baltimore, MD 21231
USA
<hverheul@jhmi.edu>

[2]VUmc Cancer Center Amsterdam
PO Box 7057
1007 MB Amsterdam
The Netherlands
<hm.pinedo@vumc.nl>

Glossary of abbreviations

5FU, 5-fluorouracil; bFGF, basic fibroblast growth factor; GI, gastrointestinal; MVD, microvessel density; PR, partial response; PDGFs, platelet derived growth factors; SD, stable disease; VEGF, vascular endothelial growth factor.

1 Introduction

Angiogenesis inhibitors have been developed for clinical use and subsequently have entered clinical trials in the past two decades. The clinical introduction has been based on preclinical experiments initiated in the beginning of the seventies by Dr. Folkman. This surgeon hypothesized that tumors need new vessels to grow and to metastasize [1]. The process of new blood vessel formation is called angiogenesis. Angiogenesis is not only required for tumor development, but is also involved in embryonic development and wound healing, and in other diseases like atherosclerosis, rheumatic disease and psoriasis [2].

Blood vessels are required for the delivery of oxygen, nutrients, and growth factors, etc., and to carry off waste products. In addition, in tumor development, metastatic cells use blood vessels to escape a primary tumor. Stimulation of new blood vessel formation is regulated by growth factors that stimulate vascular cell proliferation, migration and tube formation. On the other hand, angiogenesis inhibitors have been found to keep the vasculature quiescent by preventing vascular cell proliferation and migration. These pro- and anti-angiogenic factors have been discovered in preclinical studies [3]. The angiogenic stimulation in tumors is caused by oncogene-driven tumor expression of angiogenic factors or by downregulation of angiogenesis inhibitors by oncogenic changes.

Clinical studies that confirm the role of angiogenesis in tumor development include studies that show high expression of angiogenic factors by tumors, downregulation of angiogenesis inhibitors and the finding that highly vascularized tumors have a more progressive phenotype, including a higher metastatic rate.

The vascularity of tumors is assessed by the determination of microvessel density. In 1992, the first prospective study on tumor microvessel density (MVD) and outcome of patients showed that the MVD was an independent prognostic factor for survival and metastasis formation in breast cancer [4]. Thereafter, in many other clinical studies the MVD has been found to be of predictive value for disease outcome for several tumor types [5, 6].

The expression of angiogenic growth factors, mainly vascular endothelial growth factor (VEGF), has also been found to be predictive for survival and metastasis formation [7].

Downregulation of angiogenesis inhibitors has been detected, but these clinical studies are not as clear as in preclinical experiments. As hypothesized by Hanahan and Folkman in 1994 [8], the balance of pro- and anti-angiogenic factors determines whether tumors start to grow and disseminate. Based on the preclinical and clinical data showing that angiogenesis is required for tumor development, many pharmaceutical companies directed part of their anticancer drug development programs to develop angiogenesis inhibitors.

Many different anti-angiogenic approaches have been taken, which we discuss in this chapter. The clinical results of angiogenesis inhibitors thus far are summarized and future directions discussed. In addition, we give insight into the clinical problems that have been observed with this type of agents, including a new toxicity spectrum.

2 Preclinical background

Several growth factors are involved in new vessel formation. The most important angiogenic growth factors are VEGF, basic fibroblast growth factor (bFGF), platelet derived growth factors (PDGFs), hepatocyte growth factor and the angiopoietins [9]. Tumors have been shown to secrete some of these factors or to induce production. Based on preclinical studies, especially the corneal neovascularization assay, Folkman and Shing [10] stated that the process of angiogenesis does not occur without accurate stimuli. In the corneal neovascularization assay, a pellet with a certain angiogenic growth factor and a placebo as control is implanted in the avascular cornea of a mouse, rabbit or rat. Within a few days after implantation, neovascularization from the limbus in the direction of the pellet has been observed for several factors as named above [11].

These findings led to the opposing principle as well, namely the blocking of angiogenesis by inhibitors. Indeed, the discovery of angiogenesis inhibitors closely followed the discoveries of stimulators. Exciting was the discovery of a tumor suppressor gene that regulated the secretion of thrombospondin, an endogenous angiogenesis inhibitor present in the matrix and platelets [12]. Many endogenous inhibitors, such as the CXC-chemokine platelet factor-4, the plasminogen fragment angiostatin and an 18-kDa part of collagen XVIII, named endostatin, were discovered [13, 14]. In parallel, synthetic angiogenesis inhibitors were developed based on the biochemical pathways that were elucidated by the various groups working on angiogenesis [15]. The driving force to discover synthetic angiogenesis inhibitors was the clinical perspective that these compounds may be able to suppress human tumor development in a non-toxic way. Another strong motive was that by attacking the vasculature, chemotherapy-induced drug resistance may be circumvented, because endothelial cells are considered to be genetically more stable than tumor cells [16].

Although many different aspects in the biochemical process of angiogenesis have been elucidated, one intriguing question of how, when and why a dormant (silent) tumor becomes angiogenic has not been explained thus far. In 1996, Folkman and Hanahan [8] proposed that this switch is dependent on the balance between angiogenic stimulators and inhibitors. The cause of a switch from the anti-angiogenic state into a pro-angiogenic state in dormant tumors is presumably regulated multifactorially, and depends on genetic and environmental factors. In a transgenic mouse model of pancreatic islet carcinogenesis Hanahan and co-workers showed that after 3–4 weeks up to 50% of the islets become hyperplastic. After 10 weeks, part (8–12%) but not all of the hyperplastic islets become angiogenic by switching on angiogenesis in the normal quiescent islet capillaries. This switch is associated with further tumor expansion and is accompanied by expression of angiogenic factors, but none of these factors could specifically explain why only 8–10% of the islets become angiogenic while the other islets remain hyperplastic [17].

In another preclinical model of tumor dormancy, Udagawa et al. [18] elegantly showed that certain experimental tumors remain viable after implantation into mice, but do not progress. By transfection of these tumor cells with pro-angiogenic genes (VEGF or ras), the angiogenic balance changed and tumors started to expand.

The current dogma is that in a dormant tumor, the apoptotic rate of tumor cells outweighs the proliferation rate of these cells, while after the angiogenic switch, the tumor cell proliferation by far exceeds the apoptotic rate of the tumor cells [19].

One of the genes that may play a major role in the regulation of angiogenesis in tumors is the gene that regulates expression of the Id proteins. This family of proteins (Id1–Id4) is involved in the control of cell growth, senescence, differentiation and neoplastic transformation by preventing transcription factors from binding DNA by direct physical interaction [20]. It turned out that Id1/Id3 null mice are not viable, but by retaining one copy of Id1 or Id3 embryonic death is prevented. Interestingly, tumors hardly grow and fail to metastasize in these mice [21]. In addition, the tumors in these mice were not able to recruit circulating endothelial cells into their newly formed vasculature. However, bone marrow transplantation, with full alleles of Id1 and Id3, circumvented this problem [22]. Recently, it has been shown that Id1 represses thrombospondin expression [23], indicating that TSP1 plays a role in prevention of recruitment of circulating endothelial cells.

Although several genes may play a role in the angiogenic switch, none of them can explain why and how the switch occurs at a certain time point. One may presume that environmental factors (for example smoking) may also be a trigger causing the switch. In *in vitro* assays, hypoxia, a low pH, iron deficiency and hypoglycemia stimulate VEGF expression and subsequent endothelial cell proliferation, and may also stimulate the *in vivo* angiogenic process [24–26].

Weinberg and Hanahan [27] summarized the essential hallmarks of cancer and named sustained angiogenesis as one of them. The other essential differences of tumor cells compared to normal cells include self sufficiency in growth signals, insensitivity to growth inhibitory signals, evasion of programmed cell death, limitless replicative potential and tissue evasion and metastasis. These characteristics of tumor biology are regulated by genetic changes in the tumor cells. Both the dominantly acting oncogenes as well as the inactivation of tumor suppressor genes by a mutation are involved in the development of tumors. Inactivation of tumor suppressor genes may be caused by methylation of nucleotides in the promotor sequence that control the expression of these genes [28].

3 Clinical significance of tumor angiogenesis

Tumor dormancy is eventually the most important cause of death in cancer patients. Although initial therapy of cancer is in general adequate, 90% of cancer patients die of distant metastasis [29]. Sometimes these metastases become detectable within a few years after initial therapy, but others are found only after 15–20 years. The initial therapy including surgery, radiotherapy and sometimes systemic adjuvant therapy, cannot prevent tumor recurrence in some patients. There are at least two reasons that may explain this clinical problem. Firstly, it might well be that dormant metastasis have such a low proliferation rate that they are insensitive to the adjuvant therapy. Secondly, some of these micrometastases (sometimes single tumor cells) may not be reached by the systemic therapy because they are too far away from the blood supply or lying within fibrotic tissue [30].

A clinical example of tumor dormancy is a local recurrence of breast cancer many years after mastectomy. Such recurrences occur in 5–30% of patients. Demicheli et al. [31] found in a group of 122 breast cancer patients that long intervals between mastectomy and recurrence cannot be explained by uninterrupted constant growth of local tumor cells that were left behind after mastectomy, and confirmed these findings in a group of 1173 patients a few years later [32]. They proposed, based on statistical analysis of these 122 patients, that tumors recur after a period of tumor dormancy followed by a more rapid regrowth. A possible explanation of this phenomenon is that these dormant tumors have not yet made the switch to a pro-angiogenic phenotype and remain in an anti-angiogenic state.

In other clinical studies the importance of angiogenesis in human cancer has been confirmed by MVD and angiogenic growth factor expression, mainly VEGF. It turned out that for primary tumors, the MVD in localized areas of intense vascularization is an independent prognostic factor for overall survival and disease-free survival. This was first shown in breast cancer, and it has now been confirmed in a large variety of tumor types [5, 6].

In a recent clinical study, specific gene expression signatures in breast cancer could predict clinical outcome. Interestingly, it was clear that angiogenesis-related genes are important for clinical outcome, for example, VEGF, VEGF-receptor FLT1 and metalloproteinase MMP9 [33]. This study also confirmed that stimulation of angiogenesis in human tumors is not solely dependent on one gene-related product, but is multifactorially regulated.

4 Anti-angiogenic agents in clinical studies

Anti-angiogenic agents can be roughly categorized into four different groups depending on their mechanism of action: (1) the growth factor pathway inhibitors; (2) the direct endothelial cell cycle inhibitors; (3) agents that interfere with endothelial cell adhesion; and (4) the others. We will discuss each group separately. The growth factor pathway inhibitors include the greatest number of agents that are currently in clinical development, and are the only ones that have shown clinical significance in phase III trials; these will be discussed most extensively here.

The most promising anti-angiogenic agents that are in clinical development at this moment, are the agents that attack the VEGF pathway. Many drug companies have focused their interest on agents known to attack at least this pathway.

4.1 Angiogenic growth factor pathway inhibitors

4.1.1 Bevacizumab

Bevacizumab is a humanized antibody from a murine anti-VEGF antibody mAb A4.6.1 [34]. It is 93% human and 7% murine. It has the same affinity for VEGF as the murine antibody and causes no immune response in humans. Bevacizumab binds to all isoforms of VEGF.

In preclinical experiments, the parent murine anti-VEGF antibody as monotherapy has been shown to inhibit tumor growth and metastasis formation in several tumor models, including breast, colon and renal tumors. In addition, it reduced tumor vascularity and increased blood vessel perfusion [35].

When combined with chemotherapeutic agents, the antibody not only caused a decrease in vascular density, but an increase in tumor chemotherapy concentration. Combination with either Irinotecan, Paclitaxel, Capecitabine or Cisplatin resulted in inhibition of murine tumor growth and a prolonged survival compared to single agent therapy [34]. Furthermore, Bevacizumab in combination with Trastuzumab, an antibody used in the clinic as an inhibitor of the HER2/neu receptor and Paclitaxel had synergistic antitumor activity (preliminary data by Pegram et al., UCLA).

Clinical development of Bevacizumab started in the end of the previous century. Gordon et al. found that the maximal tolerated dose of Bevacizumab was 10 mg/kg i.v. every 2 weeks [36]. The major side effects were asthenia, headaches and nausea. In phase II studies, it showed a significant difference for time to disease progression in favor of the treatment group compared to placebo in renal cell cancer. In combination with chemotherapy, it caused a significantly longer disease-free survival in patients with advanced colorectal cancer [37, 38]. This last result has been confirmed in a large phase III trial, with Irinotecan and 5-fluorouracil (5FU) plus leucovorin as the chemotherapeutic agents, in more than 800 patients [39]. Survival of patients treated with the combination with Bevacizumab plus chemotherapy versus chemotherapy alone was 20.3 versus 15.6 months, respectively. Also overall response rate was increased from 34.8% to 44.8% in the Bevacizumab group and duration of response was significantly better in the Bevacizumab group by 3.3 months (from 7.1 to 10.4 months). The major side effects in phase II trials were hypertension, proteinuria, epistaxis, thrombosis, gastrointestinal (GI) bleeding, diarrhea and leukopenia. In the phase III trial, although there was a slight increase in diarrhea and leukopenia, no confirmation of these serious side effects were observed. The only serious concern has been a GI perforation rate of 1.5% in the Bevacizumab group compared to 0% in the control arm.

The most compelling evidence that treatment with Bevacizumab affects the human vasculature comes from the study of Willet et al [40]. In this study they treated patients with primary and non-metastatic rectal cancer with Bevacizumab alone followed by Bevacizumab plus 5FU prior to surgery. They found a significant decrease in tumor blood perfusion, tumor blood volume and after surgery in tumor vascularity. Of course, this last result may also be due or partly due to 5FU treatment.

Together these data resulted in the registration of Bevacizumab for advanced colorectal cancer in combination with chemotherapy as first-line treatment. Whether these results can be improved with other treatment strategies in colorectal cancer, for example with oxaliplatin has to be awaited. In other tumor types, like metastatic breast cancer, non-small cell lung cancer (NSCLC), renal cell cancer and pancreatic cancer, phase III trials are ongoing and the results are eagerly awaited [41, 42].

Other VEGF-attacking antibodies include HuMV833 and the soluble receptor VEGF-TRAP, which are both being investigated in phase I trials.

4.1.2 HuMV833

The antibody HuMV833, has been studied in phase I in patients with advanced solid tumors [43]. This antibody has similarities to Bevacizumab because it is also a humanized version of a mouse anti-VEGF mAb. In preclinical models it inhibited tumor growth [44]. The optimum biological active dose could not be established because of heterogeneity of the antibody uptake and clearance by different tumors.

4.1.3 VEGF-TrapR1R2

VEGF-TrapR1R2 is a derivative of the most potent VEGF binder soluble VEGFR1 [45]. The soluble form of VEGFR1 has poor pharmacokinetic characteristics especially because of its interactions with the extracellular matrix. Therefore, VEGF-Trap was engineered consisting of portions of the human VEGFR-1 and VEGFR-2 extracellular domains fused to the Fc portion of a human immunoglobulin G1, with minimal interactions with the extracellular matrix but still very potent affinity for VEGF.

In preclinical tumor models, this agent showed antitumor activity for different tumors, including ovary, lung cancer, sarcoma and melanoma murine tumor models [46]. Interestingly, in one of these models the tumor endothelial fenestrations disappeared upon treatment, and in another study systemically given VEGF-Trap reduced ascites formation in an ovarian tumor model [47].

In a phase I study in which VEGF-Trap was administered subcutaneously to 30 patients with advanced solid tumors, no antibodies against the agent have been detected, even though 14 of these patients were treated for more than 4 months [48]. The maximum tolerated dose has not yet been reached; so far the drug-related grade 3 toxicities included hypertension, proteinuria and leukopenia. Fourteen of 24 evaluable patients had stable disease (SD) for more than 10 weeks.

4.1.4 IMC-1C11

In addition to antibodies against VEGF, a chimeric antibody against the VEGFR-2 receptor has been developed, named IMC-1C11 [49]. In preclinical models it inhibited not only solid tumors but leukemia as well [50]. In a phase I study in patients with colorectal liver metastases, this antibody has been given i.v. weekly up to 4 mg/kg without grade 3 or 4 toxicity, while plasma values were reached that inhibit the kinase-insert-domain-containing receptor (KDR) *in vitro* [51]. In 7 out of 14 patients, anti-chimeric antibodies were detected.

4.1.5 SU5416, SU6668, SU011248

Another type of VEGF growth factor blockers includes the small-molecule tyrosine kinase inhibitors. These inhibitors have similar mechanisms of action. They inhibit the VEGF receptor and/or other growth factor receptors including (the PDGFR, c-KIT, FGFRs, etc.) by preventing phosphorylation of the receptor intracellularly upon binding of the growth factor extracellularly. Consequently, the intracellular signaling cascade that is normally induced by growth factors upon binding to their receptor is blocked.

Compound SU5416, administered i.v., was one of the first tyrosine kinase inhibitors against the VEGF receptor investigated [52]. Because of unexpected toxicity, especially when combined with chemotherapy (thrombosis), and because of the rapid development of a newer class of these agents that could be given orally, further clinical development of this agent was terminated [53].

The next agent of Sugen, SU6668, was an oral broad tyrosine kinase inhibitor, inhibiting the VEGFR2, PDGFR-beta, FGFR-1 and KIT [54]. Treatment with this agent resulted in serositis-like pains, fatigue and anorexia. No clinical responses were observed and to obtain stable plasma concentrations the drug had to be taken thrice daily. Because of its toxicity and the lack of response, this compound has also not been develo ped any further.

SU11248, an oral tyrosine kinase inhibitor, against FLT3, KIT, VEGF and PDGF receptors was the next compound of Sugen that reached clinical trials [55]. Preclinical studies showed a potent antitumor activity against hematological malignancies [56–58]. In a single-dose phase I trial, the activity of FLT3 phosphorylation has been studied in patients with acute myeloid leukemia with single doses from 50 to 350 mg. Phosphorylation was inhibited in 50% of patients with wild-type FLT3 and in 100% with mutated FLT3 [59]. In a continuing dosing phase I trial, grade 3 hypertension and fatigue were dose-limiting toxicities [60]. The dose that was found to be safe was 50 mg q.d. At a higher dose of 75 mg q.d., grade 4 fatigue, hypertension and cardiac failure were observed. At 50 mg q.d., grade 2 toxicities were edema, fatigue and oral ulcerations. Further clinical studies are being awaited, but the very impressive response rate of more than 20% in this trial was encouraging. In a phase I/II trial in patients with metastatic GI stromal tumors resistant for imatinib, SU11248 was administered to 98 patients daily at

50 mg q.d. for 4 weeks followed by a 2-week off drug period [61]. So far, among 48 patients for whom a response could be evaluated, 26 patients had a response [6 with partial response (PR) and 20 with SD] for >6 months. Another very promising result has been observed in patients with metastatic renal cell cancer [62]. Of 63 patients, 32 had a durable response (SD or PR) for more than 6 months. Grade 3/4 toxicities includes lymphopenia and increased lipase and amylase without clinical signs of pancreatitis, and fatigue/asthenia.

4.1.6 PTK787/ZK222584

PTK787/ZK222584 is an oral tyrosine kinase inhibitor of VEGFR-2 of Novartis [63]. It also inhibits tyrosine kinase receptors of the PDGF, c-Kit and cFms pathways, but at higher concentrations. In preclinical tumor models, it inhibited several human carcinomas including colorectal cancer and prostate cancer. One of the preclinical investigations included wound healing. It turned out that wound healing was not affected by PTK787, while tumor vascularization clearly diminished.

In two phase I studies, biological activity was observed by dynamic contrast-enhanced MRI [64]. Already 2 days after start of treatment a significant decrease in vessel perfusion was observed in patients with hepatic metastases from colorectal cancer. The maximal tolerated dose was 2000 mg daily. Currently, a phase III clinical trial in advanced colorectal cancer with chemotherapy (oxaliplatin, 5FU and leucovorin) plus or minus PTK787 has just been closed for accrual, and the results are eagerly awaited.

4.1.7 ZD6474 and AZD2171

Astra Zeneca developed two oral tyrosine kinase inhibitors (ZD6474 and AZD2171) that affect the VEGFR pathway [65]. Both agents showed clear preclinical antitumor activity and are now being evaluated in phase I trials. Both agents seem to be well tolerated. Dose limiting toxicity of ZD6474 was skin rash. This drug is now being studied in combination with docetaxel in patients with NSCLC [66]. A phase I trial of AZD2171 is currently being performed; preliminary data showed no serious toxicity up to 10 mg q.d. orally [67]. A phase I trial of AZD2171 in combination with Iressa (a tyrosine kinase inhibitor of the EGFR pathway) is also ongoing.

4.1.8 CEP-7055

This agents is a dimethylglycine ester of CEP-5241, which is also a tyrosine kinase inhibitor against the VEGFR-1 to -3 [68]. This agent has entered phase I clinical trials and showed a promising toxicity profile [69].

4.1.9 Ribozyme

Another interesting approach to interfere with the VEGF-signaling cascade has been developed by Pavco et al. [70]. These agents inactivate mRNA for the VEGFR-1or -2 by cleaving it intracellularly. The chemically stabilized synthetic ribozyme against the FLT-1 VEGFR mRNA has entered clinical trials [71]. This agent is given i.v. and could be given up to doses of 30 mg/m^2 [72]. Headache and somnolence were observed as possible related adverse events in only four patients. A clinical phase II study has been performed in which this agent was combined with chemotherapy for metastatic colorectal cancer [73].

4.2 Direct inhibitors of endothelial cells

4.2.1 Angiostatin and endostatin

Angiostatin and endostatin are both endogenous endothelial cell inhibitors that were discovered in the laboratory of Dr. Folkman [14, 74]. Despite their very promising preclinical activity, neither had a clinical activity of any importance [75]. Endostatin did cause tumor regression in several murine tumor models [76], and a combination of endostatin and angiostatin was even more active in curing mice. Whether the lack of response in humans is due to the difference between mice and men, or to drug instability when produced in large amounts, or whether there is another reason for these disappointing results remains unclear thus far.

4.2.2 ABT-510

A more promising agent that has reached the clinic, because it can be more easily manufactured, is the mimetic peptide derived from thrombospondin, ABT-510 [77]. The exact mechanism of action of thrombospondin and its mimetic peptides is unclear. However, an induction of apoptosis in endothelial cells, regulated by altered expression of the apoptotic regulatory gene products, like Bax, Bcl-2 and caspase-3, has been observed [78]. In preclinical studies, this agent showed promising antitumor activity comparable to thrombospondin itself. ABT-510 is a nonapeptide that is subcutaneously administered. In a healthy volunteer study, up to 130 mg could be administered with a linear pharmacokinetics profile and a low inter-individual variability. In a phase I trial it was safe and showed early signs of activity [77].

4.3 Agents that interfere with endothelial adhesion to the extracellular matrix

The third group of angiogenesis inhibitors includes agents that interfere with endothelial cell matrix interactions. As pointed out by Reijerkerk et al. [79], endothelial cells (and also other cells) die when they can no longer attach to their environment. Endothelial cells attach to their basement membrane through integrins. Upon interference in this attachment, the endothelial cells undergo apoptosis and die. Whether thrombospondin mimetics belong to this kind of agent is a matter of debate; however, based on these observations, the drugs vitaxin and cilengitide (EMD 121974) have been designed that interfere with this cell-basement attachment.

4.3.1 Vitaxin

Vitaxin is a humanized anti-vitronectin receptor, that showed no toxicity in phase I trials when given thrice weekly i.v. or once every 3 weeks i.v. [80, 81]. Although active in preclinical models, thus far no clinical responses of significance were observed.

4.3.2 Cilengitide

Cilengitide is a cyclic peptide that interferes with the alpha-V-beta3 and alpha-V-beta 5 integrins that are involved in endothelial cell adhesion [82]. In phase I trials this agent was well tolerated up to a dose of 1600 mg/m^2 twice weekly i.v. [83]. In one patient with a heavily pretreated head and neck cancer, this agent held the tumor stable at a dose of 600 mg/m^2 at day 1 and 4 of a 3-weekly schedule in combination with gemcitabine (1000 mg/m^2 day 1 and 8) [84].

4.4 The miscellaneous group of angiogenesis inhibitors: thalidomide, squalamine and LY317615

4.4.1 Thalidomide

Thalidomide is a widely used agent, especially in multiple myeloma patients [85]. Initially, this agent was withdrawn from the market because of deleterious teratogenic malformations in humans back in the sixties. In 1994 Thalidomide was rediscovered as an angiogenesis inhibitor [86]. The exact anti-angiogenic mechanism of Thalidomide remains unclear. At least partly it has an anti-angiogenic effect, but it has also immunomodulating activities. Preclinical studies showed activity in solid tumors [87]. Clinical studies showed high response rates in patients with multiple myeloma [88]. In solid tumors, its response rates are between 10% and 25%, rather limited as summarized by Kumar et al.

Finally, squalamine and LY 317615 are agents that are being studied clinically, but data are sparse regarding these agents thus far [89–91].

5 Toxicity and other obstacles in the clinical development of angiogenesis inhibitors

The introduction of angiogenesis inhibitors in the treatment of cancer patients has been difficult. Several hurdles had to be taken. Foremost, the thinking of clinicians had to be changed. At first clinicians had to start realizing that inhibiting angiogenesis was not going to generate rapid and major responses of tumors. Instead, one had to accept cancer as a chronic disease, that can be prohibited from progression by chronically prescribing angiogenesis inhibitors. Therefore, clinical protocols had to be designed with alternative response evaluations. While in the classical chemotherapy-based phase I and II trials at least a 25% reduction of tumor volume had to be reached before continuation of study drug supply could be prescribed, in the anti-angiogenic-based clinical trials, even a 20% progression has been introduced as SD on which continuation of the drug was made possible.

To establish methods to detect drug activity, several approaches have been taken, including measuring angiogenic growth factor levels, tumor perfusion assays by MRI and evaluation of circulating endothelial cells. All these assays were investigated as surrogate endpoints for drug activity of this new class of agents. No clear-cut assay that really predicts response towards angiogenesis inhibitors has been discovered. Thus far, as for all anticancer drugs, the only real endpoint is survival. With regard to prolongation of survival with angiogenesis inhibitors, thus far a few clinical trials of angiogenesis inhibitors have indeed showed survival benefit (as described earlier).

Another problem in the clinical development of these agents has been the whole area of drug toxicity compared to the classical chemotherapeutics. Especially, results for thrombotic and bleeding complications were telling. The first serious side effect with death due to a thrombotic complication was in the clinical trial in which SU5416 was given in combination with chemotherapy [53]. This led to the withdrawal of this drug from further clinical development. The exact mechanism through which thrombosis was induced has not been elucidated, but may have been due to the varying plasma concentrations of the inhibitor. This variation may cause intravascular problems with the normally quiescent vascular cells [92]. Another agent that has caused thrombotic complications, and has now been prescribed in combination with low molecular heparins, is Thalidomide. Increased rates of thrombosis have been observed in patients with multiple myeloma [93].

Furthermore, and possibly related to thrombosis, hypertension is frequently observed in patients treated with angiogenesis inhibitors, especially in agents interfering with the VEGF pathway. In patients treated with Bevacizumab, hypertension has been reported as an observed toxicity in up to 22% of treated patients [94]. Presumably, this may be related to the nitric oxide pathway (responsible for vasodilatation) with which these agents interfere, but, as yet, this has not been completely clarified [95].

Another expected side effect, impaired wound healing has not generated any problem thus far. In the phase III study of Bevacizumab in colorectal cancer, a higher incidence of bowel perforation has been detected. The exact cause is not clear, but it might be related to impaired ulcer healing of the stomach.

In conclusion, clinicians should be aware of these possible side effects compared to the traditional side effects induced by chemotherapeutics, but one still may consider these patterns as rather mild.

6 Future direction: angiogenesis inhibitors are of clinical importance

Ultimately, one should think ahead and consider which steps should be taken to optimize the attack against cancer. In our view, the clinical future of therapeutic anti-angiogenic agents against cancer include the following:

1) Study of combination treatments with classic chemotherapy plus anti-angiogenic agents in advanced cancer of any type to further prolong survival and disease-free survival.
2) Development of a realistic strategy for life-long non-toxic anti-angiogenic agent administration.
3) Establishment of new adjuvant treatment approaches with anti-angiogenic agents with or without combinations of chemotherapy with a curative intent.

The genomic background of tumor cells in cancer patients reflects their behavior, as has been shown by van 't Veer and others [33]. It is interesting, but not surprising, that these studies show that the expression patterns of angiogenesis-related genes are indicators for clinical outcome. These expression patterns that correlate with survival are not depicted on just one single gene product, but are multifactorially regulated. The findings mentioned above are the basis for the treatment of cancer with combination therapies. For example, by inhibiting the VEGF pathway only, most tumors will be only partly attacked and their growth only inhibited for a short period, because of other growth factor pathways. Of course, this setting differs from most preclinical models in which sometimes only one angiogenic growth factor plays a dominant role. Even in the clinical development of Imatinib (a tyrosine kinase inhibitor of the Bcr-Abl pathway in chronic myeloid leukemia and the mutated c-Kit pathway in GI stromal tumors), after initial response, resistance against this drug has been observed [96]. Studying the biological pathways that are involved in various tumor types, it becomes clear that multiple signaling proteins in the cell signaling machinery are involved in stimulation of the cell cycle in both the malignant and supporting cells of a tumor, including endothelial cells and macrophages [97]. It is hard to determine which pathways are crucial, because just overexpression of certain receptors or enzymes does not necessarily reflect their importance. For example, EGFR expression is independent of its response to blocking therapy, but mutations in the receptor indicate a responsiveness to blocking therapy [98]. In contrast, in patients with a mutated receptor, the response rate was almost 100%, while in the patients with normal EGFR, almost no response was seen. This finding, considered as one of the major findings of 2004 in anticancer science, led to a whole new area of drug targeted therapy. It is only worthwhile treating patients with EGFR inhibitors if they have a mutated form of this receptor. Presumably, this may be also true for other growth factor (receptor) pathway-interfering agents, but this has yet to be studied.

Another intriguing observation is that combination of biologicals with classic chemotherapeutic agents may enhance the chemotherapy response, even when clinical resistance against the chemotherapy has been demonstrated [99]. The combination of Cetuximab plus Irinotecan in Irinotecan-resistant patients caused 18% responses, while Cetuximab monotherapy had only a 10% response rate.

In other words, combinations of inhibitors attacking different biochemical pathways should shut down the multifactor-stimulated cascade of tumor-induced angiogenesis, and may enhance tumor responsiveness to chemotherapy. For each angiogenic factor pathway, multiple regulatory factors and intracellular signaling pathways exist. Therefore, various treatment strategies can be thought of. In contrast to some preclinical tumor models that overproduce mainly one of the angiogenic growth factors, combinations of inhibitors attacking a different biochemical pathway may halt these angiogenic biochemical processes in the clinical setting. A comparison can be made with anti-HIV treatment strategies, in which to circumvent drug resistance, at least three different biochemical pathways should be blocked to obtain sufficient anti-retroviral potency [100].

However, by targeting multiple biological pathways, the toxicity of these combinations may be synergistically increased. Normal cells in, for example, wound healing and immune reactions use the biological pathways. Therefore, these combinations should be investigated in phase I trials for optimal dosing and scheduling.

Just recently, the first data showing that the combination of an EGFR inhibitor in combination with a VEGF blocker (Erlotinib plus Bevacizumab) in patients with renal cell cancer had an 87% response rate (PD + SD) [101]. The multi-targeted Su11248 against PDGFR, VEGFR, KIT and FLT3 has a comparable response rate of 70% in metastatic renal cell cancer [62]. These data indeed confirm the importance of a multi-targeting approach.

7 Conclusion

In conclusion, because of the responses observed in phase I, II and III trials with angiogenesis inhibitors in combination with other biological agents or classic chemotherapy, there is no longer doubt that anti-angiogenic agents have become part of anticancer therapy in general. In the coming years, we should further explore the treatment strategies in which anti-angiogenic agents will add to a prolonged survival and an increase in the cure rate of cancer. In our opinion, the contribution of these agents will be tremendous.

References

1 Folkman J (1971) Tumor angiogenesis: therapeutic implications. *N Engl J Med* 285: 1182–1186

2 Folkman J (1995) Angiogenesis in cancer, vascular, rheumatoid and other disease. *Nat Med* 1: 27–31

3 Distler JH, Hirth A, Kurowska-Stolarska M, Gay RE, Gay S, Distler O (2003) Angiogenic and angiostatic factors in the molecular control of angiogenesis. *Q J Nucl Med* 47: 149–161

4 Weidner N, Folkman J, Pozza F, Bevilacqua P, Allred EN, Moore DH, Meli S, Gasparini G (1992) Tumor angiogenesis: a new significant and independent prognostic indicator in early-stage breast carcinoma. *J Natl Cancer Inst* 84: 1875–1887

5 Weidner F (1979) Comparative histological studies of regional lymph nodes of 201 melanoma patients. (Microscopic features in relation to individual age, site, and metastatic spread). *Arch Dermatol Res* 266: 161–175

6 Hasan J, Byers R, Jayson GC (2002) Intra-tumoural microvessel density in human solid tumours. *Br J Cancer* 86: 1566–1577

7 Gasparini G, Toi M, Gion M, Verderio P, Dittadi R, Hanatani M, Matsubara I, Vinante O, Bonoldi E, Boracchi P et al (1997) Prognostic significance of vascular endothelial growth factor protein in node-negative breast carcinoma. *J Natl Cancer Inst* 89: 139–147

8 Hanahan D, Folkman J (1996) Patterns and emerging mechanisms of the angiogenic switch during tumorigenesis. *Cell* 86: 353–364

9 Ribatti D, Vacca A, Presta M (2000) The discovery of angiogenic factors: a historical review. *Gen Pharmacol* 35: 227–231

10 Folkman J, Shing Y (1992) Angiogenesis. *J Biol Chem* 267: 10931–10934

11 Kenyon BM, Voest EE, Chen CC, Flynn E, Folkman J, D'Amato RJ (1996) A model of angiogenesis in the mouse cornea. *Invest Ophthalmol Vis Sci* 37: 1625–1632

12 Good DJ, Polverini PJ, Rastinejad F, Le Beau MM, Lemons RS, Frazier WA, Bouck NP (1990) A tumor suppressor-dependent inhibitor of angiogenesis in immunologically and functionally indistinguishable from a fragment of thromospondin. *Proc Natl Acad Sci USA* 87: 664–6628

13 Carmeliet P, Jain RK (2000) Angiogenesis in cancer and other diseases. *Nature* 407: 249–257

14 O'Reilly MS, Boehm T, Shing Y, Fukai N, Vasios G, Lane WS, Flynn E, Birkhead JR, Olsen BR, Folkman J (1997) Endostatin: an endogenous inhibitor of angiogenesis and tumor growth. *Cell* 88: 277–285

15 Hamby JM, Showalter HD (1999) Small molecule inhibitors of tumor-promoted angiogenesis, including protein tyrosine kinase inhibitors. *Pharmacol Ther* 82: 169–193

16 Folkman J (1996) New perspectives in clinical oncology from angiogenesis research. *Eur J Cancer* 32A: 2534–2539

17 Folkman J, Watson K, Ingber D, Hanahan D (1989) Induction of angiogenesis during the transition from hyperplasia to neoplasia. *Nature* 339: 58–61

18 Udagawa T, Fernandez A, Achilles EG, Folkman J, D'Amato RJ (2002) Persistence of microscopic human cancers in mice: alterations in the angiogenic balance accompanies loss of tumor dormancy. *FASEB J* 16: 1361–1370

19 Holmgren L, O'Reilly MS, Folkman J (1995) Dormancy of micrometastases: balanced proliferation and apoptosis in the presence of angiogenesis suppression. *Nat Med* 1: 149–153

20 Norton JD (2000) ID helix-loop-helix proteins in cell growth, differentiation and tumorigenesis. *J Cell Sci* 113: 3897–3905

21 Lyden D, Young AZ, Zagzag D, Yan W, Gerald W, O'Reilly R, Bader BL, Hynes RO, Zhuang Y, Manova K et al (1999) Id1 and Id3 are required for neurogenesis, angiogenesis and vascularization of tumour xenografts. *Nature* 401: 670–677

22 Lyden D, Hattori K, Dias S, Costa C, Blaikie P, Butros L, Chadburn A, Heissig B, Marks W, Witte L et al (2001) Impaired recruitment of bone-marrow-derived endothelial and hematopoietic precursor cells blocks tumor angiogenesis and growth. *Nat Med* 7: 1194–1201

23 Volpert OV, Pili R, Sikder HA, Nelius T, Zaichuk T, Morris C, Shiflett CB, Devlin MK, Conant K, Alani RM (2002) Id1 regulates angiogenesis through transcriptional repression of thrombospondin-1. *Cancer Cell* 2: 473–483

24 Shi Q, Le X, Wang B, Abbruzzese JL, Xiong Q, He Y, Xie K (2001) Regulation of vascular endothelial growth factor expression by acidosis in human cancer cells. *Oncogene* 20: 3751–3756

25 Shima DT, Adamis AP, Ferrara N, Yeo KT, Yeo TK, Allende R, Folkman J, D'Amore PA (1995) Hypoxic induction of endothelial cell growth factors in retinal cells: identification and characterization of vascular endothelial growth factor (VEGF) as the mitogen. *Mol Med* 1: 182–193

26 Satake S, Kuzuya M, Miura H, Asai T, Ramos MA, Muraguchi M, Ohmoto Y, Iguchi A (1998) Up-regulation of vascular endothelial growth factor in response to glucose deprivation. *Biol Cell* 90: 161–168

27 Hanahan D, Weinberg RA (2000) The hallmarks of cancer. *Cell* 100: 57–70

28 Hahn WC, Weinberg RA (2002) Rules for making human tumor cells. *N Engl J Med* 347: 1593–1603

29 Sporn MB (1997) The war on cancer: a review. *Ann N Y Acad Sci* 833: 137–146

30 Verheul HMW, Pinedo HM (1998) Clinical implications of drug resistance. In: HM Pinedo, G Giaccone (eds): . Cambridge University Press, Cambridge, 199–232

31 Demicheli R, Terenziani M, Valagussa P, Moliterni A, Zambetti M, Bonadonna G (1994) Local recurrences following mastectomy: support for the concept of tumor dormancy. *J Natl Cancer Inst* 86: 45–48

32 Demicheli R (2001) Tumour dormancy: findings and hypotheses from clinical research on breast cancer. *Semin Cancer Biol* 11: 297–306
33 van 't Veer LJ, Dai H, van de Vijver MJ, He YD, Hart AA, Mao M, Peterse HL, van der Kooy K, Marton MJ, Witteveen AT, Schreiber GJ et al (2002) Gene expression profiling predicts clinical outcome of breast cancer. *Nature* 415: 530–536
34 Ferrara N, Hillan KJ, Gerber HP, Novotny W (2004) Discovery and development of bevacizumab, an anti-VEGF antibody for treating cancer. *Nat Rev Drug Discov* 3: 391–400
35 Wildiers H, Guetens G, De Boeck G, Verbeken E, Landuyt B, Landuyt W, de Bruijn EA, van Oosterom AT (2003) Effect of antivascular endothelial growth factor treatment on the intratumoral uptake of CPT-11. *Br J Cancer* 88: 1979–1986
36 Margolin K, Gordon MS, Holmgren E, Gaudreault J, Novotny W, Fyfe G, Adelman D, Stalter S, Breed J (2001) Phase Ib trial of intravenous recombinant humanized monoclonal antibody to vascular endothelial growth factor in combination with chemotherapy in patients with advanced cancer: pharmacologic and long-term safety data. *J Clin Oncol* 19: 851–856
37 Kabbinavar F, Hurwitz HI, Fehrenbacher L, Meropol NJ, Novotny WF, Lieberman G, Griffing S, Bergsland E (2003) Phase II, randomized trial comparing bevacizumab plus fluorouracil (FU)/leucovorin (LV) with FU/LV alone in patients with metastatic colorectal cancer. *J Clin Oncol* 21: 60–65
38 Yang JC, Haworth L, Sherry RM, Hwu P, Schwartzentruber DJ, Topalian SL, Steinberg SM, Chen HX, Rosenberg SA (2003) A randomized trial of bevacizumab, an anti-vascular endothelial growth factor antibody, for metastatic renal cancer. *N Engl J Med* 349: 427–434
39 Hurwitz H, Fehrenbacher L, Novotny W, Cartwright T, Hainsworth J, Heim W, Berlin J, Baron A, Griffing S, Holmgren E et al (2004) Bevacizumab plus irinotecan, fluorouracil, and leucovorin for metastatic colorectal cancer. *N Engl J Med* 305: 2335–2342
40 Willett CG, Boucher Y, di Tomaso E, Duda DG, Munn LL, Tong RT, Chung DC, Sahani DV, Kalva SP, Kozin SV et al (2004) Direct evidence that the VEGF-specific antibody bevacizumab has antivascular effects in human rectal cancer. *Nat Med* 10: 145–147
41 Ramaswamy B, Shapiro CL (2003) Phase II trial of bevacizumab in combination with docetaxel in women with advanced breast cancer. *Clin Breast Cancer* 4: 292–294
42 Chen HX (2004) Expanding the clinical development of bevacizumab. *Oncologist* 9 Suppl 1: 27–35
43 Jayson GC, Zweit J, Jackson A, Mulatero C, Julyan P, Ranson M, Broughton L, Wagstaff J, Hakannson L, Groenewegen G et al (2002) Molecular imaging and biological evaluation of HuMV833 anti-VEGF antibody: implications for trial design of antiangiogenic antibodies. *J Natl Cancer Inst* 94: 1484–1493
44 Asano M, Yukita A, Suzuki H (1999) Wide spectrum of antitumor activity of a neutralizing monoclonal antibody to human vascular endothelial growth factor. *Jpn J Cancer Res* 90: 93–100
45 Holash J, Davis S, Papadopoulos N, Croll SD, Ho L, Russell M, Boland P, Leidich R, Hylton D, Burova E et al (2002) VEGF-Trap: a VEGF blocker with potent antitumor effects. *Proc Natl Acad Sci USA* 99: 11393–11398
46 Huang J, Frischer JS, Serur A, Kadenhe A, Yokoi A, McCrudden KW, New T, O'Toole K, Zabski S, Rudge JS et al (2003) Regression of established tumors and metastases by potent vascular endothelial growth factor blockade. *Proc Natl Acad Sci USA* 100: 7785–7790

47 Byrne AT, Ross L, Holash J, Nakanishi M, Hu L, Hofmann JI, Yancopoulos GD, Jaffe RB (2003) Vascular endothelial growth factor-trap decreases tumor burden, inhibits ascites, and causes dramatic vascular remodeling in an ovarian cancer model. *Clin Cancer Res* 9: 5721–5728
48 Dupont J, Schwartz L, Koutcher J, Spriggs D, Gordon M, Mendelson D, Murren J, Lucarelli A, Cedarbaum J (2004) Phase I and pharmacokinetic study of VEGF trap administered subcutaneously to patients with advanced solid malignancies. *Proc Am Soc Clin Oncol* 23: abstr. 3009
49 Hunt S (2001) Technology evaluation: IMC-1C11, ImClone Systems. *Curr Opin Mol Ther* 3: 418–424
50 Wang ES, Teruya-Feldstein J, Wu Y, Zhu Z, Hicklin D, Moore MA (2004) Targeting autocrine and paracrine VEGF receptor pathways inhibits human lymphoma xenografts *in vivo*. *Blood*; *in press*
51 Posey JA, Ng TC, Yang B, Khazaeli MB, Carpenter MD, Fox F, Needle M, Waksal H, LoBuglio AF (2003) A phase I study of anti-kinase insert domain-containing receptor antibody, IMC-1C11, in patients with liver metastases from colorectal carcinoma. *Clin Cancer Res* 9: 1323–1332
52 Vajkoczy P, Menger MD, Vollmar B, Schilling L, Schmiedek P, Hirth KP, Ullrich A, Fong TA (1999) Inhibition of tumor growth, angiogenesis, and microcirculation by the novel Flk-1 inhibitor SU5416 as assessed by intravital multi-fluorescence videomicroscopy. *Neoplasia* 1: 31–41
53 Kuenen BC, Rosen L, Smit EF, Parson MR, Levi M, Ruijter R, Huisman H, Kedde MA, Noordhuis P, van der Vijgh WJ et al (2002) Dose-finding and pharmacokinetic study of cisplatin, gemcitabine, and SU5416 in patients with solid tumors. *J Clin Oncol* 20: 1657–1667
54 Laird AD, Vajkoczy P, Shawver LK, Thurnher A, Liang C, Mohammadi M, Schlessinger J, Ullrich A, Hubbard SR, Blake RA et al (2000) SU6668 is a potent antiangiogenic and antitumor agent that induces regression of established tumors. *Cancer Res* 60: 4152–4160
55 O'Farrell AM, Abrams TJ, Yuen HA, Ngai TJ, Louie SG, Yee KW, Wong LM, Hong W, Lee LB, Town A et al (2003) SU11248 is a novel FLT3 tyrosine kinase inhibitor with potent activity *in vitro* and *in vivo*. *Blood* 101: 3597–3605
56 Mendel DB, Laird AD, Xin X, Louie SG, Christensen JG, Li G, Schreck RE, Abrams TJ, Ngai TJ, Lee LB, Murray LJ et al (2003) *In vivo* antitumor activity of SU11248, a novel tyrosine kinase inhibitor targeting vascular endothelial growth factor and platelet-derived growth factor receptors: determination of a pharmacokinetic/pharmacodynamic relationship. *Clin Cancer Res* 9: 327–337
57 Yee KW, Schittenhelm M, O'Farrell AM, Town AR, McGreevey L, Bainbridge T, Cherrington JM, Heinrich MC (2004) Synergistic effect of SU11248 with Cytarabine or Daunorubicin on FLT3-ITD positive leukemic cells. *Blood* 104: 4202-4209
58 Murray LJ, Abrams TJ, Long KR, Ngai TJ, Olson LM, Hong W, Keast PK, Brassard JA, O'Farrell AM, Cherrington JM et al (2003) SU11248 inhibits tumor growth and CSF-1R-dependent osteolysis in an experimental breast cancer bone metastasis model. *Clin Exp Metastasis* 20: 757–766
59 O'Farrell AM, Foran JM, Fiedler W, Serve H, Paquette RL, Cooper MA, Yuen HA, Louie SG, Kim H, Nicholas S et al (2003) An innovative phase I clinical study demonstrates inhibition of FLT3 phosphorylation by SU11248 in acute myeloid leukemia patients. *Clin Cancer Res* 9: 5465–5476

60 Fiedler W, Serve H, Dohner H, Schwittay M, Ottmann OG, O'Farrell AM, Bello CL, Allred R, Manning WC, Cherrington JM et al (2004) A phase I study of SU11248 in the treatment of patients with refractory or resistant acute myeloid leukemia (AML) or not amenable to conventional therapy for the disease. *Blood* 105: 986–993
61 Demetri GD, Desai J, Fletcher JA, Morgan JA, Fletcher CDM, Kazanovicz A, Van Den Abbeele A, Baum C, Maki R, Heinrich MC (2004) SU11248, a multi-targeted tyrosine kinase inhibitor, can overcome imatinib (IM) resistance caused by diverse genomic mechanisms in patients (pts) with metastatic gastrointestinal stromal tumor (GIST). *Proc Am Soc Clin Oncol* 23: abstr. 3001
62 Motzer RJ, Rini BI, Michaelson MD, Redman BG, Hudes GR, Wilding G, Figlin RA, Zhu J, Kim ST, Baum C (2004) SU011248, a novel tyrosine kinase inhibitor, shows antitumor activity in second-line therapy for patients with metastatic renal cell carcinoma: Results of a phase 2 trial. *Proc Am Soc Clin Oncol* 23: abstr. 4500
63 Drevs J, Muller-Driver R, Wittig C, Fuxius S, Esser N, Hugenschmidt H, Konerding MA, Allegrini PR, Wood J, Hennig J et al (2002) PTK787/ZK 222584, a specific vascular endothelial growth factor-receptor tyrosine kinase inhibitor, affects the anatomy of the tumor vascular bed and the functional vascular properties as detected by dynamic enhanced magnetic resonance imaging. *Cancer Res* 62: 4015–4022
64 Morgan B, Thomas AL, Drevs J, Hennig J, Buchert M, Jivan A, Horsfield MA, Mross K, Ball HA, Lee L et al (2003) Dynamic contrast-enhanced magnetic resonance imaging as a biomarker for the pharmacological response of PTK787/ZK 222584, an inhibitor of the vascular endothelial growth factor receptor tyrosine kinases, in patients with advanced colorectal cancer and liver metastases: results from two phase I studies. *J Clin Oncol* 21: 3955–3964
65 Wedge SR, Ogilvie DJ, Dukes M, Kendrew J, Chester R, Jackson JA, Boffey SJ, Valentine PJ, Curwen JO, Musgrove HL et al (2002) ZD6474 inhibits vascular endothelial growth factor signaling, angiogenesis, and tumor growth following oral administration. *Cancer Res* 62: 4645–4655
66 Bates D (2003) ZD-6474. AstraZeneca. *Curr Opin Investig Drugs* 4: 1468–1472
67 Medinger M, Mross K, Zirrgiebel U, Strecker R, Wheeler C, Clack G, Lewis J, Puchalski TA, Unger C, Drevs J (2004) Phase I dose escalating study of the highly potent VEGF receptor kinase inhibitor, azd2171, in patients with advanced cancers with liver metastases. *Proc Am Soc Clin Oncol* 23: abstr. 3055
68 Ruggeri B, Singh J, Gingrich D, Angeles T, Albom M, Yang S, Chang H, Robinson C, Hunter K, Dobrzanski P et al (2003) CEP-7055: a novel, orally active pan inhibitor of vascular endothelial growth factor receptor tyrosine kinases with potent antiangiogenic activity and antitumor efficacy in preclinical models. *Cancer Res* 63: 5978–5991
69 Pili R, Carducci M, Robertson PA (2003) Phase I study of the pan-VEGR tyrosine kinase inhibitor, CEP-7055, in patients with advanced malignancy. *Proc Am Soc Clin Oncol* 22: 207
70 Pavco PA, Bouhana KS, Gallegos AM, Agrawal A, Blanchard KS, Grimm SL, Jensen KL, Andrews LE, Wincott FE, Pitot PA et al (2000) Antitumor and antimetastatic activity of ribozymes targeting the messenger RNA of vascular endothelial growth factor receptors. *Clin Cancer Res* 6: 2094–2103
71 Weng DE, Usman N (2001) Angiozyme: a novel angiogenesis inhibitor. *Curr Oncol Rep* 3: 141–146

72 Sandberg JA, Parker VP, Blanchard KS, Sweedler D, Powell JA, Kachensky A, Bellon L, Usman N, Rossing T, Borden E et al (2000) Pharmacokinetics and tolerability of an antiangiogenic ribozyme (ANGIOZYME) in healthy volunteers. *J Clin Pharmacol* 40: 1462–1469

73 Venook A, Hurwitz A, Cunningham BC (2003) Relationship of clinical outcome in metastatic colorectal carcinoma to levels of soluble VEGFR-1: results of a phase II trial of a ribozyme targeting pre-mRNA of VEGR-1 (angiozyme), in combination with chemotherapy. *Proc Am Soc Clin Oncol* 22: 256

74 O'Reilly MS, Holmgren L, Shing Y, Chen C, Rosenthal RA, Moses M, Lane WS, Cao Y, Sage EH, Folkman J (1994) Angiostatin: a novel angiogenesis inhibitor that mediates the suppression of metastases by a Lewis lung carcinoma. *Cell* 79: 315–328

75 Thomas JP, Arzoomanian RZ, Alberti D, Marnocha R, Lee F, Friedl A, Tutsch K, Dresen A, Geiger P, Pluda J et al (2003) Phase I pharmacokinetic and pharmacodynamic study of recombinant human endostatin in patients with advanced solid tumors. *J Clin Oncol* 21: 223–231

76 Boehm T, Folkman J, Browder T, O'Reilly MS (1997) Antiangiogenic therapy of experimental cancer does not induce acquired drug resistance. *Nature* 390, 404–407

77 Westphal JR (2004) Technology evaluation: ABT-510, Abbott. *Curr Opin Mol Ther* 6: 451–457

78 Nor JE, Mitra RS, Sutorik MM, Mooney DJ, Castle VP, Polverini PJ (2000) Thrombospondin-1 induces endothelial cell apoptosis and inhibits angiogenesis by activating the caspase death pathway. *J Vasc Res* 37: 209–218

79 Reijerkerk A, Voest EE, Gebbink MF (2000) No grip, no growth: the conceptual basis of excessive proteolysis in the treatment of cancer. *Eur J Cancer* 36: 1695–1705

80 Patel SR, Jenkins J, Papadopolous N, Burgess MA, Plager C, Gutterman J, Benjamin RS (2001) Pilot study of vitaxin – an angiogenesis inhibitor-in patients with advanced leiomyosarcomas. *Cancer* 92: 1347–1348

81 Posey JA, Khazaeli MB, DelGrosso A, Saleh MN, Lin CY, Huse W, LoBuglio AF (2001) A pilot trial of Vitaxin, a humanized anti-vitronectin receptor (anti-alpha v beta 3) antibody in patients with metastatic cancer. *Cancer Biother Radiopharm* 16: 125–132

82 Burke PA, DeNardo SJ, Miers LA, Lamborn KR, Matzku S, DeNardo GL (2002) Cilengitide targeting of alpha(v)beta(3) integrin receptor synergizes with radioimmunotherapy to increase efficacy and apoptosis in breast cancer xenografts. *Cancer Res* 62: 4263–4272

83 Eskens FA, Dumez H, Hoekstra R, Perschl A, Brindley C, Bottcher S, Wynendaele W, Drevs J, Verweij J, van Oosterom AT (2003) Phase I and pharmacokinetic study of continuous twice weekly intravenous administration of Cilengitide (EMD 121974), a novel inhibitor of the integrins alphavbeta3 and alphavbeta5 in patients with advanced solid tumours. *Eur J Cancer* 39: 917–926

84 Raguse JD, Gath HJ, Bier J, Riess H, Oettle H (2004) Cilengitide (EMD 121974) arrests the growth of a heavily pretreated highly vascularised head and neck tumour. *Oral Oncol* 40: 228–230

85 Kumar S, Witzig TE, Rajkumar SV (2004) Thalidomide: current role in the treatment of non-plasma cell malignancies. *J Clin Oncol* 22: 2477–2488

86 D'Amato RJ, Loughnan MS, Flynn E, Folkman J (1994) Thalidomide is an inhibitor of angiogenesis. *Proc Natl Acad Sci USA* 91: 4082–4085

87 Verheul HM, Panigrahy D, Yuan J, D'Amato RJ (1999) Combination oral antiangiogenic therapy with thalidomide and sulindac inhibits tumour growth in rabbits. *Br J Cancer* 79: 114–118

88 Singhal S, Mehta J, Desikan R, Ayers D, Roberson P, Eddlemon P, Munshi N, Anaissie E, Wilson C, Dhodapkar M, Zeddis J, Barlogie B (1999) Antitumor activity of thalidomide in refractory multiple myeloma. *N Engl J Med* 134: 1565–1571

89 Sills AK Jr, Williams JI, Tyler BM, Epstein DS, Sipos EP, Davis JD, McLane MP, Pitchford S, Cheshire K, Gannon FH et al (1998) Squalamine inhibits angiogenesis and solid tumor growth *in vivo* and perturbs embryonic vasculature. *Cancer Res* 58: 2784–2792

90 Hao D, Hammond LA, Eckhardt SG, Patnaik A, Takimoto CH, Schwartz GH, Goetz AD, Tolcher AW, McCreery HA, Mamun K et al (2003) A Phase I and pharmacokinetic study of squalamine, an aminosterol angiogenesis inhibitor. *Clin Cancer Res* 9: 2465–2471

91 Keyes KA, Mann L, Sherman M, Galbreath E, Schirtzinger L, Ballard D, Chen YF, Iversen P, Teicher BA (2004) LY317615 decreases plasma VEGF levels in human tumor xenograft-bearing mice. *Cancer Chemother Pharmacol* 53: 133–140

92 Kuenen BC (2003) Analysis of prothrombotic mechanisms and endothelial perturbation during treatment with angiogenesis inhibitors. *Pathophysiol Haemost Thromb* 33 Suppl 1: 13–14

93 Zangari M, Barlogie B, Thertulien R, Jacobson J, Eddleman P, Fink L, Fassas A, Van Rhee F, Talamo G, Lee CK et al (2003) Thalidomide and deep vein thrombosis in multiple myeloma: risk factors and effect on survival. *Clin Lymphoma* 4: 32–35

94 Cobleigh MA, Langmuir VK, Sledge GW, Miller KD, Haney L, Novotny WF, Reimann JD, Vassel A (2003) A phase I/II dose-escalation trial of bevacizumab in previously treated metastatic breast cancer. *Semin Oncol* 30: 117–124

95 Kiefer FN, Neysari S, Humar R, Li W, Munk VC, Battegay EJ (2003) Hypertension and angiogenesis. *Curr Pharm Des* 9: 1733–1744

96 Xu Y, Wahner AE, Nguyen PL (2004) Progression of chronic myeloid leukemia to blast crisis during treatment with imatinib mesylate. *Arch Pathol Lab Med* 128: 980–985

97 Sullivan DC, Bicknell R (2003) New molecular pathways in angiogenesis. *Br J Cancer* 89: 228–231

98 Lynch TJ, Bell DW, Sordella R, Gurubhagavatula S, Okimoto RA, Brannigan BW, Harris PL, Haserlat SM, Supko JG, Haluska FG et al (2004) Activating mutations in the epidermal growth factor receptor underlying responsiveness of non-small-cell lung cancer to gefitinib. *N Engl J Med* 350: 2129–2139

99 Saltz LB, Meropol NJ, Loehrer PJ Sr, Needle MN, Kopit J, Mayer RJ (2004) Phase II trial of cetuximab in patients with refractory colorectal cancer that expresses the epidermal growth factor receptor. *J Clin Oncol* 22: 1201–1208

100 Weinstein MC, Goldie SJ, Losina E, Cohen CJ, Baxter JD, Zhang H, Kimmel AD, Freedberg KA (2001) Use of genotypic resistance testing to guide hiv therapy: clinical impact and cost-effectiveness. *Ann Intern Med* 134: 440–450

101 Dickler MN, Rugo HS, Caravelli J, Brogi E, Sachs D, Panageas KS, Flores S, Moasser L, Norton L, Hudis C (2004) Phase II trial of erlotinib (OSI-774), an epidermal growth factor receptor (EGFR)-tyrosine kinase inhibitor, and bevacizumab, a recombinant humanized monoclonal antibody to vascular endothelial growth factor (VEGF), in patients with metastatic breast cancer. *Proc Am Soc Clin Oncol* 23: abstr. 2001

Progress in Drug Research, Vol. 63
(R. M. Schultz, Ed.)

Epidermal growth factor receptor (EGFR) inhibitors in cancer therapy

Fortunato Ciardiello
and Ferdinando De Vita

Division of Medical Oncology
Department of Experimental and
Clinical Medicine and Surgery
"F Magrassi and A Lanzara"
Second University of Naples
Via S. Pansini 5, 80131 Napoli
Italy
<fortunato.ciardiello@unina2.it>

Glossary of abbreviations

CRC, colorectal cancer; EGFR, epidermal growth factor receptor; HNSCC, head and neck squamous cell carcinoma; ILD, interstitial lung disease; NSCLC, non-small cell lung cancer; TKIs, tyrosine kinase inhibitors.

1 Introduction

One major mechanism by which cancer cells acquire autonomous and dysregulated proliferation is the uncontrolled production of specific cell growth-promoting molecules, defined growth factors, and the abnormal, enhanced expression on their cell membrane of specific proteins, defined growth factor receptors, to which growth factors selectively bind. This interaction triggers a series of intracellular signals that ultimately lead to cancer cell proliferation, induction of angiogenesis and metastasis. G. Todaro and M. Sporn first proposed this mechanism as the hypothesis of "Autocrine secretion and malignant transformation of cells" in a landmark publication in 1980 [1]. A large body of experimental and clinical evidence has been provided on the role of different families of growth factors and their specific receptors in the development and progression of human cancers [2]. The functional activation of growth factors and receptors of the epidermal growth factor receptor (EGFR) family is a common event in the majority of human epithelial cancers [2]. Specific EGFR inhibitors have been developed as anticancer agents [3–5]. In this article we summarize the molecular basis of action of EGFR inhibitors, the clinical evidence on their anticancer activity, and we will discuss the perspectives on their use in the treatment of cancer patients.

2 EGFR in human carcinogenesis

The EGFR family consists of four related cell membrane growth factor receptors. They share the same structure: an extracellular domain that interacts with a specific ligand, a short transmembrane domain, and a tyrosine kinase domain within the cell, which is the activator of downstream intracellular signaling [6, 7]. Each receptor has a certain degree of homology with the others, but they differ in terms of ligand binding and tyrosine kinase activity. Ten different ligands (growth factors) can bind to the four EGFR family members. Among the EGFR-specific growth factors, transforming growth factor α

(TGFα) is the most frequently overexpressed growth factor in human epithelial cancers [8]. After ligand binding to a single chain EGFR, active couples of receptors (receptor dimers) are formed [6–9]. These proteins can signal within the cell by activating, through an intrinsic tyrosine kinase activity, the autophosphorylation of the same growth factor receptor. This event triggers a series of intracellular pathways that bring to the nucleus the molecular signals for activating specific gene transcription and for cell cycle progression. EGFR activation in cancer cells can be due to: (1) EGFR overexpression; (2) increased production of ligands, such as TGFα and amphiregulin; and (3) EGFR gene amplification and EGFR gene mutations [2, 8]. TGFα and EGFR overexpression are associated with a poor prognosis in different human solid tumors, including head and neck squamous cell carcinoma (HNSCC), non-small cell lung cancer (NSCLC), and colorectal cancer (CRC) [2, 8]. EGFR overexpression is also linked to the development of resistance to chemotherapy, radiotherapy, and to hormone therapy [10–13].

3 Preclinical studies with EGFR inhibitors

Twenty years ago, the laboratory of J. Mendelsohn developed a series of mouse monoclonal antibodies (mAbs) that bind to the extracellular domain of EGFR, compete with endogenous ligands for receptor binding, block ligand-induced activation of the EGFR tyrosine kinase, and inhibit the growth of human cancer cells that express a functional EGFR [14–17]. Different experimental approaches have been developed and tested in search of selective anti-EGFR drugs [3–5]. Two classes of EGFR antagonists have reached clinical development: mAbs and small-molecule inhibitors of the EGFR tyrosine kinase activity (Tabs 1 and 2). mAbs are generally directed to the extracellular domain of the EGFR to compete for ligand binding and receptor activation as EGFR blocking mAbs. These antibodies are second generation, chimeric human-mouse or humanized mAbs, since the development of human anti-mouse neutralizing antibodies precludes the repeated administration of mouse mAbs in patients [3–5]. Small-molecule tyrosine kinase inhibitors (TKIs) compete with ATP for binding to the intracellular catalytic domain of the EGFR tyrosine kinase and, thus, prevent EGFR autophosphorylation and downstream signaling. Whereas mAbs exclusively recognize the EGFR and, therefore, are highly selective for this receptor, various TKIs are also able to block other members of the EGFR family. Based on the mechanism of action,

Table 1.
Anti-EGFR monoclonal antibodies in clinical development.

Drug	Molecular properties	Target selectivity	Clinical activity in cancer types	Phase of development
Cetuximab	Human-mouse chimeric MAb mAb (IgG_1)	EGFR inhibitor	Colorectal cancer, HNSCC, NSCLC	Phase III[a]
Matuzumab	Humanized MAb mAb (IgG_1)	EGFR inhibitor	Colorectal cancer, cervical cancer, HNSCC, esophageal cancer	Phase II
Pani-tumumab	Fully human Mab ($IgG_{2\kappa}$)	EGFR inhibitor	Renal cancer, prostate cancer, pancreatic cancer, colorectal cancer, NSCLC	Phase III
hR3	Humanized mMAb (IgG_1)	EGFR inhibitor	HNSCC	Phase II

[a]Cetuximab is registered in several countries worldwide, including the USA for the treatment of advanced CRC patients refractory to previous irinotecan-based chemotherapy (alone or in combination with irinotecan).

small-molecule EGFR-TKIs can be classified in four groups depending on the reversible or irreversible inhibition of the tyrosine kinase activity and on the selectivity for only the EGFR or for also other members of the receptor family [3–5]. The mechanism of action and the biological effects of mAbs and small-molecule TKIs are not completely overlapping, with some differences that could be also clinically relevant [5, 18] (Tab. 3). However, treatment with both types of agents determines similar antitumor effects, such as: (1) inhibition of cancer cell proliferation with G_0/G_1 cell cycle arrest; (2) inhibition of angiogenic growth factor production and of tumor-induced angiogenesis; (3) inhibition of cancer cell invasion and metastasis; and (4) potentiation of antitumor activity of cytotoxic drugs and of radiotherapy. Cetuximab, the chimeric human-mouse mab derived from one of the original anti-EGFR blocking mouse mAbs generated in Mendelsohn's laboratory, induces EGFR cellular internalization and downregulation, which may contribute to growth inhibition [19, 20]. Treatment with both cetuximab and gefitinib, a small-molecule reversible EGFR-TKI, block cell cycle progression by inducing a G_1 arrest through an increase in the $p27^{kip1}$ inhibitor of cyclin-dependent ki-

Table 2.
Anti-EGFR small-molecule tyrosine kinase inhibitors in clinical development.

Drug	Molecular properties	Target selectivity	Clinical activity in cancer types	Phase of development
Gefitinib	Reversible TKI (quinazoline derivative)	EGFR inhibitor	NSCLC, HNSCC, colorectal cancer, breast cancer	Phase III[a]
Erlotinib	Reversible TKI (quinazoline derivative)	EGFR inhibitor	NSCLC, HNSCC, pancreatic cancer, colorectal cancer	Phase III[b]
Lapatinib	Reversible TKI (quinazoline derivative)	EGFR/ErbB-2 dual inhibitor	Breast cancer	Phase III
EKB-569	Irreversible TKI (Cyanoquinoline cyanoquinoline derivative)	EGFR inhibitor	Colorectal cancer, breast cancer, HNSCC, NSCLC	Phase II

[a]Gefitinib is registered in 28 countries worldwide, including the USA for the treatment of NSCLC patients refractory to previous chemotherapy (platinum-based and docetaxel-based regimens).
[b]Erlotinib is registered in the USA for the treatment of NSCLC patients following failure of platinum-base chemotherapy.

nases [21–23]. Both cetuximab and gefitinib inhibit tumor-induced angiogenesis *in vivo* by blocking cancer cell production of angiogenic factors, including TGFα, vascular endothelial growth factor (VEGF), interleukin-8 (IL-8), and basic fibroblast growth factor (bFGF) [24–30]. Increased antitumor activity has been observed with the combination of EGFR antagonists and cytotoxic drugs, including platinum derivatives, taxanes, topoisomerase I and II inhibitors, and with radiotherapy [31–46]. Gefitinib treatment inhibits ErbB-2 signaling in human breast cancer cells that co-overexpress EGFR, ErbB-2 and ErbB-3, by inducing the formation of functionally inactive EGFR/ErbB-2 and EGFR/ErbB-3 heterodimers [47–50]. In these cancer cells, gefitinib treatment causes growth inhibition, blockade of the MAPK and Akt pathways, and induction of apoptosis through a complex mechanism of interference with different EGFR family members. This effect could be particularly relevant in estrogen receptor-positive breast cancer cells, which overexpress ErbB-2 and are resistant to the antitumor activity of the anti-estrogen tamoxifen [12, 51]. In fact, it has been shown that in these cells, gefitinib treatment restores tamoxifen antitumor efficacy [51].

Table 3.
Biological and pharmacological characteristics of EGFR inhibitors.

Parameter	Blocking mAbs	Tyrosine kinase inhibitors
Route of administration	Intravenous (generally with a weekly interval dosing)	Oral (generally with a daily continous dosing)
Structure	Immunoglobulins (150–180 kDa)	Low molecular weight mass compounds (400–600 Da)
Target selectivity	Absolutely specific	Relatively specific (it may vary from one to all EGFR family receptors)
Induction of EGFR internalization and down-regulation	Yes	No (although some irreversible inhibitors, such as Carnetinib can cause receptor degradation and subsequent downregulation)
Inhibition of EGFR-dependent intracellular signaling	Yes	Yes
Activation of immune system functions (antibody-dependent cell cytotoxicity, ADCC)	Yes	No

4 Clinical studies with EGFR inhibitors

As shown in Tables 1 and 2, different EGFR-targeting agents are in advanced clinical development. These drugs have shown antitumor activity in EGFR-positive tumors, including NSCLC, HNSCC and CRC, in advanced cancer patients [4, 5]. The most extensive clinical evidence available are for an anti-EGFR mAb, cetuximab, and for two small-molecule reversible EGFR-TKIs, gefinitinib and erlotinib, and, therefore, the clinical data from large phase II studies and from randomized phase III clinical trials with these EGFR antagonists will be discussed in detail.

4.1 Cetuximab

Cetuximab treatment is generally well tolerated. The most common adverse events are skin toxicities (flushing, acne-like rash and folliculitis), fever and chills, asthenia, transient transaminase elevations and nausea [52]. For cetuximab, the recommended loading dose is 400 mg/m^2 i.v. and the weekly maintenance dose 250 mg/m^2 i.v. Phase I and II studies have shown antitumor activity of cetuximab in combination with chemotherapy or radiotherapy in three EGFR-positive cancer types: HNSCC, NSCLC and CRC [4, 5]. Cetuximab treatment has been tested in CRC patients with documented progressive and chemorefractory disease. In a phase II study, treatment with cetuximab plus irinotecan in 121 EGFR-positive advanced CRC patients, who had failed a previous treatment with irinotecan, obtained partial responses in 22.5% of patients with a median duration of response of 6 months [53]. A phase II study of cetuximab monotherapy in a similar population of 57 EGFR-positive advanced CRC patients yielded 10.5% partial responses and disease stabilization in 36.8% patients [54]. The result of a multicenter phase II study in 235 advanced CRC patients who had failed two lines of chemotherapy have confirmed a partial response rate of 12% and a disease stabilization rate of 34% [55]. A multicenter, randomized phase III study evaluated the antitumor activity of cetuximab treatment alone (111 patients) or in combination with irinotecan (218 patients) in advanced CRC patients with EGFR-positive disease which progressed on an irinotecan-containing regimen as last treatment [56]. In this heavily pretreated patient population, 261/329 (79.3%) patients received two or more types of chemotherapy before study entry. Moreover, 206/329 (62.6%) patients were also pretreated with an oxaliplatin-containing regimen. Partial responses were obtained in 22.9% patients treated with irinotecan plus cetuximab, as compared to 10.8% patients treated with cetuximab alone ($P = 0.007$). Similarly, a significantly better disease control (partial responses plus disease stabilization) was observed in the combination arm as compared to cetuximab monotherapy (55.5% *versus* 32.4%, $P < 0.001$) [56]. A significant improvement in time to disease progression was also observed in the patients treated with cetuximab plus irinotecan (hazard ratio, 0.54; 95% confidence intervals 0.42–0.71; $P < 0.001$). Collectively, these studies confirm the antitumor activity of cetuximab monotherapy in a population of heavily pretreated EGFR-positive advanced CRC patients, with a clinically relevant disease control in approximately one third of patients (10–12% partial responses plus 20–25% disease stabilization). Furthermore, treatment of these patients with cetuximab in combination with irinotecan significantly improves response rates and time to disease progression. These data are particularly relevant in advanced CRC. In fact, the most active chemotherapy combinations, such as fluoropyrimidine, irinotecan and oxaliplatin in combination or sequentially, obtain a median survival of 18–21 months in these patients. However, after failure of these drugs combinations, there are no effective treatment options. Cetuximab as monotherapy and in combination with irinotecan is a valid option in the treatment of these patients. Cetuximab has been the first anti-EGFR mAb to be approved in combination with irinotecan in several countries worldwide, including USA, for the treatment of irinotecan-resistant, EGFR-positive, advanced CRC patients. A series of randomized, phase III clinical trials of cetuximab in combination with different cytotoxic drugs are currently in progress to evaluate the efficacy of this anti-EGFR agent in the first-line treatment of advanced CRC. In this respect, recent results from two phase II study have demonstrated antitumor activity with high response rates of cetuximab in combination with 5-fluorouracil, folinic acid and irinotecan (FOLFIRI regimen), or with 5-fluorouracil, folinic acid and oxaliplatin (FOLFOX-4 regimen) in the first-line treatment of EGFR-positive advanced CRC. In 40 patients treated with FOLFIRI plus cetuximab, partial responses were reported in 43% of patients and stable disease in other 45% of patients [57]. In 42 patients treated with FOLFOX-4 plus cetuximab, complete responses were observed in 5% of patients, partial responses in 76% of patients and stable disease in 17% of patients [58].

The antitumor activity of cetuximab has been evaluated in locally advanced HNSCC patients in combination with radiotherapy as first-line treatment. In a pilot study, in 16 patients with locally advanced HNSCC, 13 patients achieved a complete response, and two patients had a partial response [59]. The median duration of response was 28 months with 1- and 2-year disease-free survival rates of 73% and 65%, respectively [59]. Although these results have been observed in a small series of patients, the expected response rate is approximately 40–50% in locally advanced HNSCC patients treated with radiotherapy alone. In this respect, the results of a multicenter, randomized phase III study evaluating the efficacy of adding cetuximab treatment to radiotherapy as first-line therapy in 424 locally advanced HNSCC have been recently presented, and have demonstrated a significant improvement in survival in those patients treated with radiotherapy plus cetuximab as compared to radiotherapy alone (median survival, 54 versus 28 months; 3-year survival, 57% versus 44%; hazard ratio, 0.71; 95% confidence intervals 0.54–0.95; $P = 0.02$) [60]. A randomized, phase III trial of cisplatin plus cetuximab or placebo in 123 chemo-naïve patients with metastatic HNSCC has been also reported [61]. A significantly higher overall response rate was observed in the cisplatin plus cetuximab arm (23% versus 9%; $P = 0.05$). Although there was a trend for a better survival in the cetuximab plus cisplatin arm (2-year survival, 29% versus 17%), no statistically significant difference in overall survival was observed. Cetuximab has also antitumor activity as monotherapy in patients with locally HNSCC refractory to platinum-based chemotherapy. No cancer-specific treatment is active in this patient population, which has a median survival of approximately 3 months. A phase II study in 103 platinum-refractory HNSCC has reported a 12.6% partial response rate plus an additional 33% disease stabilization with a medial survival of 5.9 months [62].

The combination of cetuximab with standard two-drug chemotherapy regimens, such as carboplatin-paclitaxel, carboplatin-gemcitabine and cisplatin-vinorelbine, has been evaluated in different phase II studies as first-line treatment in EGFR-positive, stages IIIB–IV NSCLC patients, with 29–35% partial response rates and median survival of 8.3–15.7 months [4, 5, 63]. However, randomized, phase III trials are necessary to define if cetuximab significantly improves the efficacy of chemotherapy in NSCLC.

4.2 Gefitinib

Phase I trials have determined gefitinib doses of 250 or 500 mg as a continuous once-daily, oral schedule [64–67]. The most frequent adverse events are diarrhea and acne-like skin rash. The antitumor activity of gefitinib alone or in combination with standard therapies such as chemotherapy, radiation therapy or hormone therapy is under active investigation in breast cancer, CRC, HNSCC, and glioblastomas [4, 5, 63]. However, in phase I clinical trials, antitumor activity has been mainly observed in patients with NSCLC [64–68]. Two large phase II trials of gefitinib monotherapy in advanced NSCLC patients who have failed one or more chemotherapy regimens have been conducted [69]. In a multicenter, European and Japanese, phase II trial of gefitinib as second- or third-line single-agent therapy (IDEAL 1 study), 210 advanced NSCLC patients, who were not selected for EGFR expression, were randomized to 250-mg or 500-mg oral daily treatment [70]. An overall response rate of 18.4% and 19% was observed in the 250- and 500-mg groups, respectively. Stable disease was obtained in 36% and 32% patients, respectively, with symptom improvements were recorded in 40.3% and 37% patients. Median progression-free survival times were 2.7 and 2.8 months, and median overall survival times were 7.6 and 8.0 months, respectively. Therefore, a 250-mg dose of gefitinib was equally active as the 500-mg dose. However, the tolerability profile was significant better with the 250-mg daily dose [70]. A parallel phase II, randomized study was conducted in the United States (IDEAL 2) in 216 unselected, symptomatic, advanced NSCLC patients who were resistant to at least two previous chemotherapy regimens, one containing a platinum derivative and one containing docetaxel [71]. Disease-specific symptoms improved in 43% of patients receiving 250 mg Gefitinib and in 35% of patients receiving 500 mg. These effects occurred rapidly in the majority of patients (i.e., within 3 weeks in 75% of responding patients). Partial responses were detected in 12% and in 9% of patients treated with 250 and 500 mg Gefitinib, respectively. One-year overall survival was 25%. In this study, the higher dose of gefitinib was again associated with worse side effects. On the basis of these clinical trials, gefitinib at a 250 mg daily dose has been licensed for platinum- and docetaxel-chemorefractory advanced NSCLC patients as a third-line treatment in 28 countries around the world, including the USA [72]. Single-agent gefitinib antitumor activity with approximately 10% partial responses, 25–30% stable disease, and with symptomatic improvement in approximately one third to half of NSCLC patients, has been confirmed by a large international extended access program that has been conducted with gefitinib, 250 mg, in advanced NSCLC patients that progressed after standard chemotherapy and/or radiation therapy [73, 74]. Moreover, gefitinib clinical activity has been reported also in elderly and/or poor-performance-status NSCLC patients [75, 76]. Gefitinib monotherapy has also shown anticancer activity against brain metastasis in advanced NSCLC patients [77, 78].

Two reports have recently shown somatic EGFR gene mutations in approximately 10% of Caucasian advanced NSCLC patients and in 15/58 advanced NSCLC patients from Japan [79–80]. These are either small, in-frame deletions or amino acid substitutions clustered in the ATP-binding pocket of the EGFR tyrosine kinase domain [79, 80]. Collectively, among 14 metastatic and chemorefractory NSCLC patients experiencing a long-lasting clinical response to gefitinib monotherapy, 13 patients had tumors with one of these somatic mutations, whereas no EGFR mutations were found in 13 patients in which gefitinib therapy failed. Lung cancer cells that possess one of these mutations have increased EGFR signaling ("gain of function" mutations) with a 50-fold increased sensitivity to gefitinib *in vitro*. These mutations probably stabilize the interaction between gefitinib and the tyrosine kinase domain, thereby enhancing the growth inhibitory effect of the drug [81].

The role of gefitinib in combination with chemotherapy has been also assessed in advanced NSCLC. Two large (1093 and 1037 patients in each trial, respectively), randomized, multicenter, double-blind, placebo-controlled, phase III trials of gefitinib (250 mg or 500 mg daily) in combination with cytotoxic agents (cisplatin/gemcitabine, INTACT 1 trial; or carboplatin/paclitaxel, INTACT 2 trial) as first-line treatment in stages IIIB–IV NSCLC patients were conducted [82, 83]. No patient selection based on EGFR expression in cancer cells was done. No difference in overall survival, as the primary endpoint of these two parallel studies, has been reported. Among the different explanations for the lack of efficacy of gefitinib plus standard double cytotoxic therapy that have been proposed [63, 84], it seems more conceivable that this is due to the high molecular and clonal heterogeneity of NSCLC cells. Only a subset of EGFR-positive NSCLC patients may have tumors that are significantly dependent upon the EGFR pathway, and who, therefore, could obtain a clinical benefit from an anti-EGFR drug [84]. This has a profound effect on the patient sample size needed to detect the clinical efficacy of an EGFR antagonist in an unselected population of NSCLC patients. Given the expected activity (approximately 30% overall response rates) of the standard two-chemotherapy drug regimens used in the INTACT trials, at least three to four times as many patients would have been required to detect the positive effect of adding gefitinib, if only a 20–30% of the total study population could benefit of the EGFR blockade [84].

Interstitial lung disease (ILD) has been identified as a possible adverse effect of gefitinib treatment. ILD was first reported in Japanese advanced NSCLC patients receiving gefitinib and who had been pretreated with chemotherapy and/or radiotherapy [85]. ILD has been observed in 291/17500 (1.7%) Japanese patients treated with gefitinib [85]. However, ILD has been observed in only 0.3% of 56000 NSCLC patients that have received Gefitinib in USA, Europe and Australia as part of an expanded access program [86]. No differences in any type of adverse pulmonary events have been observed in the double-blind, placebo-controlled, randomized INTACT 1 and 2 trials (0.9% in the placebo group as compared to 1.1% in the 250 mg/day and the 500 mg/day gefitinib groups) [82, 83]. Notably, ILD has been observed in NSCLC patients receiving standard cytotoxic treatments (1–5% incidence with chemotherapy or with radiotherapy) [86]. These data suggest that ILD is possibly occurring with a low frequency in advanced stage NSCLC patients during or after treatment with several standard treatments, and does not seems specifically linked to gefitinib treatment. A series of phase III trials are currently evaluating the role of gefitinib as an adjuvant treatment in radically resected NSCLC patients, as well as the possibility of using gefitinib as a maintenance therapy following first-line chemotherapy in advanced NSCLC patients, and the efficacy of gefitinib as compared to standard chemotherapy (docetaxel) in the treatment of platinum-resistant NSCLC patients.

4.3 Erlotinib

In phase I studies, major toxicities were diarrhea and acne-like skin rash. The recommended dose for continuous oral scheduling was 150 mg/day [87, 88]. Antitumor activity of erlotinib as single-agent therapy has been observed in heavily pretreated patients with advanced HNSCC, ovarian cancer and NSCLC [89–91]. In 57 patients with advanced NSCLC who had failed a platinum-based therapy, 1 complete response, 6 partial responses and 17 stable diseases were observed [91]. Erlotinib treatment as single agent has been evaluated in advanced NSCLC patients after failure of one or two standard chemotherapy regimens in a large (731 patients), multicenter randomized phase III clinical trial in comparison with best supportive care. The results of this study have been recently reported [92]. These patients had a metastatic NSCLC, which was treated with one standard chemotherapy regimen (50% of patients) or with two chemotherapy regimens (50% of patients). Almost all patients received a platinum-based therapy. Partial responses were observed in 9% and stable disease in 35% of the 488 erlotinib-treated patients. Erlotinib treatment significantly improved survival as compared to best supportive care (median survival, 6.7 versus 4.7 months; 1-year survival 31% versus 22%; hazard ratio, 0.73; 95% confidence intervals 0.60–0.87; $P < 0.001$). Patients treated with erlotinib also had significantly better symptom control as compared to best supportive care ($P = 0.02$) [92]. The results of this study are the first demonstration in a phase III trial of the antitumor efficacy of a small-molecule selective EGFR-TKI in the treatment of chemoresistant, advanced NSCLC patients. Based on these results, in November 2004, the FDA has licensed erlotinib for the treatment of advanced NSCLC patients following the failure of a platinum-containing chemotherapy.

The results of two large multicenter phase III studies of first-line carboplatin-paclitaxel (TRIBUTE study) or cisplatin-gemcitabine (TALENT study) with or without erlotinib in stage IIIB–IV NSCLC patients have been recently reported [93, 94]. Both studies, similar to the INTACT studies with gefitinib, have failed to show any difference in overall survival between the standard and the erlotinib-containing treatment.

5 Future directions

Targeting the EGFR is a valuable molecular approach in cancer treatment. Anti-EGFR mAbs and small-molecule TKIs have relevant clinical activity in NSCLC, HNSCC and CRC. The major challenge for the clinical use of EGFR antagonists is the appropriate selection of patients. In fact, although long-lasting therapeutic responses have been observed even in heavily pretreated, metastatic cancer patients, these responses are observed only in 10-30% patients who are treated with these drugs. It is necessary that cancer cells express functional EGFRs, but it is equally important that the EGFR-activated intracellular signal transduction machinery is intact for an optimal response to EGFR antagonists [95]. In fact, a EGFR-dependent cancer cell may escape from EGFR-targeted growth inhibition by using alternative growth factor receptor pathways, such as the insulin-like growth factor receptor I; by constitutive activation of downstream signaling effectors such as Akt and MAPK; or by enhanced production of angiogenic factors, such as VEGF [96–100]. The identification of specific EGFR gene mutations that are associated with a very high sensitivity to gefitinib treatment is the first molecular marker that could be clinically useful to select NSCLC patients [79, 80]. Clinical data suggest that gefitinib and erlotinib have greater activity in certain NSCLC histotypes, such as in adenocarcinomas and in bronchioloalveolar carcinomas and in women with a no-smoking history [101–104]. Furthermore, a higher response rate to gefitinib has been observed in Japanese NSCLC patients as compared to Caucasian patients [69, 70]. Interestingly, EGFR gene mutations that are correlated with high sensitivity to gefitinib therapy in advanced NSCLC are more frequent in women with no history of smoking and adenocarcinoma and in Japanese women [79, 80]. An acne-like rash is also considered an indirect marker of clinically activity. A retrospective analysis of four phase II studies in HNSCC, in CRC, and in pancreatic cancer has suggested that cetuximab-induced skin rash correlates with increased survival [105]. A similar observation has been reported in the randomized study evaluating cetuximab plus irinotecan in irinotecan-refractory metastatic CRC [56]. A similar retrospective analysis of acne-like rash in three phase II studies of erlotinib monotherapy in EGFR-positive patients with chemorefractory NSCLC, HNSCC and ovarian cancer has shown that skin rash severity correlates with better survival [106]. Another clinical issue is to define the effective sequences and combinations of EGFR inhibitors with cytotoxic agents and/or radiotherapy [107]. In fact, the schedules that have been tested so far in cancer patients have been based on the empiric association of a standard chemotherapy regimen with the continuous administration of an EGFR-targeting drug rather than being derived from molecular, pharmacokinetic and pharmacodynamic studies. Finally, an open question is whether anti-EGFR mAbs and small-molecule TKIs have different clinical effects. No direct comparison of these two classes of drugs has been conducted. Further, no clinical data are available on the effect of anti-EGFR mAbs in NSCLC cancer patients whose tumors harbor EGFR gene mutations.

Acknowledgements

The research program performed by the authors is supported by grants from the Associazione Italiana per la Ricerca sul Cancro (AIRC).

References

1 Sporn MB, Todaro GJ (1980) Autocrine secretion and malignant transformation of cells. *N Engl J Med* 303: 878–880
2 Salomon DS, Brandt R, Ciardiello F, Normanno N (1995) Epidermal growth factor-related peptides and their receptors in human malignancies. *Crit Rev Oncol Haematol* 19: 183–232
3 Ciardiello F, Tortora G (2001) A novel approach in the treatment of cancer: targeting the epidermal growth factor receptor. *Clin Cancer Res* 7: 2958–2970
4 Grunwald V, Hidalgo M (2003) Developing inhibitors of the epidermal growth factor receptor for cancer treatment. *J Natl Cancer Inst* 95: 851–867
5 Mendelsohn J, Baselga J (2003) Status of epidermal growth factor receptor antagonists in the biology and treatment of cancer. *J Clin Oncol* 21: 2787–2799
6 Olayioye MA, Neve RM, Lane HA, Hynes NE (2000) The ErbB signaling network: receptor heterodimerization in development and cancer. *EMBO J* 19: 3159–3167
7 Yarden Y, Sliwkowski MX (2001) Untantling the ErbB signalling network. *Nat Rev Mol Cell Biol* 2: 127–137

8 Normanno N, Bianco C, De Luca A, Maiello MR, Salomon DS (2003) Target-based agents against ErbB receptors and their ligands: a novel approach to cancer treatment. *Endocr Relat Cancer* 10: 1–21
9 Schlessinger J (2000) Cell signaling by receptor tyrosine kinases. *Cell* 103: 211–225
10 McClelland RA, Barrow D, Madden T-A et al (2001) Enhanced epidermal growth factor receptor signaling in MCF7 breast cancer cells after long-term culture in the presence of the pure antiestrogen ICI 182,780 (Faslodex). *Endocrinology* 142: 2776–2788
11 Wosikowski K, Schuuruis D, Kops GJPL, Saceda M, Bates SE (1997) Altered gene expression in drug-resistant human breast cancer cells. *Clin Cancer Res* 3: 2405–2414
12 Knowlden JM, Hutcheson IR, Jones HE et al (2003) Elevated levels of epidermal growth factor receptor/c-erbB2 heterodimers mediate an autocrine regulatory pathway in tamoxifen-resistant MCF-7 cells. *Endocrinology* 144: 1032–1044
13 Akimoto T, Hunter NR, Buchmiller L, Mason K, Ang KK, Milas L (1999) Inverse relationship between epidermal growth factor receptor expression and radiocurability of murine carcinomas. *Clin Cancer Res* 5: 2884–2890
14 Mendelsohn J (2000) Blockade of receptors for growth factors: an anticancer therapy. *Clin Cancer Res* 6: 747–753
15 Fan Z, Lu Y, Wu X, Mendelsohn J (1994) Antibody-induced epidermal growth factor receptor dimerization mediates inhibition of autocrine proliferation of A431 squamous carcinoma cells. *J Biol Chem* 269: 27595–27602
16 Fan Z, Baselga J, Masui H, Mendelsohn J (1992) Antitumor effect of anti-epidermal growth factor receptor monoclonal antibodies plus *cis*-diamminedichloroplatinum on well established A431 cell xenografts. *Cancer Res* 53: 4637–4642
17 Baselga J, Norton L, Masui H et al (1993) Antitumor effects of doxorubicin in combination with anti-epidermal growth factor receptor monoclonal antibodies. *J Natl Cancer Inst* 85: 1327–1333
18 Baselga J (2003) Targeting EGFR with MAbs versus TKIs: different mechanisms, similar endpoints. *Signal* 4: 4–6
19 Goldstein NI, Prewett M, Zuklys K, Rockwell P, Mendelsohn J (1995) Biological efficacy of a chimeric antibody to the epidermal growth factor receptor in a human tumor xenograft model. *Clin Cancer Res* 1: 1311–1318
20 Prewett M, Rothman M, Waksal H, Feldman M, Bander NH, Hicklin DJ (1998) Mouse-human chimeric anti-epidermal growth factor receptor antibody C225 inhibits the growth of human renal cell carcinoma xenografts in nude mice. *Clin Cancer Res* 4: 2957–2966
21 Wu X, Rubin M, Fan Z et al (1996) Involvement of p27kip1 in G1 arrest mediated by an anti-epidermal growth factor receptor monoclonal antibody. *Oncogene* 12: 1397–1403
22 Peng D, Fan Z, Lu Y, Deblasio T, Scher H, Mendelsohn J (1996) Anti-epidermal growth factor receptor monoclonal antibody C225 upregulates p27kip1 and induces G1 arrest in prostatic cancer cell line DU145. *Cancer Res* 56: 3666–3669
23 Di Gennaro E, Barbarino M, Bruzzese F et al *(2003)* Critical role of both p27kip1 and p21cip1/waf1 in the antiproliferative effect of ZD1839 (Iressa), an epidermal growth factor receptor tyrosine kinase inhibitor, in head and neck squamous carcinoma cells. *J Cell Physiol* 195: 139–150

24 Ciardiello F, Damiano V, Bianco R et al (1996) Antitumor activity of combined blockade of epidermal growth factor receptor and protein kinase A. *J Natl Cancer Inst* 88: 1770–1776

25 Perrotte P, Matsumoto T, Inoue K et al (1999) Anti-epidermal growth factor receptor antibody C225 inhibits angiogenesis in human transitional cell carcinoma growing orthotopically in nude mice. *Clin Cancer Res* 5: 257–265

26 Ciardiello F, Bianco R, Damiano V et al (2000) Antiangiogenic and antitumor activity of anti-epidermal growth factor receptor C225 monoclonal antibody in combination with vascular endothelial growth factor antisense oligonucleotide in human GEO colon cancer cells. *Clin Cancer Res* 6: 3739–3747

27 Bruns CJ, Harbison MT, Davis DW et al (2000) Epidermal growth factor receptor blockade with C225 plus gemcitabine results in regression of human pancreatic carcinoma growing orthotopically in nude mice by antiangiogenic mechanisms. *Clin Cancer Res* 6: 1936–1948

28 Ciardiello F, Caputo R, Bianco R et al (2001) Inhibition of growth factor production and angiogenesis in human cancer cells by ZD1839 (Iressa), a selective epidermal growth factor receptor tyrosine kinase inhibitor. *Clin Cancer Res* 7: 1459–1465

29 Hirata A, Ogawa S, Kometani T et al (2002) ZD1839 (Iressa) induces antiangiogenic effects through inhibition of epidermal growth factor receptor tyrosine kinase. *Cancer Res* 62: 2554–2560

30 Huang S-M, Li J, Harri PM (2002) Molecular inhibition of angiogenesis and metastatic potential in human squamous cell carcinomas after epidermal growth factor receptor blockade. *Mol Cancer Ther* 1: 507–514

31 Ciardiello F, Caputo R, Bianco R et al (2000) Antitumor effect and potentiation of cytotoxic drugs activity in human cancer cells by ZD-1839 (Iressa), an epidermal growth factor receptor-sensitive tyrosine kinase inhibitor. *Clin Cancer Res* 6: 2053–2063

32 Ciardiello F, Bianco R, Damiano V et al (1999) Antitumor activity of sequential treatment with topotecan and anti-epidermal growth factor receptor monoclonal antibody C225. *Clin Cancer Res* 5: 909–916

33 Inoue K, Slaton JW, Perrotte P et al (2000) Paclitaxel enhances the effects of the anti-epidermal growth factor receptor monoclonal antibody ImClone C225 in mice with metastatic human bladder transitional cell carcinoma. *Clin Cancer Res* 6: 4874–4884

34 Prewett MC, Hooper AT, Bassi R, Ellis LM, Waksal HW, Hicklin DJ (2002) Enhanced antitumor activity of anti-epidermal growth factor receptor monoclonal antibody IMC-C255 in combination with irinotecan (CPT-11) against human colorectal tumor xenografts. *Clin Cancer Res* 8: 994–1003

35 Milas L, Mason K, Hunter N et al (2000) In vivo enhancement of tumor radioresponse by C225 antiepidermal growth factor receptor antibody. *Clin Cancer Res* 6: 701–708

36 Huang SM, Bock JM, Harari PM (1999) Epidermal growth factor receptor blockade with C225 modulates proliferation, apoptosis, and radiosensitivity in squamous cell carcinomas of the head and neck. *Cancer Res* 15: 1935–1940

37 Bianco C, Bianco R, Tortora G et al (2000) Antitumor activity of combined treatment of human cancer cells with ionizing radiations and anti-epidermal growth factor receptor monoclonal antibody C225 plus type I protein kinase A antisense oligonucleotide. *Clin Cancer Res* 6: 4343–4350

38 Huang SM, Harari P (2000) Modulation of radiation response after epidermal growth factor receptor blockade in squamous cell carcinomas: inhibition of damage repair, cell cycle kinetics, and tumor angiogenesis. *Clin Cancer Res* 6: 2166–2174

39 Sirotnak FM, Zakowsky MF, Miller VA, Scher HI, Kris MG (2000) Efficacy of cytotoxic agents against human tumor xenografts is markedly enhanced by coadministration of ZD1839 (Iressa), an inhibitor of EGFR tyrosine kinase. *Clin Cancer Res* 6: 4885–4892

40 Williams K, Telfer BA, Stratford IJ, Wedge SR (2002) ZD1839 (Iressa), a specific oral epidermal growth factor receptor-tyrosine kinase inhibitor potentiates radiotherapy in a human colorectal cancer xenograft model. *Br J Cancer* 86: 1157–1161

41 Xu J-M, Azzariti A, Severino M, Lu B, Colucci G, Paradiso A (2003) Characterization of sequence-dependent synergy between ZD1839 ("Iressa") and oxaliplatin. *Biochem Pharmacol* 66: 551–563

42 Magne N, Fischel J-L, Tiffon C et al (2003) Molecular mechanisms underluing the interaction between ZD1839 ("Iressa") and cisplatin/5-fluorouracil. *Br J Cancer* 89: 585–592

43 Bianco C, Tortora G, Bianco R et al (2002) Enhancement of antitumor activity of ionizing radiation by combined treatment with the selective EGFR-tyrosine kinase inhibitor ZD1839 ('Iressa'). *Clin Cancer Res* 8: 3250–3258

44 Huang S, Li J, Harari PM (2002) Modulation of radiation response and tumor-induced angiogenesis following EGFR blockade by ZD1839 (Iressa) in human squamous cell carcinomas. *Cancer Res* 62: 4300–4306

45 She Y, Lee F, Chen J et al (2003) The epidermal growth factor receptor tyrosine kinase inhibitor ZD1839 selectively potentiates radiation response of human tumors in nude mice, with a marked improvement in therapeutic index. *Clin Cancer Res* 9: 3773–3778

46 Ciardiello F, Caputo R, Bianco R et al (2002) ZD1839 ('Iressa'), an EGFR-selective tyrosine kinase inhibitor, enhances taxane activity in bcl-2 overexpressing, multidrug-resistant MCF-7 ADR human breast cancer cells. *Int J Cancer* 98: 463–469

47 Normanno N, Campiglio M, De Luca A et al (2001) Cooperative inhibitory effect of ZD1839 (Iressa) in combination with trastuzumab (Herceptin) on human breast cancer cell growth. *Ann Oncol* 13: 65–72

48 Moulder SL, Yakes FM, Muthuswamy SK, Bianco R, Simpson JF, Arteaga CL (2001) Epidermal growth factor receptor (HER1) tyrosine kinase inhibitor ZD1839 (Iressa) inhibits HER2/*neu* (*erb*B2)-overexpressing breast cancer cells *in vitro* and *in vivo*. *Cancer Res* 61: 8887–8895

49 Anido J, Matar P, Albanell J et al (2003) ZD1839, a specific epidermal growth factor receptor (EGFR) tyrosine kinase inhibitor, induces the formation of inactive EGFR/HER2 and EGFR/HER3 heterodimers and prevents heregulin signaling in HER2-overexpressing breast cancer cells. *Clin Cancer Res* 9: 1274–1283

50 Moasser MM, Basso A, Averbuch SD, Rosen N (2001) The tyrosine kinase inhibitor ZD1839 ("Iressa") inhibits HER2-driven signaling and suppresses the growth of HER2-overexpressing tumor cells. *Cancer Res* 61: 7184–7188

51 Baselga J, Pfister D, Cooper MR et al (2000) Phase I studies of anti-epidermal growth factor receptor chimeric antibody C225 alone and in combination with cisplatin. *J Clin Oncol* 18: 904–914

52 Shou J, Massarweh S, Osborne CK et al (2004) Mechanisms of tamoxifen resistance: increased estrogen reeptor-HER2/neu cross-talk in ER/HER2-positive breast cancer. *J Natl Cancer Inst* 96: 926–935
53 Saltz L, Rubin M, Hochster H et al (2001) Cetuximab (IMC-C225) plus irinotecan (CPT-11) is active in CPT-11-refractory colorectal cancer (CRC) that expresses epidermal growth factor receptor (EGFR). *Proc Am Soc Clin Oncol* 20: abstr. 7
54 Saltz L, Meropol NJ, Loeher PJ et al (2004) Phase II trial of cetuximab in patients with refractory colorectal cancer that express the epidermal growth factor receptor. *J Clin Oncol* 22: 1201–1208
55 Lenz HJ, Mayer RJ, Gold PJ et al (2004) Activity of cetuximab in patients with colorectal cancer refractory to both irinotecan and oxaliplatin. *Proc Am Soc Clin Oncol* 23: abstr. 3510
56 Cunningham D, Humblet Y, Siena S et al (2004) A randomized comparison of cetuximab monotherapy and cetuximab plus irinotecan in irino-tecan-refractory metastatic colorectal cancer. *N Engl J Med* 351; *in press*
57 Rougier P, Rasoul J-L, Van Laethem J-L et al (2004) Cetuximab (Erbitux) combined with FOLFIRI (irinotecan plus infusional 5-FU and folinic acid given every two weeks) in patients with epidermal growth factor receptor-expressing advanced colorectal cancer *Proc Am Soc Clin Oncol* 23: abstr. 3513
58 Tabernero JM, Van Cutsem E, Sastre J et al (2004) An international phase II study of cetuximab in combination with oxaliplatin/5-fluorouracil (5FU)/folinic acid (FA) (FOLFOX-4) in the first-line treatment of patients with metastatic colorectal cancer (CRC) expressing epidermal growth factor receptor (EGFR). *Proc Am Soc Clin Oncol* 23: abstr. 3512
59 Robert F, Ezekiel MP, Spencer SA et al (2001) Phase I study of anti-epidermal growth factor receptor antibody cetuximab in combination with radiation therapy in patients with advanced head and neck cancer. *J Clin Oncol* 19: 3234–3243
60 Bonner JA, Giralt J, Harari PM et al (2004) Phase III study of high dose radiation with or without cetuximab in the treatment of locoregionally advanced squamous cell carcinoma of the head and neck (SCCHN). *Proc Am Soc Clin Oncol* 23: abstr. 5507
61 Burtness B, Li Y, Flood W et al (2002) Phase III trial comparing cisplatin (C) + placebo (P) + anti-epidermal growth factor antibody (EGFR) C225 in patients (pts) with metastatic/recurrent head and neck cancer (HNC). *Proc Am Soc Clin Oncol* 21: abstr. 901
62 Trigo J, Hitt R, Koralewski P et al (2004) Cetuximab monotherapy is active in patients with platinum-refractory recurrent/metastatic squamous cell carcinoma of the head and neck (SCCHN). *Proc Am Soc Clin Oncol* 23: abstr. 5502
63 Sridhar SS, Seymour L, Shepherd FA (2003) Inhibitors of epidermal-growth-factor receptors: a review of clinical research with a focus on non-small-cell lung cancer. *Lancet Oncol* 4: 397–406
64 Ranson M, Hammond LA, Ferry D et al (2002) ZD1839, a selective oral epidermal growth factor receptor-tyrosine kinase inhibitor, is well tolerated and active in patients with solid, malignant tumors: results of a phase I trial. *J Clin Oncol* 20: 2240–2250
65 Herbst RS, Maddox A-M, Rothenberg ML et al (2002) Selective oral epidermal growth factor receptor tyrosine inhibitor ZD1839 is generally well-tolerated and has activity

in non-small-cell lung cancer and other solid tumors: results of a phase I trial. *J Clin Oncol* 20: 3815–3828
66 Baselga J, Rischin D, Ranson M et al (2002) Phase I safety, pharmacokinetic, and pharmacodynamic trial of ZD1839, a selective oral epidermal growth factor receptor tyrosine kinase inhibitor, in patients with five selected tumor types:. *J Clin Oncol* 21: 4292–4302
67 Nakagawa K, Tamura T, Negoro S et al (2003) Phase I pharmacokinetic trial of the selective oral epidermal growth factor receptor tyrosine kinase inhibitor gefitinib ("Iressa", ZD1839) in Japanese patients with solid malignant tumors. *Ann Oncol* 14: 922–930
68 LoRusso P, Herbst RS, Rischin D et al (2003) Improvements in quality of life and disease-related symptoms in phase I trials of the selective oral epidermal growth factor receptor tyrosine kinase inhibitor ZD1839 in non-small cell lung cancer and other solid tumors. *Clin Cancer Res* 9: 2040–2048
69 Johnson DH, Arteaga CL (2003) Gefitinib in recurrent non-small cell lung cancer: an IDEAL trial? *J Clin Oncol* 21: 2227–2229
70 Fukuoka M, Yano S, Giaccone G et al (2003) Multi-institutional randomized phase II trial of gefitinib for previously treated patients with advanced non-small-cell lung cancer. *J Clin Oncol* 22: 2237–2246
71 Kris MG, Natale RB, Herbst RS et al (2003) Efficacy of gefitinib, an inhibitor of the epidermal growth factor receptor tyrosine kinase, in symptomatic patients with non-small cell lung cancer. *JAMA* 290: 2149–2158
72 Cohen MH, Williams GA, Sridhara R, Chen G, Pazdur R (2003) FDA approval summary: Gefitinib (ZD1839) (Iressa^{R}) Tablets. *Oncologist* 8: 303–306
73 Cappuzzo F, Gregorc V, Rossi E et al (2003) Gefitinib in pretreated non-small-cell lung cancer (NSCLC): analysis of efficacy and correlation with HER2 and epidermal growth factor receptor expression in locally advanced or metastatic NSCLC. *J Clin Oncol* 21: 2658–2663
74 Pallis AG, Mavroudinis D, Androulakis N et al (2003) ZD1839, a novel, oral epidermal growth factor receptor-tyrosine kinase inhibitor, as salvage treatment in patients with advanced non-small cell lung cancer. Experience from a single center participating in a compassionate use program. *Lung Cancer* 40: 301–307
75 Gridelli C, Maione P, Castaldo V, Rossi A (2003) Gefitinib in elderly and unfit patients affected by advanced non-small-cell lung cancer. *Br J Cancer* 89: 1827–1829
76 Gelibter A, Ceribelli A, Milella M et al (2003) Clinically meaningful response to the EGFR tyrosine kinase inhibitor gefitinib ("Iressa", ZD1839) in non small cell lung cancer. *J Exp Clin Cancer Res* 22: 481–485
77 Villano JL, Mauer AM, Vokes EE (2003) A case study documenting the anticancer activity of ZD1839 (Iressa) in the brain. *Ann Oncol* 14: 656–658
78 Cappuzzo F, Ardizzoni A, Soto-Parra H et al (2003) Epidermal growth factor receptor targeted therapy by ZD1839 (Iressa) in patients with brain metastases from non-small cell lung cancer (NSCLC). *Lung Cancer* 41: 227–231
79 Lynch TJ, Bell DW, Sordella R et al (2004) Activating mutations in the epidermal growth factor receptor underlying responsiveness of non-small-cell lung cancer to gefitinib. *N Engl J Med* 350: 2129–2139
80 Paez JG, Janne PA, Lee JC et al (2004) EGFR mutations in lung cancer: correlation with clinical response to gefitinib therapy. *Science* 304: 1497–1500

81 Green MR (2004) Targeting targeted therapy. *N Engl J Med* 350: 2191–2193
82 Giaccone G, Johnson DH, Manegold C et al (2004) Gefitinib in combination with gemcitabine and cispatin in advanced non-small-cell lung cancer: a phase III trial-INTACT 1. *J Clin Oncol* 22: 777–784
83 Herbst R, Giaccone G, Schiller JH et al (2004) Gefitinib in combination with paclitaxel and carboplatin in advanced non-small-cell lung cancer: a phase III trial-INTACT 2. *J Clin Oncol* 22: 785–794
84 Dancey JE, Freidin B (2003) Targeting epidermal growth factor receptor – are we missing the mark? *Lancet* 362: 62–64
85 Inoue A, Saijo Y, Maemondo M et al (2003) Severe interstitial pneumonia and Gefitinib. *Lancet* 361: 137–139
86 Soria J-C, Le Chevalier T (2003) Interstitial lung disease in NSCLC. *Signal* 4: 2–3
87 Hidalgo M, Siu LL, Nemunaitis J et al (2001) Phase I and pharmacologic study of OSI-774, an epidermal growth factor receptor tyrosine kinase inhibitor, in patients with advanced solid malignancies. *J Clin Oncol* 19: 3267–3279
88 Bulgaru AM, Mani S, Goel S, Perez-Soler R (2003) Erlotinib (Tarceva): a promising drug targeting epidermal growth factor receptor tyrosine kinase. *Expert Rev Anticancer Ther* 3: 269–279
89 Soulieres D, Senzer NN, Vokes EE et al (2001) Multicenter phase II study of erlotinib, an oral epidermal growth factor receptor tyrosine kinase inhibitor, in patients with recurrent or metastatic squamous cell carcinoma of the head and neck. *J Clin Oncol* 22: 77–85
90 Finkler N, Gordon A, Crozier M et al (2001) Phase 2 evaluation of OSI-774, a potent oral antagonist of the EGFR-TK in patients with advanced ovarian carcinoma. *Proc Am Soc Clin Oncol* 20: abstr. 831
91 Perez-Soler R, Chachoua A, Huberman M et al (2001) A phase II trial of the epidermal growth factor receptor (EGFR) tyrosine kinase inhibitor OSI-774, following platinum-based chemotherapy, in patients (pts) with advanced, EGFR-expressing, non-small cell lung cancer (NSCLC). *Proc Am Soc Clin Oncol* 20: abstr. 1235
92 Shepherd FA, Pereira J, Ciuleanu TE et al (2004) A randomized placebo-controlled trial of erlotinib in patients with advanced non-small cell lung cancer (NSCLC) following failure of first line or second line chemotherapy. A National Cancer Institute of Canada Clinical Trial Group (NCIC CTG) trial. *Proc Am Soc Clin Oncol* 23: abstr. 7022
93 Gatzemeier U, Pluzanska A, Szczesna A et al (2004) Results of a phase III trial of erlotinib (OSI-774) combined with cisplatin and gemcitabine chemotehrapy in advanced non-small cell lung cancer (NSCLC). *Proc Am Soc Clin Oncol* 23: abstr. 7010
94 Herbst RS, Prager D, Hermann R et al (2004) TRIBUTE – A phase III trial of erlotinib HCl (OSI-774) combined with carboplatin and paclitaxel chemotherapy in advanced non-small cell lung cancer (NSCLC). *Proc Am Soc Clin Oncol* 23: abstr. 7011
95 Ciardiello F, Tortora G (2003) Epidermal growth factor receptor (EGFR) as a target in cancer therapy: understanding the role of receptor expression and other molecular determniants that could influence the response to anti-EGFR drugs. *Eur J Cancer* 39: 1348–1354
96 Viloria-Petit A, Crombet T, Jothy S et al (2001) Aquired resistance to the antitumor activity of epidermal growth factor receptor-blocking antibodies *in vivo*: a role for altered tumor angiogenesis. *Cancer Res* 61: 5090–5101

97 Chakravarti A, Loeffler JS, Dyson NJ (2002) Insulin-like growth factor receptor I mediates resistance to anti-epidermal growth factor receptor therapy in primary human glioblastoma cells through continued activation of phosphoinositide 3-kinase signaling. *Cancer Res* 62: 200–207
98 Bianco R, Shin I, Ritter C et al (2003) Loss of PTEN/MMAC1/TEP in EGF receptor-expressing tumor cells counteracts the antitumor action of EGFR tyrosine kinase inhibitors. *Oncogene* 22: 2812–2822
99 She QB, Salit S, Basso A, Moasser M (2003) Resistance to Gefitinib in PTEN-null HER-overexpressing tumor cells can be overcome through restoration of PTEN function or pharmacologic modulation of constitutive phosphatidinil 3′ kinase/Akt pathway signaling. *Clin Cancer Res* 9: 4340–4346
100 Ciardiello F, Bianco R, Caputo R et al (2004) Antitumor activity of ZD6474, a small molecule VEGF receptor tyrosine kinase inhibitor, in human cancer cells with acquired resistance to EGF receptor-targeted drugs. *Clin Cancer Res* 10: 784–793
101 Wu YL, Yang X-N, Gu L-J (2003) The charactetistics of patients with non-small cell lung cancer with complete response treated with ZD1839. *Proc Am Soc Clin Oncol* 22: abstr. 2770
102 Wong N-S, Lim ST, Lim W-T, Leong S-S, Tan E-H (2003) ZD1839 is more effective in patients with non-small cell lung cancer (NSCLC) who were lifetime non-tobacco users. *Proc Am Soc Clin Oncol* 22: abstr. 2790
103 Shah NT, Miller VA, Kris MG et al (2003) Bronchioalveolar histology and smoking history predict response to gefitinib. *Proc Am Soc Clin Oncol* 22: abstr. 2524
104 Miller VA, Kris MG, Shah N et al (2004) Bronchioloalveolar pathologic subtype and smoking history predict sensitivity to gefitinib in advanced non-small-cell lung cancer. *J Clin Oncol* 22: 1103–1109
105 Saltz LB, Kies MS, Abbruzzese JL, Azarnia N, Needle M (2003) The presence and intensity of the Cetuximab-induced acne-like rash predicts increased survival in studies across multiple malignancies. *Proc Am Soc Clin Oncol* 23: abstr. 817
106 Clark GM, Perez-Soler R, Siu L, Gordon A, Santabarbara P (2003) Rash severty is predictive of increased survival with erlotinib HCl. *Proc Am Soc Clin Oncol* 22: abstr. 786
107 Arteaga CL, Baselga J (2003) Clinical trial design and endpoints for epidermal growth factor receptor-targeted therapies: implications for drug development and practice. *Clin Cancer Res* 9: 1579–89

Progress in Drug Research, Vol. 63
(R. M. Schultz, Ed.)

Cell survival signaling during apoptosis: Implications in drug resistance and anti-cancer therapeutic development

Grace Choy[1], Jun-Wei Liu[1], Dhyan Chandra[1] and Dean G. Tang[1, 2]

[1]Department of Carcinogenesis
the University of Texas M.D.
Anderson Cancer Center
Science Park-Research Division
Smithville, TX 78957, USA

[2]Program in Environmental &
Molecular Carcinogenesis
Graduate School of Biomedical
Sciences (GSBS),
Houston, TX 77030, USA
<dtang@sprd1.mdacc.tmc.edu>

Key words

Apoptosis, survival, stress, NF-κB, ROS, FOXO3a.

Glossary of abbreviations

DISC, death-inducing signaling complex; DED, death effector domain; DR, death receptor; DD, death domains; FADD, Fas-associated death domain; TRADD, TNF receptor 1-associated death domain; ROS, reactive oxygen species; Apaf-1, apoptotic protease-activating factor-1; IAP, inhibitor of apoptosis protein; ER, endoplasmic reticulum; PTP, permeability transition pore; MAPK, mitogen-activated protein kinase; BH3, Bcl-2 homology domain 3; c-FLIP, caspase-8-FLICE inhibitory protein; IKK, IκB kinase; RIP, receptor-interacting protein; PI3K, phosphatidylinositol 3-kinase; PK, protein kinase; PIP3, phosphatidylinositol 3-phosphate; PDK1, phosphoinositide-dependent protein kinase-1; SHIP-2, Src homology 2 domain containing inositol phosphatase; HSP, heat shock protein; FKHR1, Forkhead receptor-1; ERK, extracellular regulated kinase; Grb2, growth factor receptor-bound protein 2; SOS, son of sevenless; SODs, superoxide dismutases.

1 Introduction

Apoptosis is a tightly regulated mechanism used in living organisms to eliminate redundant, damaged or infected cells [1]. Apoptosis is orchestrated by pro- and anti-apoptotic factors whose fine balance would determine the fate of the distressed cell. In recent years, there have been major advances in elucidating the various molecular components of the apoptotic machinery. As the functions of various pro-death molecules are determined upon apoptotic stimulation, there is increasing evidence showing that significant cross-talk exists between the pro- and anti-apoptotic pathways in cells. The resulting balance of expression, activation and/or inhibition of pro- and anti-apoptotic factors would ultimately determine whether the cell would die or survive the external apoptotic assault. In addition, cancer cells have altered expressions or functions of genes controlling both apoptotic and survival pathways. These changes allow the cells to either escape apoptotic signals or proliferate indefinitely. Since chemotherapeutic agents, radiation and many other antineoplastic agents act primarily by inducing apoptosis, the resistance of cancer cells to apoptosis would have serious clinical implications. In this review, we first summarize the apoptotic pathways. We then discuss various survival pathways that are activated not only by pro-survival molecules but also by apoptotic stimuli. Finally, we present a model that depicts the simultaneous engagement of both pro-survival and pro-death signaling pathways by the stress signals.

2 Extrinsic and intrinsic apoptotic pathways

There are two main pathways in the execution of apoptosis upon external stimulation. These are termed the extrinsic pathway or death receptor pathway and the intrinsic or "Bcl-2 controlled" pathway [2]. Both pathways converge on the workhorses of apoptosis, the initiator and effector caspases, which carry out a proteolytic cascade that functions in dismantling cellular structures, resulting in the final demise of the cell.

All caspases are synthesized as inactive zymogens, more commonly known as procaspases, that become activated by autocatalysis or cleavage by other caspases. There are two groups within the caspase family, namely, initiator and effector caspases, and they are distinguished by the length of their prodomain [3, 4]. Initiator caspases have long prodomains which contain a protein-protein interaction platform for the recruitment of these procaspases into an activating protein complex such as the 'death-inducing signaling complex' (DISC) or the apoptosome. Initiator caspases like caspase-8 and -10 have a death effector domain (DED), while caspase-1, -2, -4, -5, -9, -11 and -12 have a caspase-activating recruitment domain (CARD). Effector caspases on the other hand do not have the long N-terminal non-enzymatic prodomain. These caspases include caspase-3, -6 and -7. They are also known as the executioner caspases because they are responsible for most cellular destruction during apoptosis.

In the extrinsic death pathway, initiator caspases like caspase-8 and -10 are recruited into the DISC, which forms upon death receptor (DR) activation by external ligands. DRs belong to the TNF super gene family with cysteine-rich extracellular domains, a transmembrane region and a cytoplasmic death domain that allows these receptors to complex with the cell's apoptotic machinery [5, 6]. Major DRs include Fas (CD95), TNFR, DR3 (Apo-3), DR4 (TRAIL-R1) and DR5 (TRAIL-R2) [7]. Once these DRs are stimulated by their respective ligands, the receptor recruits components of the DISC machinery through interaction of the death domains (DD). Among the common molecular factors is Fas-associated death domain (FADD), which functions as a critical adaptor protein to recruit caspase-8 and caspase-10 through its DED. FADD associates directly with Fas, DR4 and DR5 receptors but binds to the TNFR through association with TNF receptor 1-associated death domain (TRADD). Close proximity of caspase-8 and -10 in the DISC results in their catalytic activation presumably by an allosteric mechanism, which involves the dimerization of both caspases [8–11]. These initiator caspases, once activated, can then cleave downstream effector caspases such as caspase-3.

The intrinsic apoptotic pathway works through an important organelle, the powerhouse of the cell, the mitochondria, which contributes to apoptosis in at least three ways: release of pro-apoptotic molecules, increased production of reactive oxygen species (ROS), and impaired ATP production. The release of apoptotic factors from the mitochondria represents a critical event upon external stimulation. One of the key factors released is cytochrome c [12]. Upon its release, cytochrome c promotes the formation of a pro-apoptotic complex called apoptosome comprising apoptotic protease-activating factor-1 (Apaf-1), caspase-9 and ATP. In this complex, caspase-9 is activated through dimerization or oligomerization by an allosteric mechanism as mentioned above [8, 13]. The activated caspase-9 is then able to cleave downstream effector caspases like caspase-3.

Whether the activated caspases can degrade substrates and kill the cells is further regulated by another family of proteins, i.e., the inhibitor of apoptosis proteins or IAPs. IAPs (especially XIAP) inhibit both activated caspase-9 and caspase-3 [13]. In addition, XIAP and IAP1/2 have a carboxyl-terminal motif found in RING-finger proteins, which allow them to function as ubiquitin ligases, promoting the proteasomal degradation of bound caspases [14]. Thus to counter this, the mitochondria release, in addition to cytochrome c, other pro-apoptotic factors like second mitochondrial-derived activator of caspases (Smac/DIABLO) and Omi/HtrA2, which bind to and sequester XIAP allowing the further maturation of primed caspase-3 [15–17]. Other mitochondrial intermembrane space proteins that are pro-apoptotic and released during apoptosis include the apoptosis-inducing factor (AIF) and endonuclease G (EndoG). These factors cause apoptosis independent of caspases. AIF translocates to the nucleus and causes chromatin condensation and large-scale DNA fragmentation, while EndoG translocates into the nucleus and helps digest nuclear DNA [18, 19].

Besides mitochondrial protein release, recent findings have shown that several pro- and active caspases, including caspase-3, -9 and -8 can localize in the mitochondria [20–24]. How these mitochondrially localized caspases are generated still remains incompletely understood. It appears that the majority of the active caspase-9 and -3 in the mitochondria result from translocation from the cytosol [20]. The mitochondrially localized active caspase-3 is active in degrading cytosolic substrates, and may also participate in destroying some mitochondrial proteins [20]. The localization of active caspases on the mitochondrial outer membrane may also increase their accessibility and efficiency to cleave its substrates localized in the cytosol and other organelles like the endoplasmic reticulum (ER) [21]. For example, active caspase-8 in the mitochondria could facilitate the cleavage and subsequent insertion of t-Bid into the mitochondria to induce cytochrome c release. Active caspase-8 in the mitochondria has also been shown to cleave the ER-resident protein BAP31 to an active form, BAP20, only in mitochondria-associated ER fractions [21]. BAP20 causes Ca^{2+} release from the ER that would result in mitochondrial uptake of excessive Ca^{2+}, which then leads to mitochondrial fission, and finally the compromise of the mitochondrial integrity and function [21]. This is evidence that implicates mitochondria-ER cross-talk in apoptosis. Thus, upon apoptotic stimuli, the mitochondria might act as a cellular weapon of mass destruction containing active caspases, which would facilitate the degradation of proteins concentrated in the mitochondria or any organelle in contact with it.

The loss of mitochondrial membrane potential and the production of ROS in the mitochondria may also contribute to apoptosis. The mitochondrial membrane potential is generated by electron transport, which results in a H^+ ion gradient across the mitochondrial inner membrane. This gradient is then used by the F_0F_1-ATP synthase to produce ATP. When the membrane potential is lost during apoptosis, ATP is not synthesized, and, in addition, ROS accumulate [25]. The mitochondrial membrane potential loss is due to a permeability transition pore (PTP), which contains the inner membrane protein, adenine nucleoside translocator and the outer membrane protein, voltage-dependent anion channel (VDAC) [26, 27]. The PTP pore has been implicated in the release of mitochondrial factors upon apoptotic stimuli; in addition several members of the Bcl-2 family like Bax and Bak are found to be involved (see [28–30] for reviews).

The role of ROS in apoptosis is still not clearly understood mechanistically. There is evidence that antioxidants that counter ROS can abolish the apoptotic response of various stimuli, thus ROS can be seen as an important mediator of apoptosis [31]. In addition, anti-apoptotic Bcl-2 family members have been shown to decrease ROS production in apoptosis to protect cells from external oxidant-induced apoptosis [32, 33]. However, recent evidence highlights a specific role of ROS in redox cell signaling for proliferation that includes the activation of the transcriptional factor activator protein-1 (AP-1) through the mitogen-activated protein kinase (MAPK) family (reviewed in [34]). This ultimately leads to the transcriptional upregulation of genes involved in cellular proliferation. Thus, ROS are known to play a dual role both in mediating apoptosis as well as mitogen- or survival factor-induced cell proliferation and survival (see below).

Lastly, cross-talk between the extrinsic and intrinsic pathways exists and occurs mainly through the Bcl-2 family member, Bid. Bid is a Bcl-2 homology domain 3 (BH3) protein that is cleaved by active caspase-8 into a truncated form t-Bid. Once cleaved, this active t-Bid translocates to the mitochondria, and either directly binds to and induces the oligomerization of Bax or binds to and inactivates pro-survival Bcl-2 family proteins like Bcl-2 and Bcl-xL [35]. Since caspase-8 is the common target for DISC activation through the DRs, Bid therefore bridges the extrinsic and intrinsic pathways.

Since the ultimate goal of anti-cancer therapeutics is to efficiently kill cancer cells, current drug development centers on how to maximally activate the intrinsic and extrinsic death pathways. Strategies in development include, among others, DRs ligands such as TRAIL that preferentially kills cancer cells, drugs that target the mitochondria and facilitate the PTP opening and mitochondrial release of pro-apoptotic factors, the BH3 peptidomimetics or stabilizers, Smac peptidomimetics, chemical or small-molecule activators of apoptosome or inhibitors of IAPs, and active caspases.

3 Survival pathways

In order to gain a better perspective of how cancer cells may evade apoptosis, a brief survey of various survival pathways built into the cell would be helpful. In this section, we discuss several pro-survival pathways with an emphasis on the players, the regulation of these proteins during normal homeostasis, and the change in regulation of these molecular factors during apoptosis. This will facilitate the exploration in the last section on how these survival pathways are activated during an apoptotic onslaught. These findings highlight the fact that a cell's initial response to apoptotic stimulation is to survive.

3.1 Anti-apoptotic Bcl-2 proteins

The intrinsic apoptotic pathway is also called the Bcl-2 controlled pathway because the pro-apoptotic Bcl-2 proteins, Bax and Bak, are a gateway to the release of apoptotic factors from the mitochondria. Opposing their activation are the gatekeepers, anti-apoptotic Bcl-2 family proteins. Structurally, the Bcl-2 family members can be categorized into three groups, i.e., the multidomain anti-apoptotic and pro-apoptotic proteins and the BH3-only pro-apoptotic proteins. The multidomain anti-apoptotic Bcl-2 family members share sequence conservation in all four BH domains (i.e., BH1–BH4) and include Bcl-2, Bcl-xL, Bcl-w, Mcl-1, Boo and Bcl-B. The multidomain pro-apoptotic Bcl-2 proteins share sequence similarity in only the first three BH domains, and this group includes Bax, Bak and Bok. The BH3-only proteins, which include Bid, Bik, Bim, Bad, Bnip3, Blk, Bmf, Hrk, Noxa and Puma, exist in inactive forms during normal conditions, and become activated or induced during apoptotic stimulation. The balance of these pro- and anti-apoptotic Bcl-2 proteins contributes to the survival or death of a cell.

There are several models of how anti-apoptotic Bcl-2 family proteins promote cell survival. For example, they can bind to the BH3-only proteins, preventing them from activating the gateway proteins Bax and Bak. Anti-apoptotic Bcl-2 proteins can also directly bind to Bax or Bak preventing their activation [36, 37]. Other mechanisms also exist. For example, Bcl-2 could prevent the intracellular calcium flux, pH and ionic changes that occur early during apoptosis [38, 39] or bind to a membrane-bound protein X that is an activator of Bax and Bak oligomerization [40, 41].

Anti-apoptotic Bcl-2 proteins can regulate cell survival and be regulated in several ways. First, the localization of these proteins can affect their functions. Bcl-2 and Bcl-xL are found to localize on the mitochondrial outer membrane to inhibit the oligomerization of Bax and Bak [42]. They also localize on the ER membrane, where they may play a role in regulating calcium uptake or release during apoptosis [43]. In addition, Bcl-2 has been found to localize in the nuclear membrane and is implicated in nuclear trafficking of transcription factors such as NF-κB, AP1, CRE and NFAT [44]. Second, the anti-apoptotic Bcl-2 proteins are often overexpressed in cancer cells. Indeed,

Bcl-2 was discovered as an oncogene overexpressed in follicular lymphomas due to a translocation of the gene from chromosome 14;q32 to chromosome 18;q21 [45]. Overexpression of anti-apoptotic Bcl-2 family proteins has been shown to confer resistance to various apoptotic stimuli like radiation and chemical inducers (such as etoposide, doxorubicin and taxol) [46, 47]. Third, changes in phosphorylation can regulate the function of Bcl-2 proteins [48]. For example, phosphorylation of Bcl-2 at serine residues in some cell systems results in the loss of its anti-apoptotic functions [49, 50]. By contrast, phosphorylation of Bcl-2 at Ser70 appears to be important for its anti-apoptotic function [51]. Other studies show that phosphorylation in the unstructured loop domain of Bcl-xL and Bcl-2 diminishes their anti-apoptotic activities [52]. Lastly, Bcl-2 family members can also be regulated by post-translational modification. Studies show that cleavage of Bcl-2 by caspase-3 results in a truncated pro-apoptotic Bcl-2 protein [53]. This occurs late during apoptosis, thus playing an amplification role in the apoptotic process.

3.2 The NF-κB pathway

A classic example of the survival pathway activated by apoptotic stimuli is the activation of the NF-κB transcription factor. NF-κB is a heterodimer of p50 and p65 members of the Rel family. Under normal conditions, NF-κB is sequestered in the cytoplasm by IκBs (inhibitors of NF-κB). When NF-κB is free from bondage to IκBs, it translocates into the nucleus and transcriptionally activates various anti-apoptotic genes including IAP1/2, XIAP, Bcl-xL, caspase-8-FLICE inhibitory protein (c-FLIP), and Traf1/2 [54, 55]. These factors work in a coordinated fashion to block apoptosis at multiple steps along the apoptotic cascade. For instance, in the Fas receptor pathway, c-FLIP up-regulated by NF-κB interacts with FADD and procaspase-8 to prevent the activation of procaspase-8 [56]. IAPs bind to and inhibit the activities of activated caspases [57]. TRAF1/2 are adaptor proteins involved in the TNFR signaling pathway [58].

For NF-κB to translocate into the nucleus, IκB has to be removed. Upon apoptotic stimulation via TNFα, IκB is phosphorylated by IκB kinase (IKK). IκB is then ubiquitinated and degraded by the proteasome pathway [54]. To stop the anti-apoptotic function of NF-κB, several key components of this pathway can be degraded by caspases [59]. For example, caspases cleave RelA into a DNA-binding fragment lacking trans-activation activities [59]. Caspase-3 cleaves IκBα, creating a super repressor of NF-κB [60]. The IKK complex can also be inactivated by caspases [61]. Lastly, receptor-interacting protein (RIP) and TRAF2, both of which are involved in NF-κB activation, are also substrates of caspases [62, 63]. Thus, the NF-κB pathway is a complex interaction network integrating both pro- and anti-apoptotic signals upstream and downstream of the transcription factor NF-κB.

3.3 The PI3K/AKT pathway

Another complex survival network involves the phosphatidylinositol 3-kinase (PI3K) and AKT, a serine/threonine kinase also known as protein kinase B (PKB). AKT is activated by the presence of phosphatidylinositol 3-phosphate (PIP3), which in turn is produced by PI3K. PI3K catalyzes the phosphorylation of the D3 position on the inositol ring of lipids. The resulting PIP_3 then activates many downstream targets including AKT. Upon activation by survival signals such as insulin, AKT is recruited by PIP3 to the plasma membrane, where it is activated via sequential phosphorylation at Thr308 by phosphoinositide-dependent protein kinase-1 (PDK1) and at Ser473 position by PDK2 [64–67].

AKT is negatively regulated by lipid phosphatases like PTEN, SHIP-1 and SHIP-2 (Src homology 2 domain containing inositol phosphatase). These phosphatases control the level of PIP3 in the cytosol, thus indirectly preventing the activation of AKT [68–70]. In addition, protein phosphatase 2A (PP2A) directly dephosphorylates AKT at the Ser473 and Thr308 positions, with a higher affinity for Ser473 [71]. Carboxyl-terminal modulator protein (CTMP) is another negative AKT regulator that binds to its carboxyl terminus and prevents the phosphorylation of Ser473 and, to a lesser extent, Thr308 [72]. In contrast, heat shock protein (HSP) 90 keeps AKT active by binding to AKT and preventing dephosphorylation by PP2A [73]. HSP90 can also prevent the degradation of PDK1 by the proteasome [74].

AKT in turn activates various downstream targets that regulate apoptosis, cell cycle, DNA repair, nitric oxide production and glycogen metabolism [66]. AKT protects the cell from apoptosis by phosphorylating and inactivating various apoptotic regulators such as Bad, caspase-9 and Forkhead receptor-1 (FKHR1). AKT phosphorylation of Bad induces its interaction with 14-3-3 protein, which causes a conformational change in Bad leading to its phosphorylation by protein kinase A (PKA). This disrupts the ability of Bad to bind to Bcl-2 and Bcl-xL, thus liberating the latter to inhibit apoptosis [75]. AKT phosphorylation of FKHR1 leads to its binding to 14-3-3 proteins in the cytosol, thus preventing FKHR1 from translocating to the nucleus. This prevents FKHR1 from activating pro-apoptotic genes like Bim and FasL [76]. Similarly, AKT phosphorylation of procaspase-9 prevents its activation by the apoptosome [77]. AKT is also an indirect negative regulator of p53. It phosphorylates Mdm2, increasing its ability to translocate into the nucleus where it binds to p53 and promotes its degradation [78]. Lastly, AKT can also activate the NF-κB pathway by phosphorylating IKKα, leading to the phosphorylation and degradation of IκB [79,80]. Therefore, AKT can promote cell survival by antagonizing both the extrinsic and intrinsic apoptotic pathways.

3.4 The MAPK/ERK pathway

Extracellular regulated kinase (ERK) is a member of the MAPK family. Its activation protects a cell from apoptosis through the activation of downstream transcription factors like NF-κB, which, as mentioned above, can turn on various anti-apoptotic molecules like IAPs, TRAF1/2 and Bcl-xL [81]. The Raf/MEK/ERK pathway is also involved in cell cycle progression through the effects of cell-cycle regulatory protein induction. This pathway is activated by extracellular signals, e.g., IL-3 binding to its receptor. This recruits the adaptor protein growth factor receptor-bound protein 2 (Grb2) that in turn binds to the cytoplasmic side of cell surface receptors like EGFR and PDGFR through its Src homology 2 (SH2) domain [82]. Grb2 is constitutively bound to son of sevenless (SOS), and upon Grb2 recruitment to the plasma membrane SOS gets activated [83]. SOS is a guanine nucleotide exchange factor and, once it is activated, it exchanges the GDP for GTP on RAS [83]. This causes a conformational change in RAS and allows it to bind to an MAP kinase kinase kinase, RAF1. RAF1 is activated by binding to RAS and phosphorylates MAP kinase kinases, MEK1 and MEK2. These kinases in turn phosphorylate MAPKs, ERK1 and ERK2. Following activation, ERKs translocate into the nucleus and phosphorylate a variety of substrates. These include the 90-kDa ribosomal S6 protein kinase ($p90^{rsk}$), the cytosolic phosphatase A2 and several transcription factors like NF-κB, c-Myc, Ets, CREB and AP-1 [81].

The contributions of different MAPK family members to apoptosis have been examined by Xia and colleagues [84] in the withdrawal of nerve growth factor (NGF) from rat PC-12 pheochromocytoma cells. They showed that NGF withdrawal led to sustained activation of JNK and p38-MAPK and the inhibition of ERKs. The combined effects of dominant negative as well as constitutively activated forms of various factors in these three pathways show that the simultaneous activation of JNK and p38MAPK and the inhibition of ERK is needed for induction of apoptosis in these cells [84]. This implies that ERK is a survival factor that needs to be silenced for apoptosis to occur. JNK and p38-MAPK are both activated in cells exposed to various cellular and environmental stresses like changes in osmolarity or metabolism, DNA damage, heat shock, ischemia, inflammatory cytokines, shear stress, UV irradiation, ceramide and oxidative stresses [85–90]. Both pathways are thought to modulate signals for cellular apoptosis under various stimuli [91].

Recently, multiple studies have revealed a more direct pro-survival mechanism of the ERK pathway. Ras/Raf/MAPK/ERK activation by, e.g., serum, EGF, PDGF, insulin, integrin-mediated adhesion, or thrombin results in the phosphorylation of a critical BH3-only protein, Bim [92–99]. Phosphorylation of Bim either inhibits its interaction with Bax [92] or leads to proteosome-dependent degradation [98].

4 Cell survival signaling during apoptosis

Although great progress has been made in elucidating the core apoptotic machinery, little is known about how cells initially respond to apoptotic stimulation. For example, when a population of cycling cells is stimulated by an apoptotic signal, do they immediately enter the apoptotic mode or do they first stage a defensive response? Or do the cells simultaneously activate both pro-survival and pro-death mechanisms in response to apoptotic stimuli, and it is the balance between these two antagonizing signals that ultimately determines when and whether the stimulated cells will die? Our recent work sheds some light on these questions. We find that many stimuli cause an early mitochondrial activation characterized by a rapid induction of respiration-related proteins, including apocytochrome c and cytochrome c oxidase, which are then rapidly imported into the mitochondria to participate in the mitochondrial respiration, leading to early membrane hyperpolarization, increased oxygen consumption, and maintenance of ATP levels [100, 101]. All these responses precede the exodus of holo-cytochrome c (i.e., heme-containing cytochrome c that shuttles electrons between complex III and IV) from the mitochondria and subsequent initiation of caspase activation [101]. These observations point to the possibility that cells, upon apoptotic stimulation, perhaps rapidly mobilize defensive mechanisms to extend their survival.

Based on these earlier observations, we recently carried out more detailed experiments to address the relationship between survival and apoptosis signaling early during apoptosis induction [102]. We surprisingly find that early induction of multiple pro-survival mechanisms by apoptotic stimuli represents a rather common phenomenon.

4.1 Five classes of pro-survival mechanisms induced by apoptotic stimuli

At least five classes of pro-survival molecules are induced by apoptotic stimuli. The first class belongs to the molecules normally involved in mitochondrial respiration exemplified by cytochrome c oxidase subunits and cytochrome c [100–102]. Multiple chemotherapeutic drugs (e.g., camptothecin, teniposide), chemopreventives (e.g., butyrate, short-chain fatty acids, PPARγ agonists, retinoids), chemicals (e.g., staurosporine, Mn, NDGA), and apoptosis agents (e.g., Fas, hypoxia) have been shown to induce early mitochondrial activation characterized by cytochrome c upregulation and increased mitochondrial respiration. The upregulation of the mitochondria respiratory chain proteins and increased respiratory activity most likely represent one aspect of the global mitochondrial activation aimed, perhaps, at maintaining appropriate ATP levels critical for various cell activities as well as for cell survival. In addition to maintaining ATP levels, increased apocytochrome c in the cytosol and upregulated holocytochrome c in the mitochondria also possess anti-apoptotic and pro-survival functions [103–105].

The second class of pro-survival molecules induced or activated by apoptotic stimuli are anti-apoptotic Bcl-2 family proteins, in particular, Bcl-2 and/or Bcl-xL [102], which also function in the mitochondria. In response to DNA damage, trophic factor deprivation, and a mitochondrial toxin, Bcl-2 and/or Bcl-xL are rapidly induced [102]. The apoptotic stimuli-activated Bcl-2 and/or Bcl-xL clearly play a pro-survival role as inhibition of their upregulation using specific small interfering RNAs (siRNAs) facilitated cell death [102]. Similarly, hypoxia selectively upregulates Bcl-xL leading to generation of death-resistant cells [106]. UV irradiation eliminates Mcl-1 but also induces increased targeting of Bcl-xL to the mitochondria [107]. Moreover, various apoptotic stimuli upregulate Bcl-2 protein levels via a mechanism dependent on IRES or internal ribosomal entry site [108]. Finally, UV-A can upregulate the Bcl-xL protein levels by modulating the 3′-untranslated region [109].

The third class of pro-survival molecules is the superoxide dismutases (SODs). There are two major types of SODs, the mitochondrial MnSOD and cytosolic Cu/Zn SOD, both of which function by removing ROS, in particular, superoxide anions [110, 111]. We found that all apoptotic stimuli tested upregulate the levels of both MnSOD and Cu/ZnSOD around the same time when pro-apoptotic Bim is induced [102]. The MnSOD siRNA blocks the MnSOD induction and also enhances apoptosis [102], suggesting that the upregulated MnSOD is also serving a pro-survival function.

The fourth class of pro-survival molecules induced by apoptotic stimuli includes various chaperone and co-chaperone proteins. Multiple HSP have been shown to be cytoprotective [112–115]. We have observed that the mitochondria-localized HSP60 is rapidly upregulated and/or released from the mitochondria to the cytosol in response to apoptotic stimulation [101], presumably to extend cell survival. Mitochondrial HSP70 has been shown to interact with $p66^{Shc}$, a molecule implicated in determining the cell's lifespan, to extend cell survival in the presence of stress signals [116]. Similarly, the bacterial HSP60 (GroEL) has been shown to protect epithelial cells from apoptosis induction via activation of the ERK pathway [117].

Finally, cell-cycle inhibitors such as $p27^{KIP1}$ and $p21^{WAF-1}$ may also represent pro-survival molecules as cell cycle-arrested cells generally survive better than proliferating cells [118]. For example, $p21^{WAF-1}$ has been shown to be a critical pro-survival factor transactivated by p53 [119, 120]. Overexpression of p21 confers on colon cancer cells resistance to apoptosis induction by chemicals in both p53-depedent and p53-independent manners [121]. In contrast, decreased or loss of p21 expression sensitizes cells to apoptosis [122, 123]. Indeed, we have also observed an inverse correlation between p21 expression and apoptosis. When LNCaP cells, a p53-wt prostate cancer cell line, are stimulated with γ-irradiation (X-ray) and three chemotherapeutic drugs (i.e., etoposide, doxorubicin, and taxol), X-ray and etoposide significantly induce p21 protein expression with little cell death (evidenced by the caspase-3 activation), whereas doxorubicin and taxol do not upregulate p21, but cause obvious cell death (Fig. 1).

Other pro-survival signaling mechanisms may also exist in cells facing stress stimulation. For example, apoptotic stimulation may result in a rapid

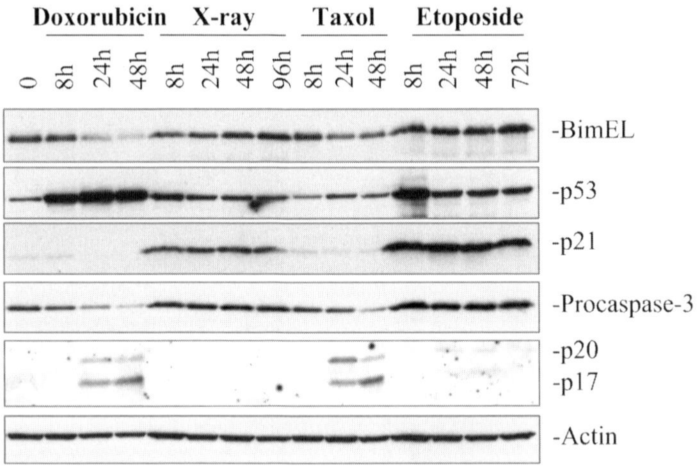

Figure 1.
p21 induction is associated with apoptosis induction. LNCaP cells were treated with doxorubicin (10 ng/ml), γ-irradiation (10 Gy X-ray), taxol (25 μM), and etoposide (50 μM) for the time intervals indicated. At the end of each time point, cells were harvested and whole cell lysates were used in Western blot (30 μg protein/lane) analysis of the molecules indicated on the right. Note that Bim was upregulated by etoposide and X-ray as previously reported [102]. P53 was upregulated by all three DNA-damaging agents (i.e., doxorubicin, X-ray, and etoposide) but p21 was induced only in X-ray and etoposide-treated cells, suggesting that p53 activation does not always lead to p21 induction.

phosphorylation of the translation initiation factor-2, leading to the cessation of *de novo* protein synthesis and providing cytoprotection [124]. Therefore, induction of pro-survival mechanisms by apoptotic stimuli seems to represent a general phenomenon. Even apoptosis induced by TNFα and Fas (see below) and death kinase PKR [125] is preceded by an early phase of NF-κB-mediated pro-survival to delay apoptosis. The induced pro-survival molecules apparently play a critical role in extending cell survival as prevention of the induction of, e.g., Bcl-2, Bcl-xL, or MnSOD by apoptotic stimuli accelerates cell death [102].

4.2 Transcription factors involved in apoptotic stimuli-activated pro-survival genes

In the above examples, the pro-survival molecules are induced either simultaneously with or slightly prior to the induction of various pro-death molecules. How are the pro-survival molecules induced by apoptotic stimuli? Our recent work demonstrates that these molecules are all induced at the transcriptional level [102], thus implicating transcription factors. Our work [102] and others' (see below) implicate master transcription factors such as NF-κB, FOXO3a, p53, Rb, E2F1, and c-Myc in regulating pro-survival and pro-death molecules (thus life and death) in stress-stimulated cells.

NF-κB undoubtedly is the most important transcription factor in mediating the pro-survival signaling in response to inflammatory, apoptotic, and stress stimulation. Although in certain circumstances NF-κB activation on some genetic backgrounds can lead to apoptosis by, e.g., stabilizing p53 [126], repressing the induction of anti-apoptotic genes [127], or entering into the mitochondria to collaborate with adenine nucleotide translocator [128], the preponderant experimental data suggest that increased NF-κB activity is associated with resistance to therapeutic agents, extended cell survival, and increased tumor development [129–136]. The pro-survival function of NF-κB is associated with its transcriptional induction of familiar pro-survival genes such as IAPs, Bcl-xL, and FLIP as well as novel pro-survival genes such as SNF1/AMP kinase-related kinase [137] and the ferritin heavy chain [138]. The essential pro-survival function of NF-κB is most vividly illustrated by the cell's response to the TNFα family proteins [139–145], although activation of this transcription factor certainly underlies cell resistance to multiple apoptotic stimuli. Upon TNFα binding to the TNFR1, two sequential signaling complexes are formed [140]. The plasma membrane-bound complex I is rapidly formed upon receptor activation and contains TNFR1, adaptor protein TRADD, death domain-containing kinase RIP1, and TRAF-2, leading to NF-κB activation. Then, complex I leaves the receptor and forms a different, long-lived complex, complex II, which localizes mainly in the cytosol and contains apoptotic proteins FADD, caspase-8, and caspase-10, in addition to TRADD, RIP1, and TRAF-2. The activation of complex II results in cell death [140]. Thus, TNFα induces the complex II-mediated apoptosis only when the complex I-initiated pro-survival signal (i.e., NF-κB) fails to be activated. Not only TNFα induces an early-phase NF-κB activation to extend cell survival, recent evidence indicates that even CD95 (Fas ligand) and TRAIL, TNFα family members conventionally thought to be solely pro-apoptotic, also activate NF-κB prior to activating the DISC and caspase-8 [139, 141–145], which explains why many cancer cells do not respond to these death ligands by undergoing apoptosis. In fact, most epithelial cancer cells appear to be so-called type II cells [139] and CD95 stimulation of these cells not only fails to kills them, but actually promotes cell migration and invasion [145], possibly through NF-κB-activated urokinase-type plasminogen activator (uPA) and the SNF1/AMP kinase-related kinase [137]. Intriguingly, unlike TNFα-mediated NF-κB activation [140], NF-κB activation by Fas is mediated through FADD, caspase-8, and RIP, and is inhibited by FLIP [143, 144]. The "paradoxical" pro-survival and pro-death functions of death ligands such as CD95 and TRAIL are not exceptions. More and more once-thought pro-apoptotic-only molecules, including the BH3-only proteins Bad [146, 147] and BNIP [148], the mitochondrial protease Omi [149], multi-BH protein Bak [150,151], and activated caspases [152,153], are found to possess apoptosis-unrelated and even pro-survival functions.

FOXO3a has recently emerged as one of the most critical regulators of cell death and survival. FOXO3a, also called FKHR-L1, is a mammalian homologue of *C. elegans* DAF-16 and one of the FOXO (Forkhead box, class O) subclass of Forkhead transcription factor family [154]. FOXO3a plays a critical role in coordinating cell survival and death and regulating stress response and longevity (reviewed in [102, 154]). The nonphosphorylated, active form of FOXO3a localizes to the cell nucleus, where it functions as a transcriptional factor to effect either cell-cycle arrest or death [76], similar to p53. Survival factors or mitogens cause the phosphorylation of FOXO3a, which promotes its interaction with 14-3-3 proteins, resulting in its exclusion from the nucleus and inhibition of target gene transcription, or promotes its proteosome-mediated degradation. FOXO3a has been shown to transcriptionally activate pro-apoptotic Bim, TRAIL and TRADD and anti-apoptotic MnSOD and cyclin-dependent kinase inhibitor $p27^{KIP1}$ [102, 154]. FOXO3a also inhibit cell-cycle progression by downregulating cyclin D1 [102, 154]. We found that FOXO3a is involved in directly regulating the apoptotic stimuli-activated Bim and MnSOD [102], two molecules that contain the FOXO3a sites in their promoter regions. Experiments using $FOXO3a^{-/-}$ MEFs indicate that MnSOD upregulation requires FOXO3a, whereas the transcriptional activation of Bim may only partially depend on FOXO3a. Interestingly, several other pro-survival molecules including Cu/ZnSOD, Bcl-2, Bcl-xL, and cytochrome c also appear to be partially regulated by FOXO3a, as their induction is also partially inhibited by dominant negative FOXO3a constructs or FOXO3a siRNA or in $FOXO3a^{-/-}$ fibroblasts [102]. Whether FOXO3a directly or indirectly regulates these molecules remains to be determined.

Other transcription factors, either individually or in combination, may also be involved in the transcriptional activation of both pro- and anti-apoptotic molecules in response to apoptotic stimulation. For example, p53 is well known to transactivate both pro-survival $p21^{WAF-1}$ [119–123] and multiple pro-apoptotic molecules such as BH3-only proteins (Bid, PUMA, and Noxa), Bax, and procaspases [155, 156]. Rb similarly regulates the transcription of multiple life-and-death gene [157]. E2F1 not only transcriptionally regulates cell cycle-related genes, but also cell death genes including Apaf-1 and caspases [158]. c-Myc has been shown to transcriptionally regulate molecules involved in cell cycle progression, survival, and death [118]. Finally, the transcription factor Nrf2 has been shown to transcriptionally activate pro-survival genes during apoptotic stimulation, in particular, during ER stress [159, 160].

Recent data also point to cross-talk between these master transcription factors. For example, activation of NF-κB can lead to decreased stabilization of p53 and therefore further enhance cell survival [129]. On the other hand, p53 activation can lead to phosphorylation of FOXO3a and its subcellular localization change, which results in inhibition of FOXO3a transcription activity [161]. Newly emerged evidence also makes the connection between FOXO3a and NF-κB. One study suggests that IκB kinase inhibits FOXO3a through physical interaction and phosphorylation independent of Akt, which promotes FOXO3a proteolysis via the ubiquitin-dependent proteasome pathway [162]. The other study suggests that FOXO3a negatively regulates NF-κB and that FOXO3a deficiency results in NF-κB hyperactivation and T cell hyperactivity [163].

4.3 Upstream activators of the apoptotic stimuli-activated transcription factors

Strikingly, our recent data show that the master transcription factors such as FOXO3a, which are causally involved in activating the apoptotic stimuli-induced pro-survival genes, are themselves induced at the transcriptional level by apoptotic stimuli with distinct mechanisms of action in several different cell types of distinct genetic backgrounds [102], suggesting that a common mechanism may likely be operating to mediate the transcriptional activation of FOXO3a. Then what signal(s) are transcriptionally activating FOXO3a and potentially other transcription factors?

Subsequent work revealed that ROS appear to function as critical apical signaling molecules to activate FOXO3a and perhaps also other multi-functional transcription factors [102]. Several pieces of evidence support this possibility. First, there is early mitochondrial activation in multiple apoptotic systems (see above), and mitochondrial activation manifested, as increased mitochondrial respiration and membrane hyperpolarization, is generally accompanied by increased ROS generation. Indeed, increased ROS are detected early upon stimulation in multiple apoptotic systems [100–102]. Increased ROS generation is not the consequence of caspase activation, at least at earlier time points [102]. Second, many of the induced anti-apoptotic molecules, including cytochrome c, Bcl-2, Bcl-xL, and SODs, are related to or induced by oxidative stress, raising the possibility that these molecules are induced by slightly increased ROS early during apoptotic stimulation to guard against further increases in ROS . Third, importantly, suppression of ROS generation by ROS inhibitors/scavengers inhibits apoptotic signal-induced upregulation of FOXO3a as well as its pro-death and pro-life targets. Conversely, artificially generated oxidative stress upregulates FOXO3a and its targets [102]. Fourth, that ROS function as signaling molecules that activate multi-functional transcription factors and ultimately determine the life and death of a cell is consistent with the well-established dual functions of ROS. Although ROS have been implicated in cell death in numerous experimental systems (e.g., [111, 164, 165]), ROS also play a critical role in signaling cell survival elicited by mitogens or survival factors (e.g., [166–168]). Finally, FOXO3a [169–172] and several other transcription factors including NF-κB [111] and p53 [111, 173] are well known to be regulated by, and also respond to, oxidative stress. For example, enforced expression of FOXO3a has been shown to confer resistance to oxidative stress [171] and protect quiescent cells from oxidative stress [170]. How ROS activate the FOXO3a is unclear at present. Recently, FOXO3a has been found to form a complex with SIRT1 (a mammalian homolog of the longevity gene Sir2) in response to oxidative stress [172]. By deacetylating FOXO3a, SIRT1 increases the ability of FOXO3a to induce cell-cycle arrest and resistance to oxidative stress and inhibits its ability to induce cell death [172].

5 A model and the implications

Our recent observations [102] and the above discussions lead us to propose that apoptotic stimuli cause an early mitochondrial activation, leading to rapid generation of ROS, which activate master transcription factors such as FOXO3a and NF-κB, which in turn activate multiple molecular targets with both pro-apoptotic and pro-survival functions (Fig. 2). This model is applicable to normal cells, as well as to transformed and cancer cells. The signaling pathways proposed seem to be activated as soon as cells sense stress, independent of how great the stress is and whether or not the final outcome is cell death [102]. It seems that the strengths and timings of the various pro-survival and pro-death signals determine the ultimate fate of the stressed cell [102]. Presumably, by integrating these signals the cell can sensitively decide whether it should continue to live or kill itself.

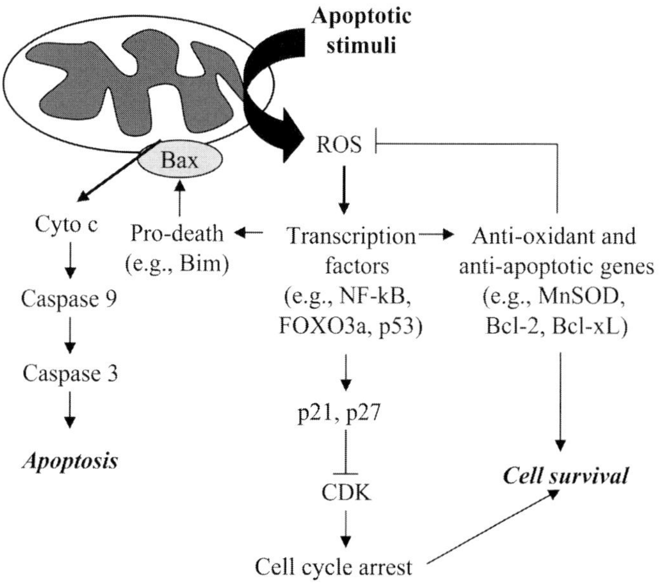

Figure 2.
A model depicting the pro-survival and pro-apoptotic signaling during apoptosis induction. Apoptotic stimuli early on induce increased mitochondrial activity leading to low-level increase in ROS production, which would activate the master transcription factors, which in turn induce the gene transcription of both pro-survival and pro-death molecules. Among the pro-survival molecules induced are anti-apoptotic Bcl-2 proteins, anti-oxidants, and negative cell-cycle regulators. The induced anti-oxidants presumably function to prevent further overproduction of ROS and preserve the mitochondrial integrity. Together with other classes of pro-survival molecules, they help to extend cell survival prior to cell demise. Therefore, it is the balance between these two opposing types of signaling mechanisms that ultimately determines whether and when the stimulated cell should die (adapted from Fig. 8 in [102]).

This model (Fig. 2) has the following important implications. First, because apoptotic stimuli activate both pro-death and pro-survival molecules, the sensitivity of any target cells, e.g., cancer cells receiving treatments, to apoptosis induction will be dictated by the balance of these two opposing signals. Furthermore, pro-survival molecules may be induced prior to induction of pro-death molecules. These considerations predict that significant cell killing will occur when, and only when, pro-apoptotic signals overwhelm the pro-survival signals or when the latter are eliminated. This prediction is consistent with the recent demonstration that apoptosis elicited by TNFα proceeds in two steps: an early step, where pro-survival signaling mediated by NF-κB dominates, and a later step, where pro-death signaling mediated by caspase-8/10 dominate. Cell death occurs only when step two is activated or when step one is inactivated [140]. Second, because cells in a tumor respond to apoptotic stimulation asynchronously and differently, some cells may preferentially upregulate pro-survival molecules, rendering them relatively resistant to further apoptotic stimulation, as often observed in therapy-resistant cancer cells. Finally, these observations suggest that the most effective anti-cancer therapies may be those that both promote apoptosis and suppress pro-survival mechanisms in cancer cells [174, 175].

Acknowledgement

The work in our lab is supported in part by NIH grants CA 90297 and AG023374, ACS grant RSG MGO-105961, DOD grant DAMD17-03-1-0137, and NIEHS grant ES07784 (D.G.T.). J.-W. Liu, D. Chandra, and G. Choy are supported by DOD Postdoctoral Traineeship Awards DAMD17-03-1-0146, DAMD17-02-0083, and PC040684, respectively.

References

1 Wang E, Marcotte R, Petroulakis E (1999) Signaling pathways for apoptosis: A racetrack for life and death. *J Cell Biochem Suppl* 32/33: 95–102
2 Sprick MR, Walczak H (2004) The interplay between the Bcl-2 family and death receptor-mediated apoptosis. *Biochim Biophys Acta* 1644: 125–132
3 Wang J, Lenardo MJ (2000) Role of caspases in apoptosis, development, and cytokine maturation revealed by homozygous gene deficiencies. *J Cell Sci* 113: 753–757
4 Salveson GS (2002) Caspases and apoptosis. *Essays Biochem* 38: 9–19
5 Gruss HJ, Dower SK (1995) Involvement in the pathology of malignant lymphomas. *Blood* 85: 3378–3404

6 Baker SJ, Reddy EP (1998) Modulation of life and death by the TNF receptor superfamily. *Oncogene* 17: 3261–3270

7 Fulda S, Debatin KM (2004) Signaling through death receptors in cancer therapy. *Curr Opin Pharmacol* 4: 327–332

8 Chang DW, Ditsworth, D, Liu H, Srinivasula SM, Alnemri ES, Yang X (2003) Oligomerization is a general mechanism for the activation of initiator and inflammatory procaspases. *J Biol Chem* 278:16466–16469

9 Chen M, Oroszo A, Spencer DM, Wang J (2002) Activation of initiator caspases through a stable dimeric intermediate. *J Biol Chem* 277: 50761–50767

10 Donepudi M, Sweeney AM, Briand C, Grutter MG (2003) Insights into the regulatory mechanism for caspase-8 activation. *Mol Cell* 11:543–549

11 Boatright KM, Renatus M, Scott FL, Sperandio S, Shin H, Pedersen IM, Ricci JE, Edris WA, Sutherlin DP, Green DR et al (2003) A unified model for apical caspase activation. *Mol Cell* 11: 529–541

12 Wang X (2001) The expanding role of mitochondria in apoptosis. *Genes Dev* 15: 2922–2933

13 Shiozaki EN, Chai J, Rigotti DJ, Riedl SJ, Srinivasula SM, Alnemri ES, Fairman R, Shi Y (2003) Mechanism of XIAP-mediated inhibition of caspase-9. *Mol Cell* 11: 519–527

14 Joazeiro CA, Weissman AM (2000) RING finger proteins: Mediators of ubiquitin ligase activity. *Cell* 102: 549–552

15 Verhagen AM, Ekert PG, Pakusch M, Silke J, Connolly LM, Reid GE, Moritz RL, Simpson RJ, Vaux DL (2000) Identification of DIABLO, a mammalian protein that promotes apoptosis by binding to an antagonizing IAP proteins. *Cell* 102: 43–53

16 Du C, Fang M, Li Y, Li L, Wang X (2000) Smac, a mitochondrial protein that promotes cytochrome c-dependent caspase activation by eliminating IAP inhibition. *Cell* 102: 33–42

17 Verhagen AM, Silke J, Ekert PG, Pakusch M, Kauffmann H, Connolly LM, Day CL, Tikoo A, Burke R, Wrobel C (2002) HtrA2 promotes cell death through its serine protease activity and its ability to antagonize inhibitor of apoptosis proteins. *J Biol Chem* 277: 445–454

18 Susin SA, Lorenzo HK, Zamzani N, Marzo I, Snow BE, Brothers GM, Mangion J, Jacotot E, Costantini P, Loeffler M et al (1999) Molecular characterization of mitochondrial apoptosis-inducing factor. *Nature* 397: 441–446

19 Li LY, Luo X, Wang X (2001) Endonuclease G is an apoptotic DNase when released from mitochondria. *Nature* 412: 95–99

20 Chandra D, Tang DG (2003) Mitochondrially localized active caspase-9 and caspase-3 result mostly from translocation from the cytosol and partly from caspase-mediated activation in the orgamelle. *J Biol Chem* 278: 17408–17420

21 Chandra D, Choy G, Deng X, Bhatia B, Daniel P, Tang DG (2004) Association of active caspase 8 with the mitochondrial membrane during apoptosis: Potential roles in cleaving BAP31 and caspase 3 and mediating mitochondrial-endoplasmic reticulum cross talk in etoposide-induced cell death. *Mol Cell Biol* 24: 6592–6607

22 Qin ZH, Wang Y, Kikly KK, Sapp E, Kegel KB, Aronin N, DiFiglia M (2001) Pro-caspase-8 is predominantly localized in mitochondria and released into cytoplasm upon apoptotic stimulation. *J Biol Chem* 276: 8079–8086

23 Stegh AH, Barnhart BC, Volkland J, Algeciras-schimnich A, Ke N, Reed JC, Peter ME (2002) Inactivation of caspase-8 on mitochondria of Bcl-xL-expressing MCT7-Fas

cells: role for the bifunctional apoptosis regulator protein. *J Biol Chem* 277: 4351–4360
24 Stegh AH, Hermann H, Lampel S, Weisenberger D, Andra K, Seper M, Wiche G, Krammer PH, Peter ME (2000) Identification of the cytolinker plectin as a major early in vivo substrate for caspase 8 during CD95- and tumor necrosis factor receptor-mediated apoptosis. *Mol Cell Biol* 20: 5665–5679
25 Zamzami N, Marchetti P, Castedo M, Decaudin D, Macho A, Hirsch T, Susin SA, Petit PX, Mignotte B, Kroemer G (1995) Sequential reduction of mitochondrial transmembrane potential and generation of reactive oxygen species in early programmed cell death. *J Exp Med* 182: 367–377
26 Gross A, McDonnell JM, Korsmeyer SJ (1999) BCL-2 family members and the mitochondria in apoptosis. *Genes Dev* 13: 1899–1911
27 Degterev A, Boyce M, Yuan J (2001) The channel of death. *J Cell Biol* 155: 695–697
28 Scorrano L, Korsmeyer SJ (2003) Mechanisms of cytochrome c release by proapoptotic BCL-2 family members. *Biochem Biophys Res Commun* 304: 437–444
29 Eposti MD, Dive C (2003) Mitochondrial membrane permeabilization by Bax/Bak. *Biochem Biophys Res Commun* 304: 455–461
30 Curtin JF, Donovan M, Cotter TG (2002) Regulation and measurement of oxidative stress in apoptosis. *J Immunol Methods* 265: 49–72
31 Li PF, Dietz R, von Harsdorf R (1999) p53 regulates mitochondrial membrane potential through reactive oxygen species and induces cytochrome c-independent apoptosis blocked by Bcl-2. *EMBO J* 18: 6027–6036
32 Gottlieb E, Van der Heiden MG, Thompson CB (2000) Bcl-x(L) prevents initial decrease in mitochondrial membrane potential and subsequent reactive oxygen species production during tumor necrosis factor alpha-induced apoptosis. *Mol Cell Biol* 20: 5680–5689
33 Behrend L, Henderson G, Zwacka RM (2003) Reactive oxygen species in oncogenic transformation *Biochem Soc Trans* 31: 1441–1444
34 Gottlieb RA (2000) Mitochondria: Execution central. *FEBS Lett* 482: 6–12
35 Li H, Zhu H, Xu CJ, Yuan J (1998) Cleavage of BID by caspase 8 mediates the mitochondrial damage in the Fas pathway of apoptosis. *Cell* 94: 491–501
36 Sattler M, Liang H, Nettesheim D, Meadows RP, Harlan JE, Eberstadt M, Yoon HS, Shuker SB, Chang BS, Minn AJ et al (1997) Structure of Bcl-xL-Bak peptide complex: Recognition between regulators of apoptosis. *Science* 275: 983–986
37 Oltvai ZN, Milliman CL, Korsmeyer SJ (1993) Bcl-2 heterodimerizes *in vivo* with a conserved homolog, Bax, that accelerates programmed cell death. *Cell* 74: 609–619
38 Matsuyama S, Reed JC (2000) Mitochondria dependent apoptosis and cellular pH damage. *Cell Death Diff* 7: 1155–1165
39 Yu SP, Canzoniero LM, Choi DW (2001) Ion homeostasis and apoptosis. *Curr Opin Cell Biol* 13: 405–411
40 Hsu YT, Youle RJ (1997) Nonionic detergents induce dimerization among members of the Bcl-2 family. *J Biol Chem* 272: 13829–13834
41 Wilson-Annan J, O'Reilly LA, Crawford SA, Hausman G, Beaumont JG, Pharma LP, Chen L, Lackman M, Lithgow, T, Hinds MG et al (2003) Proapoptotic BH3-only proteins trigger membrane integration of prosurvival Bcl-w and neutralize its activity. *J Cell Biol* 162: 877–888

42 Nakai M, Takeda A, Cleary ML, Endo T (1993) The Bcl-2 protein is inserted into the outer membrane but not into the inner membrane of rat liver mitochondria in vitro. *Biochem Biophys Res Commun* 196: 233–239

43 Distelhorst CW, Shore GC (2004) Bcl-2 and calcium: controversy beneath the surface. *Oncogene* 23: 2875–2880

44 Massaad CA, Portier BP, Taglialatela G (2004) Inhibition of transcription factor activity by nuclear compartment-associated Bcl-2. *J Biol Chem* 279: 54470–54478

45 Robertson LE, Plunkett W, McConnell K, Keating MJ, McDonnell TJ (1996) Expression in chronic lymphocytic leukemia and its correlation with the induction of apoptosis and clinical outcome. *Leukemia* 10: 456–459

46 Kitada S, Andersen J, Akar S, Zapata JM, Takayama S, Krajewski S, Wang H-G, Zhang X, Bullrich F, Croce CM (1998) Expression of apoptosis-regulating proteins in chronic lymphocytic leukemia: correlations with in vitro and in vivo chemoresponses. *Blood* 91: 3379–3389

47 McDonnell TJ, Beham A, Sarkiss M, Andersen MM, Lo P (1996) Importance of Bcl-2 family in cell death regulation. *Experentia* 52: 1008–1017

48 Pratesi G, Perego P, Zunino F (2001) Role of Bcl-2 and its post-transcriptional modification in response to antitumor therapy. *Biochem Pharmacol* 61: 381–386

49 Haldar S, Jena N, Croce CM (1995) Inactivation of Bcl-2 by phosphorylation. *Proc Natl Acad Sci USA* 92: 4507–4511

50 Haldar S, Chintapalli J, Croce CM (1996) Taxol induces Bcl-2 phosphorylation and death of prostate cancer cells. *Cancer Res* 56: 1253–1255

51 Ito T, Deng X, Carr B, May WS (1997) Bcl-2 phosphorylation required for its anti-apoptotic function. *J Biol Chem* 272: 11671–11673

52 Chang BS, Minn AJ, Muchmore SW, Fesik SW, Thompson CB (1997) Identification of a novel regulatory domain in Bcl-X(L) and Bcl-2. *EMBO J* 16: 968–977

53 Kirsch DG, Doseff A, Chau BN, Lim DS, de Souza-Pinto NC, Hansford R, Kastan MB, Lazebnik YA, Hardwick JM (1999) Caspase-3-dependent cleavage of Bcl-2 promotes release of cytochrome c. *J Biol Chem* 274: 21155–21161

54 Karin M, Lin A (2002) NF-κB at the crossroads of life and death. *Nat Immunol* 3: 221–227

55 Lin A, Karin M (2003) NF-κB in cancer: a marked target. *Semin Cancer Biol* 13: 107–114

56 Micheau O, Lens S, Gaide O, Alevizopoulos K, Tschopp J (2001) NF-κB signals induce the expression of c-FLIP. *Mol Cell Biol* 21: 5299–5305

57 Deveraux QL, Roy N, Stennicke HR, Van Arsdale T, Zhou Q, Srinivasula SM, Alnemri ES, Salvesen GS, Reed JC (1998) IAPs block apoptotic events induced by caspase-8 and cytochrome c by direct inhibition of distinct caspases. *EMBO J* 17:2215–2223

58 Baldwin AS Jr (1996) The NF-kappa B and I kappa B proteins: new discoveries and insights. *Annu Rev Immunol* 14:649–683

59 Levkau B, Scatena M, Giachelli CM, Ross R, Raines EW (1999) Apoptosis overrides survival signals through a caspase-mediated dominant-negative NF-kappa B loop. *Nat Cell Biol* 1: 227–233

60 Reuther JY, Baldwin AS Jr (1999) Apoptosis promotes a caspase-induced amino-terminal truncation of IkappaBalpha that functions as a stable inhibitor of NF-kappaB. *J Biol Chem* 274: 20664–20670

61 Tang G, Yang J, Minemoto Y, Lin A (2001) Blocking caspase-3-mediated proteolysis of IKKbeta suppresses TNF-alpha-induced apoptosis. *Mol Cell* 8:1005–1016

62 Hong SY, Yoon WH, Park JH, Kang SG, Ahn JH, Lee TH (2000) Involvement of two NF-kappa B binding elements in tumor necrosis factor alpha -, CD40-, and epstein-barr virus latent membrane protein 1-mediated induction of the cellular inhibitor of apoptosis protein 2 gene. *J Biol Chem* 275: 18022–18028

63 Arch RH, Gedrich RW, Thompson CB (2000) Translocation of TRAF proteins regulates apoptotic threshold of cells. *Biochem Biophys Res Commun* 272: 936–945

64 Datta SR, Brunet A, Greenberg ME (1999) Cellular survival: a play in three Akts. *Genes Dev* 13: 2905–2927

65 Hill MM, Hemmings BA (2002) Inhibition of protein kinase B/Akt. implications for cancer therapy. *Pharmacol Ther* 93: 243–251

66 Vivanco I, Sawyers CL (2002) The phosphatidylinositol 3-Kinase AKT pathway in human cancer. *Nat Rev Cancer* 2: 489–501

67 Troussard AA, Mawji NM, Ong C, Mui A, St-Arnaud R, Dedhar S (2003) Conditional knock-out of integrin-linked kinase demonstrates an essential role in protein kinase B/Akt activation. *J Biol Chem* 278: 22374–22378

68 Damen JE, Liu L, Rosten P, Humphries RK, Jefferson AB, Majerus PW, Krystal G (1996) The 145-kDa protein induced to associate with Shc by multiple cytokines is an inositol tetraphosphate and phosphatidylinositol 3,4,5-triphosphate 5-phosphatase. *Proc Natl Acad Sci USA* 93: 1689–1693

69 Stambolic V, Suzuki A, de la Pompa JL, Brothers GM, Mirtsos C, Sasaki T, Ruland I, Penninger JM, Siderovski DP, Mak TW (1998) Negative regulation of PKB/Akt-dependent cell survival by the tumor suppressor PTEN. *Cell* 95: 29–39

70 Wisniewski D, Strife A, Swenseman S, Erdjument-Bromage H, Geromanos S, Kavanaugh WM, Tempst P, Clarkson B (1999) A novel SH2-containing phosphatidylinositol 3,4,5-trisphosphate 5-phosphatase (SHIP2) is constitutively tyrosine phosphorylated and associated with src homologous and collagen gene (SHC) in chronic myelogenous leukemia progenitor cells. *Blood* 93: 2707–2720

71 Andjelkovic M, Maira S-M, Cron P, Parker PJ, Hemmings BA (1999) Domain swapping used to investigate the mechanism of protein kinase B regulation by 3-phosphoinositide-dependent protein kinase 1 and Ser473 kinase. *Mol Cell Biol* 19: 5061–5072

72 Maira SM, Galetic I, Brazil DP, Kaech S, Ingley E, Thelen M, Hemmings BA (2001) Carboxyl-terminal modulator protein (CTMP), a negative regulator of PKB/Akt and v-Akt at the plasma membrane. *Science* 294: 374–380

73 Sato S, Fujita N, Tsuruo T (2000) Modulation of Akt kinase activity by binding to Hsp90. *Proc Natl Acad Sci USA* 97: 10832–10837

74 Fujita N, Sato S, Ishida A, Tsuruo T (2002) Involvement of Hsp90 in signaling and stability of 3-phosphoinositide-dependent kinase-1. *J Biol Chem* 277:10346–10353

75 Hermeking H (2003) The 14-3-3 cancer connection. *Nat Rev Cancer* 3: 942–943

76 Brunet A, Bonni A, Zigmond MJ, Lin MZ, Juo P, Hu LS, Anderson MJ, Arden KC, Blenis J, Greenberg ME (1999) Akt promotes cell survival by phosphorylating and inhibiting a Forkhead transcription factor. *Cell* 96: 857–868

77 Cardone MH, Roy N, Stennicke HR, Salvesen GS, Franke TF, Stanbridge E, Frisch S, Reed JC (1998) Regulation of cell death protease caspase-9 by phosphorylation. *Science* 282: 1318–3121

78 Sordet O, Khan Q, Kohn KW, Pommier Y (2003) Apoptosis induced by topoisomerase inhibitors. *Curr Med Chem Anticancer Agents* 3: 271–290

79 Ozes ON, Mayo LD, Gustin JA, Pfeffer SR, Pfeffer LM, Donner DB (1999) NF-kappaB activation by tumour necrosis factor requires the Akt serine-threonine kinase. *Nature* 401: 82–85
80 Romashkova JA, Makarov SS (1999) NF-kappaB is a target of AKT in anti-apoptotic PDGF signalling. *Nature* 401: 86–90
81 Chang F, Steelman LS, Shelton JG, Lee JT, Navolanic PM, Blalock WL, Franklin R, McCubrey JA (2003) Regulation of cell cycle progression and apoptosis by the Ras/Raf/ERK pathway. *Int J Oncol* 22:469–480
82 Lowenstein EJ, Daly RJ, Batzer AG, Li W, Margolis B, Lammers R, Ullrich A, Skolnik EY, Bar-Sagi D, Schlessinger J (1992) The SH2 and SH3 domain-containing protein GRB2 links receptor tyrosine kinases to ras signaling. *Cell* 70:431–442
83 Chardin P, Camonis JH, Gale NW, van Aelst L, Schlessninger J, Wigler MH, Bar-Sagi D (1993) Human SOS1: a guanine nucleotide exchange factor for Ras that binds to GRB2. *Science* 260: 1338–1343
84 Xia Z, Dickens M, Raingeaurd J, Davis RJ, Greenberg ME (1995) Opposing effects of ERK and JNK-p38 MAP kinases on apoptosis. *Science* 270: 1326–1331
85 Seger R, Krebs EG (1995) The MAPK signaling cascade. *FASEB J* 9: 726–735
86 Tibbles LA and Woodgett JR (1999) The stress-activated protein kinase pathways. *Cell Mol Life Sci* 55: 1230–1254
87 Widmann C, Gibson S, Jarpe MB, Johnson GL (1999) Mitogen-activated protein kinase: conservation of a three-kinase module from yeast to human. *Physiol Rev* 79: 143–180
88 Chang L, Karin M (2001) Mammalian MAP kinase signalling cascades. *Nature* 410: 37–40
89 Johnson GL, Lapadat R (2002) Mitogen-activated protein kinase pathways mediated by ERK, JNK, and p38 protein kinases. *Science* 298: 1911–1912
90 Dent P, Yacoub A, Fisher PB, Hagan MP, Grant S (2003) MAPK pathways in radiation responses. *Oncogene* 22: 5885–5896
91 Wada T, Penninger JM (2004) Mitogen-activated protein kinases in apoptosis regulation. *Oncogene* 23: 2838–2849
92 Harada H, Quearry B, Ruiz-Vela A, Korsmeyer SJ (2004) Survival factor-induced extracellular signal-regulated kinase phosphorylates BIM, inhibiting its association with BAX and proapoptotic activity. *Proc Natl Acad Sci USA* 101:15313–15317
93 Marani M, Hancock D, Lopes R, Tenev T, Downward J, Lemoine NR (2004). Role of Bim in the survival pathway induced by Raf in epithelial cells. *Oncogene* 23: 2431–2441
94 Wang P, Gilmore AP, Streuli CH (2004) Bim is an apoptosis sensor that responds to loss of survival signals delivered by epidermal growth factor but not those provided by integrins. *J Biol Chem* 279: 41280–41285
95 Chalmers CJ, Balmanno K, Hadfield K, Ley R, Cook SJ (2003) Thrombin inhibits Bim (Bcl-2-interacting mediator of cell death) expression and prevents serum-withdrawal-induced apoptosis via protease-activated receptor 1. *Biochem J* 375: 99–109
96 Reginato MJ, Mills KR, Paulus JK, Lynch DK, Sgroi DC, Debnath J, Muthuswamy SK, Brugge JS (2003) Integrins and EGFR coordinately regulate the pro-apoptotic protein Bim to prevent anoikis. *Nat Cell Biol* 5: 733–740
97 Molton SA, Todd DE, Cook SJ (2003) Selective activation of the c-Jun N-terminal kinase (JNK) pathway fails to elicit Bax activation or apoptosis unless the phosphoinositide 3'-kinase (PI3K) pathway is inhibited. *Oncogene* 22: 4690–4701

98 Ley R, Balmanno K, Hadfield K, Weston C, Cook SJ (2003) Activation of the ERK1/2 signaling pathway promotes phosphorylation and proteasome-dependent degradation of the BH3-only protein, Bim. *J Biol Chem* 278: 18811–18816

99 Weston CR, Balmanno K, Chalmers C, Hadfield K, Molton SA, Ley R, Wagner EF, Cook SJ (2003) Activation of ERK1/2 by deltaRaf-1:ER* represses Bim expression independently of the JNK or PI3K pathways. *Oncogene* 22: 1281–1293

100 Joshi B, Li L, Taffe BG, Zhu Z, Wahl S, Tian H-S, Ben-Josef E, Taylor JD, Porter AT, Tang DG (1999) Apoptosis induction by a novel anti-prostate cancer compound, BMD188 (a fatty acid-containing hydroxamic acid), requires the mitochondrial respiratory chain. *Cancer Res* 59: 4343–4355

101 Chandra D, Liu JW, Tang DG (2002) Early mitochondrial activation and cytochrome c up-regulation during apoptosis. *J Biol Chem* 277: 50842–50854

102 Liu J-W, Chandra D, Rudd MD, Butler AP, Pallotta V, Brown D, Coffer PJ, Tang DG (2005) Induction of pro-survival molecules by apoptotic stimuli: Involvement of FOXO3a and ROS. *Oncogene* 24: 2020–2031

103 Martin AG, Fearnhead HO (2002) Apocytochrome c blocks caspase-9 activation and Bax-induced apoptosis. *J Biol Chem* 277: 50834–50841

104 Zhao Y, Wang Z-B, Xu J-X (2003) Effect of cytochrome c on the generation and elimination of O_2^- and H_2O_2 in mitochondria. *J Biol Chem* 278: 2356–2360

105 Martin AG, Nguyen J, Wells JA, Fearnhead HO (2004) Apo cytochrome c inhibits caspases by preventing apoptosome formation. *Biochem Biophys Res Commun* 319: 944–950

106 Dong Z, Wang J (2004) Hypoxia selection of death-resistant cells: A role for Bcl-xL. *J Biol Chem* 279: 9215–9221

107 Nijhawan D, Fang M, Traer E, Zhong Q, Gao W, Du F, Wang X (2003) Elimination of Mcl-1 is required for the initiation of apoptosis following ultraviolet irradiation. *Genes Dev* 17: 1475–1486

108 Sherrill KW, Byrd MP, Van Eden ME, Lloyd RE (2004) BCL-2 translation is mediated via internal ribosome entry during cell stress. *J Biol Chem* 279: 29066–29074

109 Bachelor MA, Bowden TG (2004) Ultraviolet A-induced modulation of Bcl-XL by p38 MAPK in Human Keratinocytes. Post-transcriptional regulation through the 3'-untranslated region. *J Biol Chem* 279: 42658–42668

110 Kinnula VL, Crapo JD (2003) Superoxide dismutases in the lung and human lung diseases. *Am J Respir Crit Care Med* 167: 1600–1619

111 Mikkelsen RB, Wardman P (2003) Biological chemistry of reactive oxygen and nitrogen and radiation-induced signal transduction mechanisms. *Oncogene* 22: 5734–5754

112 Chen J-G, Yang C-PH, Cammer M, Horwitz SB (2003) Gene expression and mitotic exit induced by microtubule-stabilizing drugs. *Cancer Res* 63: 7891–7899

113 Takayama S, Reed JC, Homma S (2003) Heat-shock proteins as regulators of apoptosis. *Oncogene* 22: 9041–9047

114 Parcellier A, Schmitt E, Gurbuxani S, Seigneurin-Berny D, Pance A, Chantome A, Plenchette S, Khochbin S, Solary E, Garrido C (2003) HSP27 is a ubiquitin-binding protein involved in I-kappaBalpha proteasomal degradation. *Mol Cell Biol* 23: 5790–5802

115 Garrido C, Solary E (2003) A role of HSPs in apoptosis through "protein triage"? *Cell Death Differ* 10: 619–620

116 Parcellier A, Gurbuxani S, Schmitt E, Solary E, Garrido C, Orsini F, Migliaccio E, Moroni M, Contrusi C, Raker VA et al (2004) The life span determinant p66^{Shc} localizes to mitochondria where it associates with mitochondrial heat shock protein 70 and regulates transmembrane potential. *J Biol Chem* 279: 25689–25695
117 Zhang L, Pelech S, Uitto V-J (2004) Bacterial Gro-EL heat shock protein 60 protects epithelial cells from stress-induced death through activation of ERK and inhibition of caspase 3. *Exp Cell Res* 292: 231–240
118 Green DR, Evan GI (2001). A matter of life and death. *Cancer Cell* 1: 19–30
119 Shibue T, Takeda K, Oda E, Tanaka H, Murasawa H, Takaoka A, Morishita Y, Akira S, Taniguchi T, Tanaka N (2003) Integral role of Noxa in p53-mediated apoptotic response. *Genes Dev* 17: 2233–2238
120 Yu J, Wang Z, Kinzler KW, Vogelstein B, Zhang L (2003) PUMA mediates the apoptotic response to p53 in colorectal cancer cells. *Proc Natl Acad Sci USA* 100: 1931–1936
121 Mahyar-Roemer M, Roemer K (2001) p21 Waf/Cip1 can protect human colon carcinoma cells against p53-dependent and p53-independent apoptosis induced by natural chemopreventive and therapeutic agents. *Oncogene* 20: 3387–3398
122 Javelaud D, Besancon F (2002) Inactivation of p21^{WAF-1} sensitizes cells to apoptosis via an increase of both p14^{ARF} and p53 levels and alteration of the Bax/Bcl-2 ratio. *J Biol Chem* 277: 37949–37954
123 Spierings GE, de Vries E, Stel AJ, Riestap NT, Vellenga E, de Jong S (2004) Low p21$^{Waf1/Cip1}$ protein level sensitizes testicular germ cell tumor cells to Fas-mediated apoptosis. *Oncogene* 23: 4862–4872
124 Lu PD, Jousse C, Marciniak SJ, Zhang Y, Novoa I, Scheuner D, Kaufman RJ, Ron D, Harding HP (2004) Cytoprotection by pre-emptive conditional phosphorylation of translation initiation factor 2. *EMBO J* 23: 169–179
125 Donze O, Deng J, Curran J, Sladek R, Picard D, Sonerberg N (2004) The protein kinase PKR: a molecular clock that sequentially activates survival and death programs. *EMBO J* 23: 564–571
126 Fujioka S, Schmidt C, Sclabas GM, Li Z, Lelicano H, Peng B, Yao A, Niu J, Zhang W, Evans DB et al (2004) Stabilization of p53 is a novel mechanism for proapoptotic function of NF-κB. *J Biol Chem* 279: 27549–27559
127 Campbell KJ, Rocha S, Perkins ND (2004) Active repression of antiapoptotic gene expression by RelA(p65) NF-κB. *Mol Cell* 13: 853–865
128 Zamora M, Merono C, Vinas O, Mampel T (2004) Recruitment of NF-κB into mitochondria is involved in adenine nucleotide translocase 1 (ANT1)-induced apoptosis. *J Biol Chem* 279: 38415–38423
129 Tergaonkar V, Pando M, Vafa O, Wahl G, Verma I (2002) p53 stabilization is decreased upon NFκB activation: a role for NFκB in acquisition of resistance to chemotherapy. *Cancer Cell* 1: 493–503
130 Jang J-H, Surh Y-J (2004) Bcl-2 attenuation of oxidative cell death is associated with up-regulation of γ-glutamylcysteine ligase via constitutive NF-κB activation. *J Biol Chem* 279: 38779–38786
131 Mabuchi S, Ohmichi M, Nishio Y, Hayasaka T, Kimura A, Ohta T, Saito M, Kawagoe J, Takahashi K, Yada-Hashimoto N et al (2004) Inhibition of NFκB increases the efficacy of cisplatin in *in vitro* and *in vivo* ovarian cancer models. *J Biol Chem* 279: 23477–23485

132 Balkwill F, Coussens LM (2004) Cancer: an inflammatory link. *Nature* 431: 405–406
133 Pikarsky E, Porat RM, Stein I, Abramovitch R, Amit S, Kasem S, Gutkovich-Pyest E, Urieli-Shoval S, Galun E, Ben-Neriah Y (2004) NF-kappaB functions as a tumour promoter in inflammation-associated cancer. *Nature* 431: 461–466
134 Clevers H (2004) At the crossroads of inflammation and cancer. *Cell* 118: 671–674
135 Luo JL, Maeda S, Hsu LC, Yagita H, Karin M (2004) Inhibition of NF-kappaB in cancer cells converts inflammation-induced tumor growth mediated by TNFalpha to TRAIL-mediated tumor regression. *Cancer Cell* 6: 297–305
136 Aggarwal BB (2004) Nuclear factor-kappaB: the enemy within. *Cancer Cell* 6: 203–208
137 Legembre P, Schickel R, Barnhart BC, Peter ME (2004) Identification of SNF1/AMP kinase-related kinase as an NF-B-regulated anti-apoptotic kinase involved in CD95-induced motility and invasiveness. *J Biol Chem* 279: 46742–46747
138 Pham CG, Bubici C, Zazzeroni F, Papa S, Jones J, Alvarez K, Jayawardena S, De Smaele E, Cong R, Beaumont C et al (2004) Ferritin heavy chain upregulation by NF-B inhibits TNF-induced apoptosis by suppressing reactive oxygen species. *Cell* 119: 529–542
139 Algeciras-Schmnich A, Pietras EM, Barnhart BC, Legembre P, Vijayan S, Holbeck SL, Peter ME (2003) Two CD95 tumor classes with different sensitivities to antitumor drugs. *Proc Natl Acad Sci USA* 100: 11445–11450
140 Micheau O, Tschopp J (2003) Induction of TNF receptor I-mediated apoptosis via two sequential signaling complexes. *Cell* 114**:** 181–190
141 Ehrhardt H, Fulda S, Schmid I, Hiscott J, Debatin K-M, Jeremias I (2003) TRAIL induced survival and proliferation in cancer cells resistant towards TRAIL-induced apoptosis mediated by NF-κB. *Oncogene* 22: 3842–3852
142 Huerta-Yepez S, Vega M, Jazirehi A, Garban H, Hongo F, Cheng G, Bonaivida B (2004) Nitric oxide sensitizes prostate carcinoma cell lines to TRAIL-mediated apoptosis via inactivation of NF-κB and inhibition of Bcl-xL expression. *Oncogene* 23: 4993–5003
143 Kreuz S, Siegmund D, Rumpf J-J, Samel D, Leverkus M, Janssen O, Hacker G, Dittrich-Breiholz O, Kracht M, Scheurich P et al (2004) NF-κB activation by Fas is mediated through FADD, caspase-8, and RIP and is inhibited by FLIP. *J Cell Biol* 166: 369–380
144 Imamura R, Konaka K, Matsumoto N, Hasegawa M, Fukui M, Mukaida N, Kinoshita T, Suda T (2004) Fas ligand induces cell-autonomous NF-κB activation and interleukin-8 production by a mechanism distinct from that of tumor necrosis factor-α. *J Biol Chem* 279: 46415–46423
145 Barnhart BC, Legenbre P, Pietras E, Bubici C, Franzoso G, Peter ME (2004) CD95 ligand induces motility and invasiveness of apoptosis-resistant tumor cells. *EMBO J* 23: 3175–3185
146 Danial NN, Gramm CF, Scorrano L, Zhang CY, Kraus S, Ranger AM, Datta SR, Greenberg ME, Licklider LJ, Lowell BB et al (2003) BAD and glucokinase reside in a mitochondrial complex that integrates glycolysis and apoptosis. *Nature* 424: 952–956
147 Seo SY, Chen Y, Ivanovska I, Ranger AM, Hong SJ, Dwason VL, Korsmeyer SJ, Bellows DS, Fannjiang Y, Hardwick JM (2004) BAD is a pro-survival factor prior to activation of its proapoptotic function. *J Biol Chem* 279: 42240–42249
148 Nakajima, K, Hirose H, Taniguchi M, Kurashina H, Arasaki K, Nagahama M, Tani K, Yamamoto A, Tagaya M (2004) Involvement of BNIP1 in apoptosis and endoplasmic reticulum membrane fusion. *EMBO J* 23: 3216–3226

149 Jones JM, Datta P, Srinivasula SM, Ji W, Gupta S, Zhang Z, Davies E, Hajnoczky G, Saunders TL, Van Keuren ML et al (2003) Loss of Omi mitochondrial protease activity causes the neuromuscular disorder of mnd2 mutant mice. *Nature* 425: 721–727
150 Cheng EH-Y, Sheiko TV, Fisher JK, Craigen WJ, Korsmeyer SJ (2003) VDAC2 inhibits BAK activation and mitochondrial apoptosis. *Science* 301: 513–517
151 Fannjiang Y, Kim CH, Huganir RL, Zou S, Lindsten T, Thompson CB, Mito T, Traystman RJ, Larsen T, Griffin DE et al (2003) BAK alters neuronal excitability and can switch from anti- to pro-death function during postnatal development. *Dev Cell* 4: 575–585
152 Yang L, Cao Z, Yan H, Wood WC (2003) Coexistence of high levels of apoptotic signaling and inhibitor of apoptosis proteins in human tumor cells: implication for cancer specific therapy. *Cancer Res* 63: 6815–6824
153 Newton K, Strasser A (2003) Caspases signal not only apoptosis but also antigen-induced activation in cells of the immune system. *Genes Dev* 17: 819–825
154 Birkenkamp KU, Coffer PJ (2003) FOXO transcription factors as regulators of immune homeostasis: Molecules to die for? *J Immunol* 171: 1623–1629
155 El-Deiry W (2003) The role of p53 in chemosensitivity and radisensitivity. *Oncogene* 22: 7486–7495
156 Fridman JS, Lowe SW (2003) Control of apoptosis by p53. *Oncogene* 22: 9030–9040
157 Chau BN, Wang YJ (2003) Coordinated regulation of life and death by RB. *Nat Rev Cancer* 3: 130–138
158 Bell LA, Ryan KM (2003) Life and death decisions by E2F-1. *Cell Death Differ* 10: 1–6
159 Dhakshinamoorthy S, Porter AG (2004) Nitric oxide-induced transcriptional up-regulation of protective genes by Nrf2 via the antioxidant response element counteracts apoptosis of neuroblastoma cells. *J Biol Chem* 279: 20096–20107
160 Cullinan SB, Diehl JA (2004) ERK-dependent activation of Nrf2 contributes to redox homeostasis and cell survival following endoplasmic reticulum stress. *J Biol Chem* 279: 20108–20117
161 You H, Jang Y, You-Ten AI, Okada H, Liepa J, Wakeham A, Zaugg K, Mak TW (2004) p53-dependent inhibition of FKHRL1 in response to DNA damage through protein kinase SGK1. *Proc Natl Acad Sci USA* 101: 14057–14062
162 Hu MC, Lee DF, Xia W, Golfman LS, Ou-Yang F, Yang JY, Zou Y, Bao S, Hanada N, Saso H et al (2004) IkappaB kinase promotes tumorigenesis through inhibition of forkhead FOXO3a. *Cell* 117: 225–237
163 Lin L, Hron JD, Peng SL (2004) Regulation of NF-kappaB, Th activation, and autoinflammation by the forkhead transcription factor Foxo3a. *Immunity* 21: 203–213
164 Huang H-L, Fang L-W, Lu S-P, Chou C-K, Luh T-Y, Lai M-Z (2003) DNA-damaging reagents induce apoptosis through reactive oxygen species-dependent Fas aggregation. *Oncogene* 22: 8168–8177
165 Katoh I, Tomimori Y, Ikawa Y, Kurata S (2004) Dimerization and processing of procaspase-9 by redox stress in mitochondria. *J Biol Chem* 279: 15515–15523
166 Sattler M, Winkler T, Verma S, Byrne CH, Shrikhande G, Salgia R, Griffin JD (1999) Hematopoietic growth factors signal through the formation of reactive oxygen species. *Blood* 93: 2928–2935
167 Sundaresan M, Yu ZX, Ferrons VJ, Irani K, Finkel T (1995) Requirement for generation of H_2O_2 for platelet-derived growth factor signal transduction. *Science* 270: 296–299

168 Vaquero EC, Edderkaoui M, Pandol SJ, Gukovsky I, Gukovskaya AS (2004) Reactive oxygen species produced by NAD(P)H oxidase inhibit apoptosis in pancreatic cancer cells. *J Biol Chem* 279: 34643–34654

169 Furukawa-Hibi Y, Yoshida-Araki K, Ohta T, Ikeda K, Motoyama N (2002) FOXO Forkhead transcription factors induce G_2-M checkpoint in response to oxidative stress. *J Biol Chem* 277: 26729–26732

170 Kops GJPL, Dansen TB, Polderman PE, Saarloos I, Wirtz KWA, Coffer PJ, Huang T-T, Bos JL, Medema RH, Burgering BMT (2002) Forkhead transcription factor FOXO3a protects quiescent cells from oxidative stress. *Nature* 419: 316–321

171 Nemoto S, Finkel T (2002) Redox regulation of forkhead proteins through a *p66shc*-dependent signaling pathway. *Science* 295: 2450–2452

172 Brunet A, Sweeney LB, Sturgill JF, Chua KF, Greer PL, Lin Y, Tran H, Ross SE, Mostoslavsky R, Cohen HY et al (2004) Stress-dependent regulation of FOXO transcription factors by the SIRT1 deacetylase. *Science* 303: 2011–2015

173 Macip S, Igarashi M, Berggren P, Yu J, Lee SW, Aaronson SA (2003) Influence of induced reactive oxygen species in p53-mediated cell fate decisions. *Mol Cell Biol* 23: 8576–8585

174 McCormick F (2004) Survival pathways meet their ends. *Nature* 428: 267–269

175 Wendel H-G, de Stanchina E, Fridman JS, Malina A, Ray S, Kogan S, Cordon-Cardo C, Pelletier J, Lowe SW (2004) Survival signaling by Akt and eIF4E in oncogenesis and cancer therapy. *Nature* 428: 332–337

Progress in Drug Research, Vol. 63
(R. M. Schultz, Ed.)

Targeted histone deacetylase inhibition for cancer prevention and therapy

Carlo Palmieri, R. Charles Coombes and David M. Vigushin

Department of Cancer Medicine
7th Floor MRC Cyclotron Building
Imperial College London
Hammersmith Hospital Campus
Du Cane Road
London W12 0NN, UK
<d.vigushin@imperial.ac.uk

Key words

Histone deacetylase, acetylation, differentiation, gene expression, chromatin; cancer.

Glossary of abbreviations

AML, acute myeloid leukemia; Aoe, 2*S*,9*S*,-2-amino-8-oxo-9,10-epoxy-decanoyl; APL, acute promyelocytic leukemia; ATRA, all-*trans*-retinoic acid; CBP, CREB-binding protein; CHAP, cyclic hydroxamic acid-containing peptide; CREB, cyclic AMP response element-binding; ERα, estrogen receptor α; HATs, histone acetyltransferases; HDACs, histone deacetylases; HDLP, histone deacetylase-like protein; MEF2, myocyte enhancer factor 2; N-CoR, nuclear co-repressor; PLZF, promyelocytic leukemia zinc finger protein; PML, promyelocytic leukemia protein; RAR, retinoic acid receptor; Rb, retinoblastoma; SAHA, suberoylanilide hydroxamic acid; TSA, trichostatin A.

1 Chromatin remodeling

Eukaryotic DNA is packaged into chromatin whose basic unit is the nucleosome. Each nucleosome contains 145 bp of DNA tightly wrapped around a core histone octamer comprising two heterodimers of H2A and H2B flanking a central heterotetramer of H3 and H4. Reversible post-translational acetylation and deacetylation of nucleosome core histones can alter the conformation of chromatin and regulate gene transcription [1]. Core histones are subject to a number of enzyme-catalyzed post-translational modifications including phosphorylation, methylation, ubiquitination, and ADP-ribosylation but acetylation has been the most extensively studied [2]. Global cellular acetylation status is determined by the dynamic equilibrium between the catalytic activity of two enzyme families; the histone acetyltransferases (HATs) and histone deacetylases (HDACs) [3, 4]. The ε-amino groups of lysines near the *N* termini of histones are substrates for HATs and HDACs. Covalent modification of histones appears to constitute a histone code, which serves as an epigenetic marker for regulation of gene expression by providing recognition sites for transcriptional activators or repressors. In general, transcriptionally active genes are associated with highly acetylated core histones, whereas transcriptional repression is associated with low levels of histone acetylation. Within the nucleosome, positively charged hypoacetylated histones are tightly bound to the phosphate backbone of DNA, maintaining chromatin in a transcriptionally silent state. At neutral pH lysine has a positively charged ammonium group, but addition of an acetyl group generates an uncharged amide, which reduces the affinity of histones and in particular histone tails for DNA. Acetylation disrupts the higher order structure of chromatin to form euchromatin, enhancing access of transcription factors, transcriptional regulatory complexes and RNA polymerases to promoter regions of DNA. Acetylated lysine residues also interact with specific bromodomains in proteins that regulate transcription, and with chromatin-remodeling engines that initiate conformation changes in chromatin. Conversely, histone deacetylation restores the positive charge on lysine residues of core histones, allowing chromatin to condense into a tightly supercoiled, transcriptionally silent higher order conformation known as heterochromatin [5–7].

2 Histone acetyltransferases

A relationship between histone acetylation and transcriptional activation was first proposed in 1966 [8], but the underlying molecular mechanisms have only recently come to light. There are at least four families of transcriptional co-activator proteins with intrinsic HAT activity in mammalian cells [4, 9, 10]. These include GCN5 closely related to the yeast transcriptional activator Gcn5 [11]; cyclic AMP response element-binding (CREB) protein CBP/p300 and p300/CBP-associated factor (P/CAF) [12]; TAFIIp250, a component of the basic transcription complex TFIIE [13]; and SRC-1 and ACTR, which are co-activators for ligand-dependent nuclear receptors [14]. HATs are recruited to promoters by DNA-bound transcription factors [15]. The acetylation of histone-tail lysine residues by HATs preferentially occurs on specific lysine substrates [2, 15]. HATs function in association with protein complexes that may contain other HATs, transcription co-activators and co-repressors. Multiple associations within these complexes may confer specificity in the regulation of gene expression. HATs also target non-histone protein substrates, in particular transcription factors such as p53, GATA-1, E2F, estrogen receptor α (ERα), androgen receptor and glucocorticoid receptor with variable functional effects [15, 16]. Indeed, increasing numbers of proteins other than histones are now known to be modified by acetylation [17].

3 Histone deacetylases

Transcriptional co-repressors function in large multisubunit protein complexes with HDAC enzymes [4, 9, 10]. Transcriptional repression is in part due to recruitment of HDAC complexes to gene promoters. HDACs are highly conserved throughout evolution from archaea to humans. Eighteen mammalian HDAC enzymes have been identified, and these can be divided into three classes based on sequence homology with yeast counterparts. Class I HDACs are homologs of the yeast transcriptional regulator RPD3, and include HDAC1, HDAC2, HDAC3, HDAC8 and HDAC11 [18, 19]. Class II HDACs are homologs of yeast HDA1 that are involved in cellular differentiation, and include HDAC4, HDAC5, HDAC6, HDAC7 HDAC9 and HDAC10 [20–27]. The sirtuins, of which there are seven, are members of a third class of HDACs which are homologous to yeast Sir2 [28]. Class I and II HDACs utilize a zinc-catalyzed mechanism for deacetylase activity, whereas the sirtuins require nicotinamide adenine dinucleotide (NAD) for deacetylase activity [29].

HDAC1 and HDAC2 are components of the large multisubunit protein complexes mSin3 and Mi2. HDAC-mSin3 complexes can then be recruited to transcription factors including unliganded nuclear receptors [30, 31], methyl CpG-binding protein 2 (MeCP2) [32–34], and p53 [35]. The co-repressors nuclear co-repressor (N-CoR) and silencing mediator for retinoid and thyroid receptors (SMRT) interact with HDAC1 and HDAC2 through the mSin3 complex [30, 31, 36, 37]. Other proteins that interact with HDAC1 and HDAC2 through the Mi2 or nucleosome remodeling and histone deacetylase complex (NuRD) are involved in gene silencing by DNA methylation [38]. HDACs are known to deacetylate non-histone protein substrates, and thereby modulate the activity of transcription factors such as p53 [39], TFIIE and TFIIF [40], GATA-1 [41] and ERα [42]. Class I HDACs also regulate cell cycle gene transcription by binding the E2F transcription factor to repress transcription through an association with the retinoblastoma (Rb) protein [43, 44]. Phosphorylation of Rb can disrupt the interaction with class I HDACs, and phosphorylation of HDAC1/2 can disrupt complexes formed with co-repressors such as mSin3 [45]. Relief of histone deacetylation and transcriptional repression may, therefore, be regulated not only by recruitment of HAT complexes, but also by phosphorylation of HDAC complexes.

Like class I HDACs, members of the class II family exist in complexes with SMRT/N-CoR co-repressors. Indeed, the deacetylase activity of HDAC4/5 may

Table 1.
The human HDAC family.

HDAC Group	Yeast HDAC	Human HDAC	Protein length (aa)	Deacetylase mechanism
Class I	RPD3	HDAC1	482	Zn^{2+} dependent
		HDAC2	488	
		HDAC3	428	
		HDAC8	377	
		HDAC11	347	
Class II	HDA1	HDAC4	1084	Zn^{2+} dependent
		HDAC5	1122	
		HDAC6	1215	
		HDAC7	912	
		HDAC9	1011	
		HDAC10	669	
Class III	SIR2	SIRT1	747	NAD^{+} dependent
	HST1	SIRT2	373	
	HST2	SIRT3	399	
	HST3	SIRT4	314	
	HST4	SIRT5	310	
		SIRT6	355	
		SIRT7	400	

in part arise from the class I HDAC3 in SMRT/N-CoR-containing HDAC complexes [46, 47]. In contrast to class I HDACs, the class II enzymes HDAC4, HDAC5, HDAC6 and HDAC7 are regulated by nucleocytoplasmic shuttling, often in relation to cellular differentiation [23, 48, 49]. Class II HDACs interact with human myocyte enhancer factor 2 (MEF2) transcription factors and with 14-3-3 chaperone proteins in the regulation of myocyte differentiation [22, 50–52]. Subcellular localization of class II HDACs is phosphorylation dependent [45]. HDAC4 also undergoes post-translational modification by SUMO-1 (a small ubiquitin-like modifier) [53]. Unlike polyubiquitination, sumoylation does not target a protein for proteasomal degradation but rather appears to mediate protein-protein interactions, subcellular compartmentalization and protein stability. Sumoylation is necessary for nuclear retention of HDAC4 and desumoylation is required for its nuclear export. Sumoylation may be an important regulatory mechanism for transcriptional repression by other class I and II HDACs [53].

The mammalian Sir2 gene family has seven members that share a conserved core domain. SIRT1 is the best characterized of the human Sir2 orthologs, and appears to act as a positive effector of cell growth. SIRT1 interacts with, deacetylates, and represses the transcriptional activity of p53 [54–57], promyelocytic leukemia protein (PML) nuclear bodies [57, 58], BCL6 [59], and the TAF_I68 subunit of the RNA polymerase I complex [60]. Upregulation of SIRT1 activity may, therefore, function to inhibit cellular senescence. A SIRT1 knockout mouse model showed that SIRT1 is important in embryonic development [61, 62], and recent data indicate that it negatively regulates skeletal muscle differentiation by deacetylating MyoD. Less is known about the function of the other six mammalian sirtuins [63].

4 Aberrant acetylation in cancer

Mutations in HAT genes that disrupt HAT activity have been found in various human cancers, both epithelial and hematological [38, 64–66]. Missense mutations in the p300 gene or encoding truncated p300 protein have been identified in colorectal and gastric tumors [67, 68]. Rubinstein-Taybi syndrome is a developmental disorder characterized by CBP mutation that inactivates its HAT activity, and affected individuals are at increased risk of cancer as well as formation of keloid, a hyperproliferative response of fibroblasts to dermal injury [69]. Loss of heterozygosity of the p300 gene is common in glioblastomas, and loss of heterozygosity at the CBP locus occurs in hepatocellular carcinomas [70]. Translocations resulting in in-frame fusions of the p300 or CBP genes with other genes are well known in acute myeloid leukemia (AML), myelodysplastic syndrome, and treatment-related AML [71–75].

Alterations in HDAC genes have not been identified in human malignancies. However, HDACs are associated with well-characterized oncogenes or tumor suppressor genes [38]. In proliferating cells, Myc/Max heterodimers enhance transcription of genes that stimulate proliferation and are regulated by E-box promoter elements such as E2F [76]. In differentiating cells, however, Mad/Max heterodimers repress growth stimulatory genes by recruitment of an HDAC-mSin3 complex [77]. The most common abnormality in this pathway in human malignancy is c-Myc overexpression, which prevents Mad/Max heterodimerization, thereby blocking transcriptional repression by Mad leading to uncontrolled proliferation [78]. c-Ski is a component of the HDAC-N-CoR-mSin3 complex and its oncogenic form, v-Ski, can transform cells by blocking Mad-transcriptional repression, even without c-Myc overexpression [79]. Disruption of the HDAC-mSin3 complex is, therefore, likely to be important in oncogenesis.

Abnormalities in the Myc/Mad pathway are common in human cancers, but the Rb/E2F pathway is disrupted in almost every human malignancy [80]. The Rb gene is deleted or mutated in many solid tumors [38]; carcinoma of the cervix is frequently associated with human papilloma viruses that express E7 oncoprotein, which binds Rb to disrupt interaction with E2F and class I HDACs [43], and there are genetic aberrations that result in constitutively phosphorylated and inactive Rb [81].

Gene silencing by HDACs is an important pathogenic mechanism in acute promyelocytic leukemia (APL) [82]. APL is most frequently associated with a chromosomal translocation t(15;17) that fuses the retinoic acid receptor (RAR)-α and transcription factor PML genes. The resultant fusion protein PML-RAR-α acts as an oncoprotein, recruiting HDAC activity to repress RAR-regulated gene transcription and block myeloid cell maturation [83, 84]. RAR-α and retinoid X-receptor (RXR) heterodimers recruit the transcriptional co-repressor N-CoR-mSin3-HDAC complex. This co-repressor complex normally dissociates in the presence of retinoic acid, and is replaced by a co-activator complex with HAT activity [83]. However, in the case of PML-RAR-α, RAR-α no longer responds to physiological concentrations of retinoic acid, and acts as a constitutive transcriptional repressor to block normal differentiation of promyelocytes, thereby leading to APL. Pharmacological doses of all-*trans*-retinoic acid (ATRA) can overcome the maturation block and induce differentiation of the malignant APL cells. APL will eventually become resistant to ATRA but co-treatment with an HDAC inhibitor can restore sensitivity to retinoids [82, 83, 85]. Less commonly, APL may result from the translocation t(11;17) that fuses RAR-α to the promyelocytic leukemia zinc finger protein PLZF. PLZF-RAR-α is completely insensitive to ATRA, probably because PLZF also binds the N-CoR-mSin3-HDAC co-repressor complex. PLZF-RAR-α therefore binds co-repressors at two domains, one of which is insensitive to retinoic acid. However, concurrent HDAC inhibition can restore sensitivity of PLZF-RAR-α to ATRA and allow the APL cells to differentiate [82, 83, 85].

Aberrant transcriptional repression by HDACs has also been implicated in lymphoma and in certain types of AML. For example, in certain types of non-Hodgkin's lymphoma, overexpression of the transcriptional repressor LAZ3/BCL6 (lymphoma-associated zinc finger-3/B-cell lymphoma 6) leads to lymphoid oncogenesis [86]. AML M2 subtype is associated with a t(8;21) chromosomal translocation, which produces an AML1-ETO fusion protein that is a potent dominant transcriptional repressor through recruitment of HDAC activity [74, 87, 88]. HDAC inhibition can relieve ETO-mediated transcriptional repression and induce differentiation of the AML1-ETO cells [89]. These observations underscore the significance of HDAC-mediated gene silencing in human oncogenesis, and suggest that HDAC inhibitors may have utility in the treatment of hematological malignancies.

5 Histone deacetylase inhibitors

A number of structurally diverse natural and synthetic HDAC inhibitors have been identified. These may be classified according to their chemical structure as depicted in Figure 1: (a) hydroxamic acids (such as trichostatin A, TSA [90, 91]; oxamflatin [92]; NVP-LAQ824 [93]; and hydroxamic acid-based hybrid polar compounds like suberoylanilide hydroxamic acid, SAHA [94] and pyroxamide [95]); (b) cyclic tetrapeptides with the epoxyketone-containing amino acid (2*S*,9*S*)-2-amino-8-oxo-9,10-epoxy-decanoyl (Aoe) (such as trapoxin A and B [96], Cyl-1 and Cyl-2 [97], HC-toxin [98], WF-3161 [99], chlamydocin [100]); (c) cyclic tetrapeptides without Aoe (such as apicidin [101] and the depsipeptide FK-228, formerly known as FR-901228 [102]); (d) short-chain and aromatic fatty acids (such as butyrate [103], 4-phenybutyrate [104] and valproic acid [105]); (e) benzamides (such as MS-275 [106]); and (f) miscellaneous compounds (such as depudecin [107]).

TSA and its glucopyranosyl derivative trichostatin C were first isolated from cultures of *Streptomyces hygroscopicus* as antifungal antibiotics active against *Trichophyton* species [90, 108]. Many years later, the trichostatins were shown to have potent anti-proliferative and differentiating activity at nanomolar concentrations against Friend murine erythroleukemia cells in culture [109]. TSA was orders of magnitude more potent than dimethyl sulfoxide and sodium butyrate [110]. The natural configuration of TSA is (R)-TSA, and (S)-TSA is 70-fold less biologically active [111]. The extreme potency and chiral specificity of (R)-TSA suggested that the compound binds to a specific molecular target. TSA was active in normal and tumor cell lines, arresting the growth of rat fibroblast cells in G_1 and G_2 phases of the cell cycle [112]. Nuclear histones from TSA-treated cells were highly acetylated due to reduced deacetylation [91]. TSA was a potent, reversible, non-competitive in-

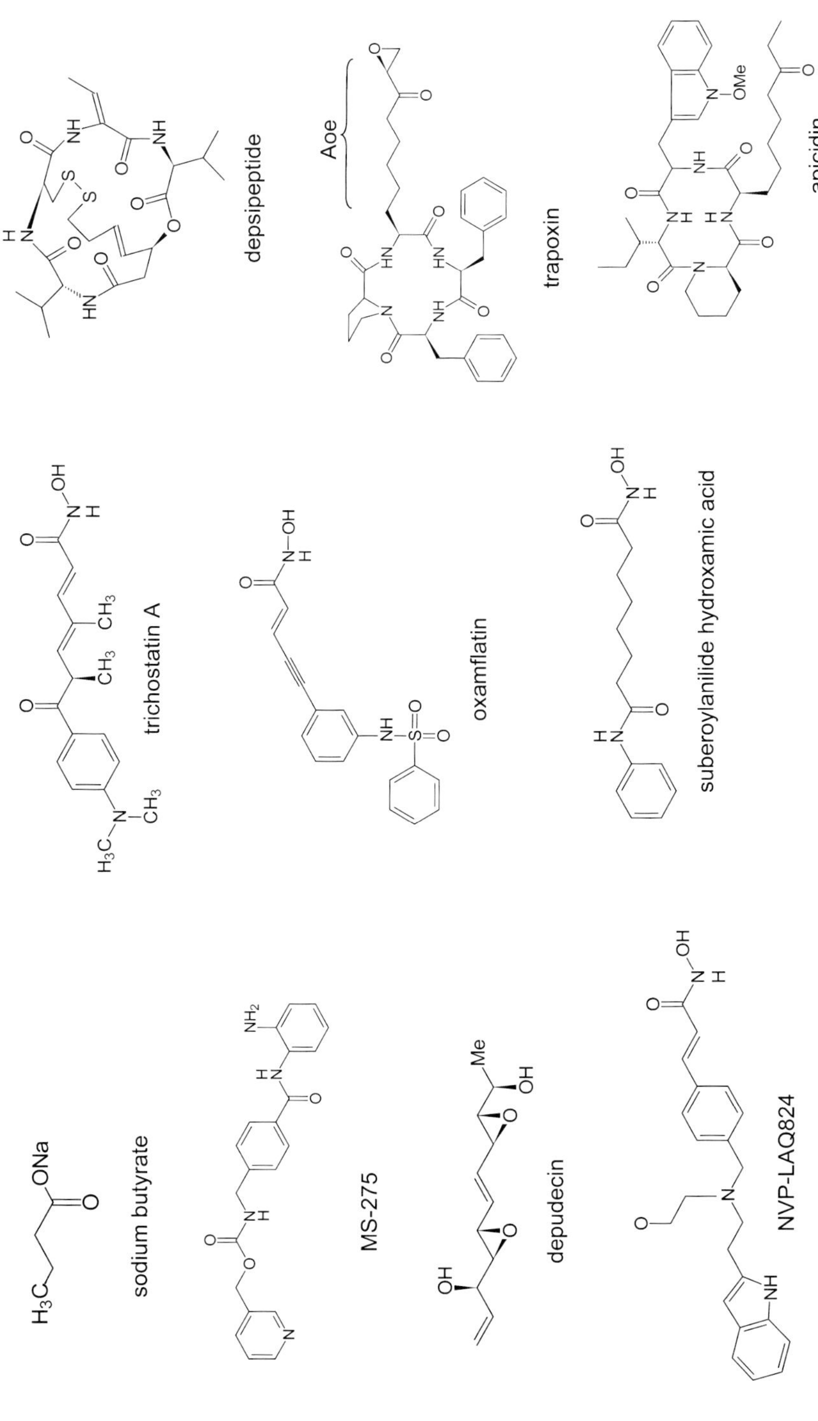

Figure 1.
Structures of selected histone deacetylase inhibitors described in the text.

hibitor of partially purified mouse HDAC with a K_i of 3.4 nM close to the effective cellular anti-proliferative concentration. The K_i was 10-fold higher for HDAC from a cell line that was resistant to TSA, suggesting that HDAC was the likely primary target of TSA [91]. Before the discovery and biological characterization of TSA, sodium butyrate was known to be a non-competitive inhibitor of HDAC but lacked potency and specificity [113, 114]. Isolation of TSA and characterization of its extremely potent and specific HDAC inhibitory activity was therefore a significant advance.

Trapoxins A and B were isolated as metabolites of the fungus *Helioma ambiens* that could induce morphological reversion of v-*sis*-transformed fibroblast cells in culture [115]. Trapoxins have a cyclic tetrapeptide structure consisting of two L-phenylalanine residues and the unusual amino acid Aoe, which has an epoxyketone [96]. Trapoxin at low nanomolar concentrations was found to induce histone hyperacetylation in mammalian cells and irreversibly inhibit histone deacetylation in partially purified enzyme preparations [96]. The epoxyketone is the only chemically reactive functional group in trapoxin, and reduction of the epoxide abolishes biological activity, suggesting a covalent interaction between the epoxide and a nucleophilic residue in the active site of HDAC [96]. Although deacetylase activity had first been identified in crude nuclear extracts 30 years before isolation of trapoxin, molecular characterization of HDAC proved elusive. The total syntheses of trapoxin B and K-trap, in which a phenylalanine residue of trapoxin is replaced by a protected lysine, allowed affinity purification of two nuclear proteins with sequence homology to the yeast transcriptional regulator RPD3. Full-length cDNA encoding the catalytic subunit of human HDAC1 could then be cloned and pure recombinant HDAC1 expressed and characterized for the first time [18].

Several other natural product HDAC inhibitors have subsequently been isolated. Apicidin is a cyclic tetrapeptide metabolite of the fungus *Fusarium sp.* first identified by its anti-protozoal activity [101]. Unlike other natural cyclopeptides, apicidin lacks Aoe, and is a reversible HDAC inhibitor at low nanomolar concentrations [116]. An ethylketone moiety is thought to be the functionally active moiety in apicidin. The depsipeptide FK-228 isolated from *Chromobacterium violaceum* is another cyclopeptide without Aoe that reversibly inhibits HDAC at nanomolar concentrations [102]. Depudecin is a metabolite of the fungus *Alternaria brassicicola* characterized by an unusual chemical structure with two epoxides and six chiral centers in an 11-carbon chain [117, 118]. Depudecin is an irreversible HDAC inhibitor with micromolar potency [107].

An increasing number of synthetic and natural product analog HDAC inhibitors have been reported. Many are hydroxamic acids such as oxamflatin, an aromatic sulfonamide HDAC inhibitor [92], SAHA, the prototype synthetic hydroxamic acid-based hybrid polar compound [94], NVP-LAQ824 [93] and PXD-101 [119], all of which inhibit HDAC with nanomolar potency. MS-275 is a benzamide derivative that inhibits HDAC at micromolar concentrations [106].

The X-ray crystal structure of the HDAC catalytic core has been solved to atomic resolution by crystallization of the histone deacetylase-like protein HDLP [120], and more recently by crystallization of human HDAC8 [121, 122]. HDLP from the hyperthermophilic bacterium *Aquifex aerolicus* shares a 375-amino acid region of sequence homology with human HDAC1, and has deacetylase activity for histones that can be inhibited by TSA. Co-crystallization studies of HDLP with TSA or SAHA and HDAC8 with four structurally diverse hydroxamate inhibitors has shed light on the catalytic mechanism of HDACs and inhibition by small molecules. The catalytic core has a single α/β domain and the active site consists of a tubular pocket with a zinc-binding site and two aspartate-histidine charge-relay systems. TSA and SAHA act as substrate mimics; the aliphatic chain and hydroxamic acid of each inhibitor are analogous to the lysine side chain and acetyl group of the substrate, respectively. These inhibitors bind inside the pocket by inserting the aliphatic chain into the tube, making contact with residues at the rim, walls, and at the bottom where the hydroxamic acid co-ordinates zinc in a bidentate fashion. Chelation of zinc by the hydroxamic acid group is the main mechanism of HDAC enzyme inhibition. In the case of TSA, the dimethylaminophenyl group acts as a cap to pack the inhibitor at the rim of the tubular active site pocket. Structural homology of HDLP and HDAC8 as well as mutagenesis and sequence data indicate that HDLP and class I and II mammalian HDACs all share a conserved deacetylase core domain and identical zinc-dependent catalytic machinery [120–122].

TSA competes with trapoxin for binding to HDAC1, suggesting that the aliphatic side chain of Aoe acts as an analog of the lysine substrate, presumably alkylating a conserved charge-relay histidine residue in the catalytic center [18]. To test this hypothesis, a novel cyclic tetrapeptide analog of trapoxin, in which the epoxyketone has been replaced by a hydroxamic acid moiety has been synthesized [123]. This cyclic hydroxamic acid-containing peptide (CHAP)1 is a hybrid of TSA and trapoxin that reversibly inhibited HDAC1 at nanomolar concentrations, as opposed to the irreversible mode of HDAC inhibition by trapoxin. The aliphatic short-chain fatty acid sodium butyrate is an HDAC inhibitor at millimolar concentrations, but an analog of trapoxin B in which the epoxyketone is replaced by a carboxylic acid side chain inhibits HDAC1 with an IC_{50} (50% inhibitory concentration) of 100 nM. These observations are consistent with the hypothesis that the cyclic tetrapeptide is a cap group acting to pack the inhibitor at the rim of the active site pocket [120].

Hydroxamic acids are the zinc-binding groups in the majority of HDAC inhibitors reported to date. However, hydroxamic acids are subject to glucuronidation, sulfation and enzymatic hydrolysis, and the hydroxamic acid group in matrix metalloproteinase inhibitors has been associated with poor pharmacokinetic properties. It has therefore become desirable to identify HDAC inhibitors containing alternative zinc-binding functional groups. A number of small molecule nonhydroxamate HDAC inhibitors have been described including *o*-aminoanilides [124–126], electrophilic ketones [127–129], bromoacetamides [130], semicarbazides [130] and *N*-formyl hydroxylamines [131], but all have reduced potency compared to hydroxamate inhibitors. However, SAHA analogs in which the hydroxamic acid is replaced by a thiol [132] or mercaptoacetamide [133] are potent HDAC inhibitors with comparable activity to SAHA.

Yeast experiments in which specific HDACs were deleted or knocked down indicate that RPD3, SIR2 and HDA1 are likely to have distinct functions related to cell cycle progression, amino acid synthesis, and carbohydrate transport and metabolism, respectively [134]. There is increasing evidence to support distinct biological roles for each of the mammalian HDACs, and it is probable that inhibition of specific members of the HDAC family will have specific functional consequences, such as on gene expression, regulation of the cell cycle, proliferation, differentiation and apoptosis. As a result, there is substantial interest in developing compounds that selectively inhibit individual HDAC enzymes or with specificity for class I or class II HDACs. This has proved difficult since recombinant HDACs often have poor enzymatic activity, and in cells HDACs function in large multisubunit protein complexes [135].

TSA is a relatively non-selective inhibitor of HDAC1, HDAC4 and HDAC6 [123]. In contrast, trapoxin B inhibited HDAC1 and HDAC4 at subnanomolar concentrations, but HDAC6 was highly resistant. Less striking resistance for HDAC6 was also seen with CHAP1 and with CHAP counterparts to other natural cyclopeptides containing Aoe. TSA is a simple analog of acetyl-lysine with a small cap group, which may explain its lack of selectivity for class I and II HDACs. Cyclic tetrapeptides make more extensive contacts at the rim of the active site pocket and in the shallow grooves surrounding the pocket entrance, which might confer a degree of selectivity. HDAC6 is primarily cytoplasmic, co-localizes with the microtubule-associated dynein motor complex, and shuttles into the nucleus in response to cellular differentiation stimuli [23, 136]. HDAC6 is unique in having two functional catalytic domains [137, 138] that deacetylate histones as well as α-tubulin. Tubacin is a selective inhibitor of HDAC6 [125].

A screen for HDAC8 inhibitors identified Scriptaid, SB-429201, and SB-379872-A, which is a specific but relatively weak inhibitor of HDAC8 [17]. MS-275 inhibits HDAC1 and HDAC3, but is inactive against HDAC8 [139]. The depsipeptide FK-228 has activity against the class I enzymes HDAC1 and HDAC2, but class II enzymes HDAC4 and HDAC6 are resistant [140].

The X-ray crystal structure of the SIRT2 catalytic core has been solved [29]. In yeast and nematodes, the homolog Sir2 is a transcriptional repressor at telomeres and ribosomal RNA gene clusters that regulate the life span of these organisms [29]. Discovery of small molecules that inhibit the deacetylase activity of the Sir2 family, such as splitomicin, indicates that the sirtuins maintain transcriptional silencing in non-dividing cells [141]. Sirtinol is another inhibitor that interferes with body axis formation in *Arabidopsis.* Nicotinamide is an inhibitor of SIRT1, a negative regulator of p53, promoting p53-dependent apoptosis in mammalian cells [55, 56]. Small molecule activators of SIRT1 have also been identified, including quercetin, piceatannol, and the more potent resveratrol which is a polyphenol found in red wine. Resveratrol increases survival of human tumor cell lines following DNA damage and reduces acetylation of p53 at lysine 382, which is a known substrate of SIRT1 [142].

6 Biological properties of histone deacetylase inhibitors

The consequences of HDAC inhibition in cultured mammalian cells include reversion of transformed morphology and inhibition of cell proliferation by induction of cell cycle arrest in the G_1/S and/or G_2/M phase, and differentiation and/or apoptosis of tumor cell lines. Growth inhibition has been documented in virtually all transformed cell types, including cell lines arising from both epithelial and hematological tumors.

Malignant transformation usually alters cellular morphology and cytoskeletal architecture [143] with a characteristic loss of actin stress fibers [144]. HDAC inhibition can re-organize the actin-containing microfilament system, revert the morphological changes of cellular transformation induced by oncogenes such as v-*sis*, v-*src*, and v-*ras*, and induce morphological and biochemical differentiation of tumor cell lines [96, 145]. Detransforming activity is suppressed by both actinomycin D and cycloheximide, indicating that both mRNA and *de novo* protein synthesis are required [118]. Gelsolin is an actin-binding protein that maintains the actin cytoskeleton, and gelsolin protein levels are reduced in many transformed cell lines and tumor tissues [146]. In response to HDAC inhibition, derepression of the gelsolin gene results in increased levels of expression of gelsolin mRNA and protein, which correlate with reversion of transformed morphology and induction of a differentiated phenotype [145, 147]. The detransforming effects of HDAC inhibitors are suppressed after microinjection of anti-gelsolin antibodies, underscoring the relevance of gelsolin to the transformed phenotype [107].

Recruitment of HDAC activity is central to the control of cell proliferation by the Myc/Mad and Rb/E2F pathways. HDAC inhibition might, therefore, be predicted to prevent cell cycle arrest. Paradoxically, HDAC inhibitors induce cell cycle arrest, which can be explained by upregulation of *CDKN1A* [148] and downregulation of cyclins D and A. The *CDKN1A* gene encodes $p21^{WAF/CIP1}$, a tumor suppressor protein and cyclin-dependent kinase (CDK) inhibitor that binds and inhibits the activity of CDKs, leading to hypophosphorylation of Rb and inhibition of S-phase progression [148]. In normal cells, $p21^{WAF/CIP1}$ is induced by p53 in response to DNA damage, hence the terminology WAF or CIP1 (wild-type p53-activated factor or CDK inhibitor protein-1) [149]. HDAC inhibitors act directly on an Sp-1 site in the *CDKN1A* gene promoter, upregulating *CDKN1A* gene transcription [150–152]. Induction of *CDKN1A* is required for G_1/S phase arrest in response to HDAC inhibition. The favorable association between a diet high in fiber and a reduced incidence of colon cancer is thought to result from upregulation of $p21^{WAF/CIP1}$ expression in the colon by short-chain fatty acid products of fiber fermentation [38, 148]. HDAC inhibitor treatment of cells deficient in

CDKN1A leads to an accumulation of cells with 4*n* DNA content and sensitization to apoptosis [153–155]. Untransformed human fibroblasts and some tumor cell lines treated with HDAC inhibitors arrest in G_2/M with little or no apoptosis [156]. However, most tumor cells that do not arrest in G_1/S phase in response to HDAC inhibition replicate their DNA and undergo apoptosis (reviewed in [157]).

HDAC inhibition induces accumulation of hyperacetylated histones in most regions of chromatin, but only ~2% of genes show a twofold or more change in the level of mRNA transcripts [158]. The basis for this selectivity is not clear. Genes that are upregulated by HDAC inhibitors in transformed cells include *CDKN1A, CDKN2A* (which encodes $p16^{INK4A}$) and the genes for cyclin E and thioredoxin-binding protein 2 (*TBP2*), which are all regulators of cell proliferation as well as the putative tumor suppressor gelsolin [159–162]. TSA has also been shown to induce upregulation of the telomerase catalytic subunit *TERT* in normal human cell lines [163]. Several of the genes upregulated in response to HDAC inhibition have Sp-1 sites in their promoters, including *CDKN1A, TERT* and *TBP2*. Specific sites in the promoter region of genes may be important in the selective effects of HDAC inhibitors on gene transcription [159, 163].

HDAC inhibitors induce transcription of a subset of genes such as $p21^{WAF/CIP1}$ but repress transcription of an equal or larger number of genes, such as *CCND1* which encodes cyclin D1. The mechanisms of gene repression are incompletely understood, and may include recruitment or activation of co-repressors or acetylation of non-histone protein substrates. Transcription factors in particular are important targets for acetylation with varying functional effects. Acetylation enhances activity of the tumor suppressor p53 [164, 165], the Kruppel-like factor EKLF [166], and the erythroid differentiation factor GATA-1 [41], but represses transcriptional activity of T cell factor. Acetylation of the co-activator ACTR inhibits ligand-induced nuclear receptor signaling [167]. Studies in our laboratory indicate that ERα is acetylated in an MCF-7 breast adenocarcinoma cell line and hyperacetylated in response to TSA treatment [168]. Another group has reported that acetylation of lysine residues in the hinge/ligand binding domain of ERα suppresses ligand sensitivity and regulates transcriptional activation by HDAC inhibitors [42]. Conservation of the acetylated ERα motif in other nuclear receptors suggests that direct acetylation may play an important role in the regulation of nuclear receptor signaling [42, 169].

HDAC inhibitors affect regulation of several important cellular proteins at both transcriptional and post-translational levels. Our group has shown that TSA represses ERα and cyclin D1 transcription and promotes ubiquitin-dependent proteasomal degradation of cyclin D1 in the MCF-7 breast cancer cell line, leading to G_1/S phase cell cycle arrest [170]. FK-228 was reported to acetylate Hsp90 in lung cancer cells, destabilizing the chaperone complex of Hsp90 with client proteins that include c-erbB2, c-Raf-1, and mutant p53, and targeting them for degradation via the proteasome [171]. NVP-LAQ824 has been shown to promote proteasomal degradation of c-erbB2 in human breast cancer cell lines [172], and induce degradation of Bcr-Abl in chronic myelogenous leukemia blast crisis cells [173].

HDAC inhibitors induce apoptosis in human tumor cell lines by activating both death receptor and intrinsic apoptotic pathways [174–179]. Untransformed normal cells are resistant to HDAC inhibitor induced apoptosis. The absence of a G_2 checkpoint in tumor cells may account for the selective apoptotic response [156]. Normal human fibroblasts or melanocytes treated with hydroxamic acid-based hybrid polar compounds do not undergo apoptosis at doses that are toxic to transformed cell lines [180, 181]. Breast cancer cells treated with FK-228 undergo apoptosis associated with p53-independent expression of $p21^{WAF/CIP1}$, phosphorylation and inactivation of the anti-apoptotic protein Bcl-2 [182]. Other studies suggest that apoptosis induced by HDAC inhibitors is mediated by upregulation of c-Myc, gelsolin or pro-apoptotic proteins such as Bax [145, 152, 183–186]. Enhanced production of reactive oxygen species has been shown to play a role in the apoptotic response to SAHA [187, 188] and MS-275 [189]. Interestingly, apoptosis of human lung cancer cells induced by TSA or FK-228 was greatly augmented by the DNA methyltransferase inhibitor 5-aza-2′-deoxycytidine (DAC) [190]. DNA methylation status is an important determinant of chromatin structure and function, and methylated DNA is transcriptionally repressed [32, 33, 191, 192]. Concurrent treatment of cells with TSA and DAC can restore expression of methylated tumor suppressor genes [193]. However, in ERα-negative breast cancer cell lines, TSA alone is sufficient to derepress the methylated ERα gene [194]. The combination of DAC and an HDAC inhibitor FK-228 has also been used to augment the expression of tumor antigens for adoptive immunotherapy [195].

HDAC inhibitors can inhibit hypoxia induced angiogenesis. In bovine aortic endothelial cells, FK-228 blocked hypoxia-induced cell proliferation, invasion, migration, adhesion and tube formation [196]. Expression of angiogenic-stimulating factors such as vascular endothelial growth factor (VEGF) was downregulated, while levels of angiogenic-inhibiting factors such as the hypoxia sensor von Hippel Lindau were upregulated, suggesting that inhibition of angiogenesis by HDAC inhibitors was at the transcriptional level [196].

The potential clinical utility of HDAC inhibitors has been broadened by the recent observation that these compounds can sensitize tumor cell lines to other anticancer drugs. Pretreatment with either TSA or SAHA enhanced the cytotoxicity of etoposide, ellipticine, doxorubicin, and cisplatin in D54 and U118 glioblastoma, MCF-7 breast carcinoma and RKO colon carcinoma cell lines in culture [197]. NVP-LAQ824 sensitized human breast cancer cells that overexpress c-erbB2 to apoptosis induced by trastuzumab, taxotere, gemcitabine, and epothilone B [172]. HDAC inhibitors can also restore sensitivity of tumor cells that are resistant to chemotherapeutics. For example, imatinib-resistant Bcr-Abl-positive chronic myelogenous leukemia cells were sensitized to imatinib by co-treatment with SAHA [198]. In another study, TSA treatment sensitized ERα-negative breast cancer cells to tamoxifen probably by upregulating ERβ activity [199]. Augmentation of HDAC inhibitor induced tumor cell apoptosis by concurrent administration of a demethylating drug is another important strategy for cancer therapy.

7 Antitumor effects of HDAC inhibitors in preclinical models

The short-chain fatty acids sodium butyrate, sodium phenylbutyrate, its metabolic precursor sodium phenylacetate, and the lipophilic prodrug, pivaloyloxymethyl butyrate all have antitumor activity in animal models of solid and hematological cancers at relatively high doses that are associated with significant toxicity [103, 200].

Other more potent HDAC inhibitors have been shown to inhibit tumor growth when administered by various routes at doses that cause little or no toxicity in experimental models. FK-228 administered by intraperitoneal injection prolonged survival in syngeneic mouse leukemias and melanomas, and had potent antitumor activity against MCF-7 breast and A549 lung tumor xenografts [201]. Administered by intravenous injection, FK-228 was active in syngeneic murine colon carcinoma, reticulum cell sarcoma and fibrosarcoma models, and against human lung and stomach carcinoma xenografts [201]. FK-228 or ATRA were active against APL in a murine model, and the combination was synergistic [202]. Oxamflatin increased survival of mice with syngeneic melanomas at non-toxic doses [92]. The benzamide MS-275 administered orally was effective in nude mouse xenografts models of leukemia, colorectal, gastric, ovarian and pancreatic tumors. Dose-limiting toxicities included weight loss and poor general appearance, but MS-275 had antitumor activity without toxicity at half the maximum tolerated dose [106]. TSA was reported to be inactive against a human melanoma xenograft mouse model [180]. However, our group observed that TSA administered by subcutaneous injection had potent antitumor activity without toxicity *in vivo* in the *N*-methyl-*N*-nitrosourea carcinogen-induced rat mammary cancer model. Induction of differentiation was the likely mechanism of antitumor activity [168]. Another study reported that TSA inhibits hypoxia-induced angiogenesis *in vivo* in the Lewis lung carcinoma model [203]. SAHA and other hydroxamic acid-based hybrid polar compounds exhibit antitumor activity without apparent toxicity in human melanoma [180] and androgen-independent prostate tumor xenografts models [204], as well as preventive activity in carcinogen-induced rat mammary [205] and murine lung carcinoma models [204]. The cyclic hydroxamic acid-containing peptide CHAP31 had potent antitumor efficacy against syngeneic murine melanomas and human breast, lung, melanoma and gastric tumor xenografts. CHAP31 was considerably more stable in cell culture than either TSA or trapoxin, and effective plasma concentrations were maintained for several hours after intravenous administration in the rat. However, the therapeutic index of CHAP31 was low and significant weight loss occurred at effective antitumor doses, limiting its potential for clinical drug development [206].

8 HDAC inhibitors in clinical development

Phase I clinical and pharmacokinetic studies of sodium butyrate and sodium phenylbutyrate have been performed in cancer patients despite the limitations of low potency and lack of specificity of these compounds [207, 208]. Oral or intravenous dosing can achieve millimolar or high micromolar peak plasma concentrations. Prolonged intravenous infusion of sodium phenylbutyrate resulted in potentially therapeutic steady-state circulating concentrations, but was complicated by somnolence and confusion [209]. Sodium butyrate and phenylbutyrate are well absorbed from the gastrointestinal tract, but oral doses of several grams per day are needed to achieve biologically active plasma concentrations of 0.5 mM. Toxicity at these doses included nausea, vomiting, confusion, edema, fatigue, hyperuricemia and hypocalcemia [210]. Sodium butyrate induced partial remission of AML [211], and sodium phenylbutyrate in combination with ATRA was effective in one patient with relapsed APL unresponsive to retinoids [104] but not in a larger study. Histone hyperacetylation in normal peripheral blood mononuclear cells or bone marrow, or in tumor tissues, can provide a useful pharmacodynamic marker in clinical studies of HDAC inhibitors. Histone hyperacetylation was detectable in both bone marrow and peripheral blood mononuclear cells during sodium phenylbutyrate treatment of the patient with APL [104].

In a phase I study, pivaloyloxymethyl butyrate was well tolerated at doses of up to 3.3 g/day when given by intravenous infusion on days 1–5 in a 21-day treatment cycle. Toxicity was confined to fatigue, nausea and dysgeusia. One patient with non-small cell lung cancer had an objective response [212]. In a non-randomized phase II study of 47 patients with non-small cell lung cancer, pivaloyloxymethyl butyrate was well tolerated at 2.34 g/m^2/day administered by intravenous infusion daily for 3 days in a 21-day cycle. Three patients (6.4%) had a partial tumor response and 14 patients (30%) had stabilization of disease for more than 12 weeks [213]. In preclinical studies, pivaloxyloxymethyl butyrate had synergistic activity in combination with cytotoxic drugs. A randomized phase II study comparing taxotere with the combination of pivaloxyloxymethyl butyrate and taxotere is currently underway in patients with non-small cell lung cancer [213].

The short-chain fatty acid valproic acid and its sodium salt have long been used as antiepileptic drugs, but recently were found to inhibit HDAC at millimolar or high micromolar concentrations [214]. Like other short-chain fatty acid HDAC inhibitors, valproic acid lacks potency and specificity. Millimolar concentrations of valproic acid are required to inhibit proliferation of the MCF-7 breast cancer cell line (D.M. Vigushin, unpublished observation), while the effective anti-epileptic plasma concentration is in the micromolar range. Metabolic disturbances and other serious dose-related toxicities may preclude administration of valproic acid at potentially therapeutic anticancer doses.

Several potent and specific HDAC inhibitors are in early phase clinical development as potential treatments for solid and hematological cancers. FK-228 is one of the first potent compounds to enter clinical trials and is currently in phase II development [215]. Preclinical studies in rodents showed that peak circulating levels in excess of those predicted to be therapeutic *in vitro* could be achieved with single intravenous or oral doses of FK-228, and could be sustained with intravenous infusion [216]. Significant cardiac and catheter-site-related toxicity occurred in preclinical models, but FK-228 has been well tolerated in patients with manageable hematological (neutropenia, thrombocytopenia) and non-hematological (nausea/vomiting, fatigue, ECG changes, hypocalcemia) toxicity [217]. In a phase I and pharmacokinetic study, escalating doses of FK-228 were delivered as a 4-hour intravenous infusion on days 1 and 5 every 21 days [217]. The maximum tolerated dose was 17.8 mg/m^2; serum from patients treated at this dose arrested proliferation of PC3 cells in culture and histone hyperacetylation was detectable in peripheral blood mononuclear cells, indicating that biologically active circulating concentrations of FK-228 were achieved. In phase I and II studies, FK-228 had antitumor activity against renal cell carcinoma [217], peripheral and cutaneous T cell lymphomas, and chronic lymphocytic leukemia [215].

SAHA is in phase II development and is reported to be active in solid tumors and Hodgkin's disease at non-toxic doses [16]. Histone hyperacetylation in tumor biopsy specimens and peripheral mononuclear cells was detectable at subtherapeutic doses. SAHA had good oral bioavailability and early phase clinical studies were reported to be ongoing in patients with both solid tumors and hematological cancers [16]. In phase I studies, the closely related compound pyroxamide caused severe fatigue and hepatotoxicity when administered by the prolonged intravenous infusion required to achieve potentially therapeutic circulating concentrations of the drug [16].

MS-275 is in phase II development, but to date there have been no published reports of its toxicity or efficacy. Acetyldinaline (CI-994) is an orally bioavailable HDAC inhibitor in early phase clinical development as a potential anticancer drug. In phase I trials the drug was well tolerated, penetrated into cerebrospinal fluid, and had antitumor efficacy against non-small cell lung and renal cell carcinomas [218]. Phase II studies of CI-994 monotherapy resulted in low response rates, and further clinical development has therefore been in combination with cytotoxic drugs. A recent phase I study reported manageable toxicity and promising antitumor activity for CI-994 administered in combination with carboplatin and paclitaxel to patients with advanced solid tumors [219].

There remain a number of unanswered questions regarding the optimal evaluation and utilization of HDAC inhibitors for cancer prevention and treatment. Tumor regression is unlikely to be the best biological endpoint for clinical studies of antitumor efficacy. Pharmacodynamic markers such as histone hyperacetylation in peripheral mononuclear cells and pharmacokinetic endpoints that relate to target inhibition in preclinical models may provide a better guide to plasma levels required for biological activity in patients. Future studies will define the role of combination therapies with HDAC inhibitors and other anticancer drugs that exhibit synergistic or additive activities. HDAC inhibitors are an exciting class of relatively non-toxic drugs that have potential utility for the treatment of solid and hematological malignancies.

References

1. Pazin MJ, Kadonaga JT (1997) What's up and down with histone deacetylation and transcription? *Cell* 89: 325–328
2. Strahl BD, Allis CD (2000) The language of covalent histone modifications. *Nature* 403: 41–45
3. Struhl K (1998) Histone acetylation and transcriptional regulatory mechanisms. *Genes Dev* 12: 599–606
4. Kouzarides T (1999) Histone acetylases and deacetylases in cell proliferation. *Curr Opin Genet Dev* 9: 40–48
5. Grunstein M (1997) Histone acetylation in chromatin structure and transcription. *Nature* 389: 349–352
6. Davie JR (1998) Covalent modifications of histones: expression from chromatin templates. *Curr Opin Genet Dev* 8: 173–178
7. Davie JR, Spencer VA (1999) Control of histone modifications. *J Cell Biochem Suppl*: 141–148
8. Allfrey VG (1966) Structural modifications of histones and their possible role in the regulation of ribonucleic acid synthesis. *Proc Can Cancer Conf* 6: 313–335
9. Kuo MH, Allis CD (1998) Roles of histone acetyltransferases and deacetylases in gene regulation. *Bioessays* 20: 615–626
10. Bannister AJ, Miska EA (2000) Regulation of gene expression by transcription factor acetylation. *Cell Mol Life Sci* 57: 1184–1192
11. Brownell JE, Zhou J, Ranalli T, Kobayashi R, Edmondson DG, Roth SY, Allis CD (1996) Tetrahymena histone acetyltransferase A: a homolog to yeast Gcn5p linking histone acetylation to gene activation. *Cell* 84: 843–851
12. Ogryzko VV, Schiltz RL, Russanova V, Howard BH, Nakatani Y (1996) The transcriptional coactivators p300 and CBP are histone acetyltransferases. *Cell* 87: 953–959
13. Mizzen CA, Yang XJ, Kokubo T, Brownell JE, Bannister AJ, Owen-Hughes T, Workman J, Wang L, Berger SL, Kouzarides T et al (1996) The TAF(II)250 subunit of TFIID has histone acetyltransferase activity. *Cell* 87: 1261–1270

14 Spencer TE, Jenster G, Burcin MM, Allis CD, Zhou J, Mizzen CA, McKenna NJ, Onate SA, Tsai SY et al (1997) Steroid receptor coactivator-1 is a histone acetyltransferase. *Nature* 389: 194–198

15 Roth SY, Denu JM, Allis CD (2001) Histone acetyltransferases. *Annu Rev Biochem* 70: 81–120

16 Marks P, Rifkind RA, Richon VM, Breslow R, Miller T, Kelly WK (2001) Histone deacetylases and cancer: causes and therapies. *Nat Rev Cancer* 1: 194–202

17 McLaughlin F, La Thangue NB (2004) Histone deacetylase inhibitors open new doors in cancer therapy. *Biochem Pharmacol* 68: 1139–1144

18 Taunton J, Hassig CA, Schreiber SL (1996) A mammalian histone deacetylase related to the yeast transcriptional regulator Rpd3p. *Science* 272: 408–411

19 Gao L, Cueto MA, Asselbergs F, Atadja P (2002) Cloning and functional characterization of HDAC11, a novel member of the human histone deacetylase family. *J Biol Chem* 277: 25748–25755

20 Rundlett SE, Carmen AA, Kobayashi R, Bavykin S, Turner BM, Grunstein M (1996) HDA1 and RPD3 are members of distinct yeast histone deacetylase complexes that regulate silencing and transcription. *Proc Natl Acad Sci USA* 93: 14503–14508

21 Wang AH, Bertos NR, Vezmar M, Pelletier N, Crosato M, Heng HH, Th'ng J, Han J, Yang XJ (1999) HDAC4, a human histone deacetylase related to yeast HDA1, is a transcriptional corepressor. *Mol Cell Biol* 19: 7816–7827

22 Grozinger CM, Schreiber SL (2000) Regulation of histone deacetylase 4 and 5 and transcriptional activity by 14-3-3-dependent cellular localization. *Proc Natl Acad Sci USA* 97: 7835–7840

23 Verdel A, Curtet S, Brocard MP, Rousseaux S, Lemercier C, Yoshida M, Khochbin S (2000) Active maintenance of mHDA2/mHDAC6 histone-deacetylase in the cytoplasm. *Curr Biol* 10: 747–749

24 Kao HY, Downes M, Ordentlich P, Evans RM (2000) Isolation of a novel histone deacetylase reveals that class I and class II deacetylases promote SMRT-mediated repression. *Genes Dev* 14: 55–66

25 Dressel U, Bailey PJ, Wang SC, Downes M, Evans RM, Muscat GE (2001) A dynamic role for HDAC7 in MEF2-mediated muscle differentiation. *J Biol Chem* 276: 17007–17013

26 Gray SG, Ekstrom TJ (2001) The human histone deacetylase family. *Exp Cell Res* 262: 75–83

27 Kao HY, Lee CH, Komarov A, Han CC, Evans RM (2002) Isolation and characterization of mammalian HDAC10, a novel histone deacetylase. *J Biol Chem* 277: 187–193

28 Imai S, Armstrong CM, Kaeberlein M, Guarente L (2000) Transcriptional silencing and longevity protein Sir2 is an NAD-dependent histone deacetylase. *Nature* 403: 795–800

29 Finnin MS, Donigian JR, Pavletich NP (2001) Structure of the histone deacetylase SIRT2. *Nat Struct Biol* 8: 621–625

30 Alland L, Muhle R, Hou H, Jr., Potes J, Chin L, Schreiber-Agus N, DePinho RA (1997) Role for N-CoR and histone deacetylase in Sin3-mediated transcriptional repression. *Nature* 387: 49–55

31 Heinzel T, Lavinsky RM, Mullen TM, Soderstrom M, Laherty CD, Torchia J, Yang WM, Brard G, Ngo SD, Davie JR et al (1997) A complex containing N-CoR, mSin3 and histone deacetylase mediates transcriptional repression. *Nature* 387: 43–48

32 Jones PL, Veenstra GJ, Wade PA, Vermaak D, Kass SU, Landsberger N, Strouboulis J, Wolffe AP (1998) Methylated DNA and MeCP2 recruit histone deacetylase to repress transcription. *Nat Genet* 19: 187–191
33 Nan X, Ng HH, Johnson CA, Laherty CD, Turner BM, Eisenman RN, Bird A (1998) Transcriptional repression by the methyl-CpG-binding protein MeCP2 involves a histone deacetylase complex. *Nature* 393: 386–389
34 Wade PA, Jones PL, Vermaak D, Veenstra GJ, Imhof A, Sera T, Tse C, Ge H, Shi YB, Hansen JC et al (1998) Histone deacetylase directs the dominant silencing of transcription in chromatin: association with MeCP2 and the Mi-2 chromodomain SWI/SNF ATPase. *Cold Spring Harb Symp Quant Biol* 63: 435–445
35 Murphy M, Ahn J, Walker KK, Hoffman WH, Evans RM, Levine AJ, George DL (1999) Transcriptional repression by wild-type p53 utilizes histone deacetylases, mediated by interaction with mSin3a. *Genes Dev* 13: 2490–2501
36 Hassig CA, Fleischer TC, Billin AN, Schreiber SL, Ayer DE (1997) Histone deacetylase activity is required for full transcriptional repression by mSin3A. *Cell* 89: 341–347
37 Zhang Y, Iratni R, Erdjument-Bromage H, Tempst P, Reinberg D (1997) Histone deacetylases and SAP18, a novel polypeptide, are components of a human Sin3 complex. *Cell* 89: 357–364
38 Cress WD, Seto E (2000) Histone deacetylases, transcriptional control, and cancer. *J Cell Physiol* 184: 1–16
39 Juan LJ, Shia WJ, Chen MH, Yang WM, Seto E, Lin YS, Wu CW (2000) Histone deacetylases specifically down-regulate p53-dependent gene activation. *J Biol Chem* 275: 20436–20443
40 Imhof A, Yang XJ, Ogryzko VV, Nakatani Y, Wolffe AP, Ge H (1997) Acetylation of general transcription factors by histone acetyltransferases. *Curr Biol* 7: 689–692
41 Boyes J, Byfield P, Nakatani Y, Ogryzko V (1998) Regulation of activity of the transcription factor GATA-1 by acetylation. *Nature* 396: 594–598
42 Wang C, Fu M, Angeletti RH, Siconolfi-Baez L, Reutens AT, Albanese C, Lisanti MP, Katzenellenbogen BS, Kato S, Hopp T et al (2001) Direct acetylation of the estrogen receptor alpha hinge region by p300 regulates transactivation and hormone sensitivity. *J Biol Chem* 276: 18375–18383
43 Brehm A, Miska EA, McCance DJ, Reid JL, Bannister AJ, Kouzarides T (1998) Retinoblastoma protein recruits histone deacetylase to repress transcription. *Nature* 391: 597–601
44 Magnaghi-Jaulin L, Groisman R, Naguibneva I, Robin P, Lorain S, Le Villain JP, Troalen F, Trouche D, Harel-Bellan A (1998) Retinoblastoma protein represses transcription by recruiting a histone deacetylase. *Nature* 391: 601–605
45 Galasinski SC, Resing KA, Goodrich JA, Ahn NG (2002) Phosphatase inhibition leads to histone deacetylases 1 and 2 phosphorylation and disruption of corepressor interactions. *J Biol Chem* 277: 19618–19626
46 Guenther MG, Barak O, Lazar MA (2001) The smrt and n-cor corepressors are activating cofactors for histone deacetylase 3. *Mol Cell Biol* 21: 6091–6101
47 Fischle W, Dequiedt F, Hendzel MJ, Guenther MG, Lazar MA, Voelter W, Verdin E (2002) Enzymatic activity associated with class II HDACs is dependent on a multiprotein complex containing HDAC3 and SMRT/N-CoR. *Mol Cell* 9: 45–57
48 Khochbin S, Verdel A, Lemercier C, Seigneurin-Berny D (2001) Functional significance of histone deacetylase diversity. *Curr Opin Genet Dev* 11: 162–166

49 Miska EA, Langley E, Wolf D, Karlsson C, Pines J, Kouzarides T (2001) Differential localization of HDAC4 orchestrates muscle differentiation. *Nucleic Acids Res* 29: 3439–3447

50 Miska EA, Karlsson C, Langley E, Nielsen SJ, Pines J, Kouzarides T (1999) HDAC4 deacetylase associates with and represses the MEF2 transcription factor. *EMBO J* 18: 5099–5107

51 Sparrow DB, Miska EA, Langley E, Reynaud-Deonauth S, Kotecha S, Towers N, Spohr G, Kouzarides T, Mohun TJ (1999) MEF-2 function is modified by a novel co-repressor, MITR. *EMBO J* 18: 5085–5098

52 McKinsey TA, Zhang CL, Lu J, Olson EN (2000) Signal-dependent nuclear export of a histone deacetylase regulates muscle differentiation. *Nature* 408: 106–111

53 Kirsh O, Seeler JS, Pichler A, Gast A, Muller S, Miska E, Mathieu M, Harel-Bellan A, Kouzarides T, Melchior F et al (2002) The SUMO E3 ligase RanBP2 promotes modification of the HDAC4 deacetylase. *EMBO J* 21: 2682–2691

54 Luo J, Su F, Chen D, Shiloh A, Gu W (2000) Deacetylation of p53 modulates its effect on cell growth and apoptosis. *Nature* 408: 377–381

55 Vaziri H, Dessain SK, Ng Eaton E, Imai SI, Frye RA, Pandita TK, Guarente L, Weinberg RA (2001) hSIR2(SIRT1) functions as an NAD-dependent p53 deacetylase. *Cell* 107: 149–159

56 Luo J, Nikolaev AY, Imai S, Chen D, Su F, Shiloh A, Guarente L, Gu W (2001) Negative control of p53 by Sir2alpha promotes cell survival under stress. *Cell* 107: 137–148

57 Langley E, Pearson M, Faretta M, Bauer UM, Frye RA, Minucci S, Pelicci PG, Kouzarides T (2002) Human SIR2 deacetylates p53 and antagonizes PML/p53-induced cellular senescence. *EMBO J* 21: 2383–2396

58 Seeler JS, Dejean A (1999) The PML nuclear bodies: actors or extras? *Curr Opin Genet Dev* 9: 362–367

59 Bereshchenko OR, Gu W, Dalla-Favera R (2002) Acetylation inactivates the transcriptional repressor BCL6. *Nat Genet* 32: 606–613

60 Muth V, Nadaud S, Grummt I, Voit R (2001) Acetylation of TAF(I)68, a subunit of TIF-IB/SL1, activates RNA polymerase I transcription. *EMBO J* 20: 1353–1362

61 McBurney MW, Yang X, Jardine K, Bieman M, Th'ng J, Lemieux M (2003) The absence of SIR2alpha protein has no effect on global gene silencing in mouse embryonic stem cells. *Mol Cancer Res* 1: 402–409

62 Cheng HL, Mostoslavsky R, Saito S, Manis JP, Gu Y, Patel P, Bronson R, Appella E, Alt FW, Chua KF (2003) Developmental defects and p53 hyperacetylation in Sir2 homolog (SIRT1)-deficient mice. *Proc Natl Acad Sci USA* 100: 10794–10799

63 Blander G, Guarente L (2004) The Sir2 family of protein deacetylases. *Annu Rev Biochem* 73: 417–435

64 Urnov FD, Wolffe AP (2001) Chromatin remodeling and transcriptional activation: the cast (in order of appearance). *Oncogene* 20: 2991–3006

65 Mahlknecht U, Hoelzer D (2000) Histone acetylation modifiers in the pathogenesis of malignant disease. *Mol Med* 6: 623–644

66 Timmermann S, Lehrmann H, Polesskaya A, Harel-Bellan A (2001) Histone acetylation and disease. *Cell Mol Life Sci* 58: 728–736

67 Giles RH, Peters DJ, Breuning MH (1998) Conjunction dysfunction: CBP/p300 in human disease. *Trends Genet* 14: 178–183

68 Gayther SA, Batley SJ, Linger L, Bannister A, Thorpe K, Chin SF, Daigo Y, Russell P, Wilson A, Sowter HM et al (2000) Mutations truncating the EP300 acetylase in human cancers. *Nat Genet* 24: 300–303
69 Murata T, Kurokawa R, Krones A, Tatsumi K, Ishii M, Taki T, Masuno M, Ohashi H, Yanagisawa M, Rosenfeld MG et al (2001) Defect of histone acetyltransferase activity of the nuclear transcriptional coactivator CBP in Rubinstein-Taybi syndrome. *Hum Mol Genet* 10: 1071–1076
70 Sakai K, Nagahara H, Abe K, Obata H (1992) Loss of heterozygosity on chromosome 16 in hepatocellular carcinoma. *J Gastroenterol Hepatol* 7: 288–292
71 Borrow J, Stanton VP Jr, Andresen JM, Becher R, Behm FG, Chaganti RS, Civin CI, Disteche C, Dube I, Frischauf AM et al (1996) The translocation t(8;16)(p11;p13) of acute myeloid leukaemia fuses a putative acetyltransferase to the CREB-binding protein. *Nat Genet* 14: 33–41
72 Liang J, Prouty L, Williams BJ, Dayton MA, Blanchard KL (1998) Acute mixed lineage leukemia with an inv(8)(p11q13) resulting in fusion of the genes for MOZ and TIF2. *Blood* 92: 2118–2122
73 Rowley JD, Reshmi S, Sobulo O, Musvee T, Anastasi J, Raimondi S, Schneider NR, Barredo JC, Cantu ES, Schlegelberger B et al (1997) All patients with the T(11;16)(q23;p13.3) that involves MLL and CBP have treatment-related hematologic disorders. *Blood* 90: 535–541
74 Fenrick R, Hiebert SW (1998) Role of histone deacetylases in acute leukemia. *J Cell Biochem Suppl* 31: 194–202
75 Pandolfi PP (2001) Transcription therapy for cancer. *Oncogene* 20: 3116–3127
76 Sears R, Ohtani K, Nevins JR (1997) Identification of positively and negatively acting elements regulating expression of the E2F2 gene in response to cell growth signals. *Mol Cell Biol* 17: 5227–5235
77 McArthur GA, Laherty CD, Queva C, Hurlin PJ, Loo L, James L, Grandori C, Gallant P, Shiio Y, Hokanson WC et al (1998) The Mad protein family links transcriptional repression to cell differentiation. *Cold Spring Harb Symp Quant Biol* 63: 423–433
78 Dang CV (1999) c-Myc target genes involved in cell growth, apoptosis, and metabolism. *Mol Cell Biol* 19: 1–11
79 Nomura T, Khan MM, Kaul SC, Dong HD, Wadhwa R, Colmenares C, Kohno I, Ishii S (1999) Ski is a component of the histone deacetylase complex required for transcriptional repression by Mad and thyroid hormone receptor. *Genes Dev* 13: 412–423
80 Sellers WR, Kaelin WG Jr (1997) Role of the retinoblastoma protein in the pathogenesis of human cancer. *J Clin Oncol* 15: 3301–3312
81 Hall M, Peters G (1996) Genetic alterations of cyclins, cyclin-dependent kinases, and Cdk inhibitors in human cancer. *Adv Cancer Res* 68: 67–108
82 Lin RJ, Nagy L, Inoue S, Shao W, Miller WH Jr, Evans RM (1998) Role of the histone deacetylase complex in acute promyelocytic leukaemia. *Nature* 391: 811–814
83 Grignani F, De Matteis S, Nervi C, Tomassoni L, Gelmetti V, Cioce M, Fanelli M, Ruthardt M, Ferrara FF, Zamir I et al (1998) Fusion proteins of the retinoic acid receptor-alpha recruit histone deacetylase in promyelocytic leukaemia. *Nature* 391: 815–818
84 Grignani F, Valtieri M, Gabbianelli M, Gelmetti V, Botta R, Luchetti L, Masella B, Morsilli O, Pelosi E, Samoggia P et al (2000) PML/RAR alpha fusion protein expression in normal human hematopoietic progenitors dictates myeloid commitment and the promyelocytic phenotype. *Blood* 96: 1531–1537

85 He LZ, Guidez F, Tribioli C, Peruzzi D, Ruthardt M, Zelent A, Pandolfi PP (1998) Distinct interactions of PML-RARalpha and PLZF-RARalpha with co-repressors determine differential responses to RA in APL. *Nat Genet* 18: 126–135
86 Dhordain P, Lin RJ, Quief S, Lantoine D, Kerckaert JP, Evans RM, Albagli O (1998) The LAZ3(BCL-6) oncoprotein recruits a SMRT/mSIN3A/histone deacetylase containing complex to mediate transcriptional repression. *Nucleic Acids Res* 26: 4645–4651
87 Kitabayashi I, Yokoyama A, Shimizu K, Ohki M (1998) Interaction and functional cooperation of the leukemia-associated factors AML1 and p300 in myeloid cell differentiation. *EMBO J* 17: 2994–3004
88 Wang J, Hoshino T, Redner RL, Kajigaya S, Liu JM (1998) ETO, fusion partner in t(8;21) acute myeloid leukemia, represses transcription by interaction with the human N-CoR/mSin3/HDAC1 complex. *Proc Natl Acad Sci USA* 95: 10860–10865
89 Wang J, Saunthararajah Y, Redner RL, Liu JM (1999) Inhibitors of histone deacetylase relieve ETO-mediated repression and induce differentiation of AML1-ETO leukemia cells. *Cancer Res* 59: 2766–2769
90 Tsuji N, Kobayashi M, Nagashima K, Wakisaka Y, Koizumi K (1976) A new antifungal antibiotic, trichostatin. *J Antibiot (Tokyo)* 29: 1–6
91 Yoshida M, Kijima M, Akita M, Beppu T (1990) Potent and specific inhibition of mammalian histone deacetylase both *in vivo* and *in vitro* by trichostatin A. *J Biol Chem* 265: 17174–17179
92 Kim YB, Lee KH, Sugita K, Yoshida M, Horinouchi S (1999) Oxamflatin is a novel antitumor compound that inhibits mammalian histone deacetylase. *Oncogene* 18: 2461–2470
93 Remiszewski SW, Sambucetti LC, Bair KW, Bontempo J, Cesarz D, Chandramouli N, Chen R, Cheung M, Cornell-Kennon S, Dean K et al (2003) *N*-hydroxy-3-phenyl-2-propenamides as novel inhibitors of human histone deacetylase with *in vivo* antitumor activity: discovery of (2E)-*N*-hydroxy-3-[4-[[(2-hydroxyethyl)[2-(1H-indol-3-yl)-ethyl]amino]methyl]phenyl]-2-propenamide (NVP-LAQ824). *J Med Chem* 46: 4609–4624
94 Richon VM, Emiliani S, Verdin E, Webb Y, Breslow R, Rifkind RA, Marks PA (1998) A class of hybrid polar inducers of transformed cell differentiation inhibits histone deacetylases. *Proc Natl Acad Sci USA* 95: 3003–3007
95 Butler LM, Webb Y, Agus DB, Higgins B, Tolentino TR, Kutko MC, LaQuaglia MP, Drobnjak M, Cordon-Cardo C, Scher HI et al (2001) Inhibition of transformed cell growth and induction of cellular differentiation by pyroxamide, an inhibitor of histone deacetylase. *Clin Cancer Res* 7: 962–970
96 Kijima M, Yoshida M, Sugita K, Horinouchi S, Beppu T (1993) Trapoxin, an antitumor cyclic tetrapeptide, is an irreversible inhibitor of mammalian histone deacetylase. *J Biol Chem* 268: 22429–22435
97 Hirota A, Suzuki A, Aizawa K, Tamura S (1974) Mass spectrometric determination of amino acid sequence in Cyl-2, a novel cyclotetrapeptide from *Cylindrocladium scoparium*. *Biomed Mass Spectrom* 1: 15–19
98 Kawai M, Rich DH, Walton JD (1983) The structure and conformation of HC-toxin. *Biochem Biophys Res Commun* 111: 398–403
99 Umehara K, Nakahara K, Kiyoto S, Iwami M, Okamoto M, Tanaka H, Kohsaka M, Aoki H, Imanaka H (1983) Studies on WF-3161, a new antitumor antibiotic. *J Antibiot (Tokyo)* 36: 478–483

100 Closse A, Huguenin R (1974) Isolation and structural clarification of chlamydocin. *Helv Chim Acta* 57: 533–545

101 Darkin-Rattray SJ, Gurnett AM, Myers RW, Dulski PM, Crumley TM, Allocco JJ, Cannova C, Meinke PT, Colletti SL, Bednarek MA et al (1996) Apicidin: a novel antiprotozoal agent that inhibits parasite histone deacetylase. *Proc Natl Acad Sci USA* 93: 13143–13147

102 Nakajima H, Kim YB, Terano H, Yoshida M, Horinouchi S (1998) FR901228, a potent antitumor antibiotic, is a novel histone deacetylase inhibitor. *Exp Cell Res* 241: 126–133

103 Newmark HL, Lupton JR, Young CW (1994) Butyrate as a differentiating agent: pharmacokinetics, analogues and current status. *Cancer Lett* 78: 1–5

104 Warrell RP Jr, He LZ, Richon V, Calleja E, Pandolfi PP (1998) Therapeutic targeting of transcription in acute promyelocytic leukemia by use of an inhibitor of histone deacetylase. *J Natl Cancer Inst* 90: 1621–1625

105 Phiel CJ, Zhang F, Huang EY, Guenther MG, Lazar MA, Klein PS (2001) Histone deacetylase is a direct target of valproic acid, a potent anticonvulsant, mood stabilizer, and teratogen. *J Biol Chem* 25: 25

106 Saito A, Yamashita T, Mariko Y, Nosaka Y, Tsuchiya K, Ando T, Suzuki T, Tsuruo T, Nakanishi O (1999) A synthetic inhibitor of histone deacetylase, MS-27–275, with marked *in vivo* antitumor activity against human tumors. *Proc Natl Acad Sci USA* 96: 4592–4597

107 Kwon HJ, Owa T, Hassig CA, Shimada J, Schreiber SL (1998) Depudecin induces morphological reversion of transformed fibroblasts via the inhibition of histone deacetylase. *Proc Natl Acad Sci USA* 95: 3356–3361

108 Tsuji N, Kobayashi M (1978) Trichostatin C, a glucopyranosyl hydroxamate. *J Antibiot (Tokyo)* 31: 939–944

109 Yoshida M, Nomura S, Beppu T (1987) Effects of trichostatins on differentiation of murine erythroleukemia cells. *Cancer Res* 47: 3688–3691

110 Yoshida M, Horinouchi S, Beppu T (1995) Trichostatin A and trapoxin: novel chemical probes for the role of histone acetylation in chromatin structure and function. *Bioessays* 17: 423–430

111 Yoshida M, Hoshikawa Y, Koseki K, Mori K, Beppu T (1990) Structural specificity for biological activity of trichostatin A, a specific inhibitor of mammalian cell cycle with potent differentiation- inducing activity in Friend leukemia cells. *J Antibiot (Tokyo)* 43: 1101–1106

112 Yoshida M, Beppu T (1988) Reversible arrest of proliferation of rat 3Y1 fibroblasts in both the G1 and G2 phases by trichostatin A. *Exp Cell Res* 177: 122–131

113 Cousens LS, Gallwitz D, Alberts BM (1979) Different accessibilities in chromatin to histone acetylase. *J Biol Chem* 254: 1716–1723

114 Kruh J (1982) Effects of sodium butyrate, a new pharmacological agent, on cells in culture. *Mol Cell Biochem* 42: 65–82

115 Itazaki H, Nagashima K, Sugita K, Yoshida H, Kawamura Y, Yasuda Y, Matsumoto K, Ishii K, Uotani N, Nakai H et al (1990) Isolation and structural elucidation of new cyclotetrapeptides, trapoxins A and B, having detransformation activities as antitumor agents. *J Antibiot (Tokyo)* 43: 1524–1532

116 Han JW, Ahn SH, Park SH, Wang SY, Bae GU, Seo DW, Kwon HK, Hong S, Lee HY, Lee YW et al (2000) Apicidin, a histone deacetylase inhibitor, inhibits proliferation of tumor cells via induction of p21WAF1/Cip1 and gelsolin. *Cancer Res* 60: 6068–6074

117 Oikawa T, Onozawa C, Inose M, Sasaki M (1995) Depudecin, a microbial metabolite containing two epoxide groups, exhibits anti-angiogenic activity *in vivo*. *Biol Pharm Bull* 18: 1305–1307
118 Shimada J, Kwon HJ, Sawamura M, Schreiber SL (1995) Synthesis and cellular characterization of the detransformation agent, (-)-depudecin. *Chem Biol* 2: 517–525
119 Plumb JA, Finn PW, Williams RJ, Bandara MJ, Romero MR, Watkins CJ, La Thangue NB, Brown R (2003) Pharmacodynamic response and inhibition of growth of human tumor xenografts by the novel histone deacetylase inhibitor PXD101. *Mol Cancer Ther* 2: 721–728
120 Finnin MS, Donigian JR, Cohen A, Richon VM, Rifkind RA, Marks PA, Breslow R, Pavletich NP (1999) Structures of a histone deacetylase homologue bound to the TSA and SAHA inhibitors. *Nature* 401: 188–193
121 Vannini A, Volpari C, Filocamo G, Casavola EC, Brunetti M, Renzoni D, Chakravarty P, Paolini C, De Francesco R, Gallinari P et al (2004) Crystal structure of a eukaryotic zinc-dependent histone deacetylase, human HDAC8, complexed with a hydroxamic acid inhibitor. *Proc Natl Acad Sci USA* 101: 15064–15069
122 Somoza JR, Skene RJ, Katz BA, Mol C, Ho JD, Jennings AJ, Luong C, Arvai A, Buggy JJ, Chi E et al (2004) Structural snapshots of human HDAC8 provide insights into the class I histone deacetylases. *Structure (Camb)* 12: 1325–1334
123 Furumai R, Komatsu Y, Nishino N, Khochbin S, Yoshida M, Horinouchi S (2001) Potent histone deacetylase inhibitors built from trichostatin A and cyclic tetrapeptide antibiotics including trapoxin. *Proc Natl Acad Sci USA* 98: 87–92
124 Suzuki T, Ando T, Tsuchiya K, Fukazawa N, Saito A, Mariko Y, Yamashita T, Nakanishi O (1999) Synthesis and histone deacetylase inhibitory activity of new benzamide derivatives. *J Med Chem* 42: 3001–3003
125 Wong JC, Hong R, Schreiber SL (2003) Structural biasing elements for in-cell histone deacetylase paralog selectivity. *J Am Chem Soc* 125: 5586–5587
126 Haggarty SJ, Koeller KM, Wong JC, Butcher RA, Schreiber SL (2003) Multidimensional chemical genetic analysis of diversity-oriented synthesis-derived deacetylase inhibitors using cell-based assays. *Chem Biol* 10: 383–396
127 Frey RR, Wada CK, Garland RB, Curtin ML, Michaelides MR, Li J, Pease LJ, Glaser KB, Marcotte PA, Bouska JJ et al (2002) Trifluoromethyl ketones as inhibitors of histone deacetylase. *Bioorg Med Chem Lett* 12: 3443–3447
128 Wada CK, Frey RR, Ji Z, Curtin ML, Garland RB, Holms JH, Li J, Pease LJ, Guo J, Glaser KB et al (2003) Alpha-keto amides as inhibitors of histone deacetylase. *Bioorg Med Chem Lett* 13: 3331–3335
129 Vasudevan A, Ji Z, Frey RR, Wada CK, Steinman D, Heyman HR, Guo Y, Curtin ML, Guo J, Li J et al (2003) Heterocyclic ketones as inhibitors of histone deacetylase. *Bioorg Med Chem Lett* 13: 3909–3913
130 Suzuki T, Nagano Y, Matsuura A, Kohara A, Ninomiya S, Kohda K, Miyata N (2003) Novel histone deacetylase inhibitors: design, synthesis, enzyme inhibition, and binding mode study of SAHA-based non-hydroxamates. *Bioorg Med Chem Lett* 13: 4321–4326
131 Wu TY, Hassig C, Wu Y, Ding S, Schultz PG (2004) Design, synthesis, and activity of HDAC inhibitors with a N-formyl hydroxylamine head group. *Bioorg Med Chem Lett* 14: 449–453

132 Suzuki T, Kouketsu A, Matsuura A, Kohara A, Ninomiya S, Kohda K, Miyata N (2004) Thiol-based SAHA analogues as potent histone deacetylase inhibitors. *Bioorg Med Chem Lett* 14: 3313–3317

133 Suzuki T, Matsuura A, Kouketsu A, Nakagawa H, Miyata N (2005) Identification of a potent non-hydroxamate histone deacetylase inhibitor by mechanism-based drug design. *Bioorg Med Chem Lett* 15: 331–335

134 Bernstein BE, Tong JK, Schreiber SL (2000) Genomewide studies of histone deacetylase function in yeast. *Proc Natl Acad Sci USA* 97: 13708–13713

135 Curtin M, Glaser K (2003) Histone deacetylase inhibitors: the Abbott experience. *Curr Med Chem* 10: 2373–2392

136 Kawaguchi Y, Kovacs JJ, McLaurin A, Vance JM, Ito A, Yao TP (2003) The deacetylase HDAC6 regulates aggresome formation and cell viability in response to misfolded protein stress. *Cell* 115: 727–738

137 Grozinger CM, Hassig CA, Schreiber SL (1999) Three proteins define a class of human histone deacetylases related to yeast Hda1p. *Proc Natl Acad Sci USA* 96: 4868–4873

138 Verdel A, Khochbin S (1999) Identification of a new family of higher eukaryotic histone deacetylases. Coordinate expression of differentiation-dependent chromatin modifiers. *J Biol Chem* 274: 2440–2445

139 Hu E, Dul E, Sung CM, Chen Z, Kirkpatrick R, Zhang GF, Johanson K, Liu R, Lago A, Hofmann G et al (2003) Identification of novel isoform-selective inhibitors within class I histone deacetylases. *J Pharmacol Exp Ther* 307: 720–728

140 Furumai R, Matsuyama A, Kobashi N, Lee KH, Nishiyama M, Nakajima H, Tanaka A, Komatsu Y, Nishino N, Yoshida M et al (2002) FK228 (depsipeptide) as a natural prodrug that inhibits class I histone deacetylases. *Cancer Res* 62: 4916–4921

141 Bedalov A, Gatbonton T, Irvine WP, Gottschling DE, Simon JA (2001) Identification of a small molecule inhibitor of Sir2p. *Proc Natl Acad Sci USA* 98: 15113–15118

142 Howitz KT, Bitterman KJ, Cohen HY, Lamming DW, Lavu S, Wood JG, Zipkin RE, Chung P, Kisielewski A, Zhang LL et al (2003) Small molecule activators of sirtuins extend *Saccharomyces cerevisiae* lifespan. *Nature* 425: 191–196

143 Wahrman MZ, Gagnier SE, Kobrin DR, Higgins PJ, Augenlicht LH (1985) Cellular and molecular changes in 3T3 cells transformed spontaneously or by DNA transfection. *Tumour Biol* 6: 41–56

144 Wang E, Goldberg AR (1976) Changes in microfilament organization and surface topogrophy upon transformation of chick embryo fibroblasts with Rous sarcoma virus. *Proc Natl Acad Sci USA* 73: 4065–4069

145 Hoshikawa Y, Kwon HJ, Yoshida M, Horinouchi S, Beppu T (1994) Trichostatin A induces morphological changes and gelsolin expression by inhibiting histone deacetylase in human carcinoma cell lines. *Exp Cell Res* 214: 189–197

146 Kwiatkowski DJ (1988) Predominant induction of gelsolin and actin-binding protein during myeloid differentiation. *J Biol Chem* 263: 13857–13862

147 Tanaka M, Mullauer L, Ogiso Y, Fujita H, Moriya S, Furuuchi K, Harabayashi T, Shinohara N, Koyanagi T, Kuzumaki N (1995) Gelsolin: a candidate for suppressor of human bladder cancer. *Cancer Res* 55: 3228–3232

148 Archer SY, Meng S, Shei A, Hodin RA (1998) p21(WAF1) is required for butyrate-mediated growth inhibition of human colon cancer cells. *Proc Natl Acad Sci USA* 95: 6791–6796

149 Di Leonardo A, Linke SP, Clarkin K, Wahl GM (1994) DNA damage triggers a prolonged p53-dependent G1 arrest and long-term induction of Cip1 in normal human fibroblasts. *Genes Dev* 8: 2540–2551

150 Xiao H, Hasegawa T, Isobe K (1999) Both Sp1 and Sp3 are responsible for p21waf1 promoter activity induced by histone deacetylase inhibitor in NIH3T3 cells. *J Cell Biochem* 73: 291–302

151 Sowa Y, Orita T, Minamikawa S, Nakano K, Mizuno T, Nomura H, Sakai T (1997) Histone deacetylase inhibitor activates the WAF1/Cip1 gene promoter through the Sp1 sites. *Biochem Biophys Res Commun* 241: 142–150

152 Sowa Y, Orita T, Hiranabe-Minamikawa S, Nakano K, Mizuno T, Nomura H, Sakai T (1999) Histone deacetylase inhibitor activates the p21/WAF1/Cip1 gene promoter through the Sp1 sites. *Ann N Y Acad Sci* 886: 195–199

153 Sandor V, Senderowicz A, Mertins S, Sackett D, Sausville E, Blagosklonny MV, Bates SE (2000) P21-dependent g(1)arrest with downregulation of cyclin D1 and upregulation of cyclin E by the histone deacetylase inhibitor FR901228. *Br J Cancer* 83: 817–825

154 Burgess AJ, Pavey S, Warrener R, Hunter LJ, Piva TJ, Musgrove EA, Saunders N, Parsons PG, Gabrielli BG (2001) Up-regulation of p21(WAF1/CIP1) by histone deacetylase inhibitors reduces their cytotoxicity. *Mol Pharmacol* 60: 828–837

155 Vrana JA, Decker RH, Johnson CR, Wang Z, Jarvis WD, Richon VM, Ehinger M, Fisher PB, Grant S (1999) Induction of apoptosis in U937 human leukemia cells by suberoylanilide hydroxamic acid (SAHA) proceeds through pathways that are regulated by Bcl-2/Bcl-XL, c-Jun, and p21CIP1, but independent of p53. *Oncogene* 18: 7016–7025

156 Qiu L, Burgess A, Fairlie DP, Leonard H, Parsons PG, Gabrielli BG (2000) Histone deacetylase inhibitors trigger a G2 checkpoint in normal cells that is defective in tumor cells. *Mol Biol Cell* 11: 2069–2083

157 Johnstone RW (2002) Histone-deacetylase inhibitors: novel drugs for the treatment of cancer. *Nat Rev Drug Discov* 1: 287–299

158 Van Lint C, Emiliani S, Verdin E (1996) The expression of a small fraction of cellular genes is changed in response to histone hyperacetylation. *Gene Expr* 5: 245–253

159 Huang L, Pardee AB (2000) Suberoylanilide hydroxamic acid as a potential therapeutic agent for human breast cancer treatment. *Mol Med* 6: 849–866

160 Sambucetti LC, Fischer DD, Zabludoff S, Kwon PO, Chamberlin H, Trogani N, Xu H, Cohen D (1999) Histone deacetylase inhibition selectively alters the activity and expression of cell cycle proteins leading to specific chromatin acetylation and antiproliferative effects. *J Biol Chem* 274: 34940–34947

161 Richon VM, Sandhoff TW, Rifkind RA, Marks PA (2000) Histone deacetylase inhibitor selectively induces p21WAF1 expression and gene-associated histone acetylation. *Proc Natl Acad Sci USA* 97: 10014–10019

162 Mielnicki LM, Ying AM, Head KL, Asch HL, Asch BB (1999) Epigenetic regulation of gelsolin expression in human breast cancer cells. *Exp Cell Res* 249: 161–176

163 Takakura M, Kyo S, Sowa Y, Wang Z, Yatabe N, Maida Y, Tanaka M, Inoue M (2001) Telomerase activation by histone deacetylase inhibitor in normal cells. *Nucleic Acids Res* 29: 3006–3011

164 Sakaguchi K, Herrera JE, Saito S, Miki T, Bustin M, Vassilev A, Anderson CW, Appella E (1998) DNA damage activates p53 through a phosphorylation-acetylation cascade. *Genes Dev* 12: 2831–2841

165 Liu L, Scolnick DM, Trievel RC, Zhang HB, Marmorstein R, Halazonetis TD, Berger SL (1999) p53 sites acetylated *in vitro* by PCAF and p300 are acetylated *in vivo* in response to DNA damage. *Mol Cell Biol* 19: 1202–1209

166 Zhang W, Bieker JJ (1998) Acetylation and modulation of erythroid Kruppel-like factor (EKLF) activity by interaction with histone acetyltransferases. *Proc Natl Acad Sci USA* 95: 9855–9860

167 Chen H, Lin RJ, Xie W, Wilpitz D, Evans RM (1999) Regulation of hormone-induced histone hyperacetylation and gene activation via acetylation of an acetylase. *Cell* 98: 675–686

168 Vigushin DM, Ali S, Pace PE, Mirsaidi N, Ito K, Adcock I, Coombes RC (2001) Trichostatin A is a histone deacetylase inhibitor with potent antitumor activity against breast cancer *in vivo*. *Clin Cancer Res* 7: 971–976

169 Fu M, Wang C, Zhang X, Pestell RG (2004) Acetylation of nuclear receptors in cellular growth and apoptosis. *Biochem Pharmacol* 68: 1199–1208

170 Alao JP, Lam EW, Ali S, Buluwela L, Bordogna W, Lockey P, Varshochi R, Stavropoulou AV, Coombes RC, Vigushin DM (2004) Histone deacetylase inhibitor trichostatin A represses estrogen receptor alpha-dependent transcription and promotes proteasomal degradation of cyclin D1 in human breast carcinoma cell lines. *Clin Cancer Res* 10: 8094–8104

171 Yu X, Guo ZS, Marcu MG, Neckers L, Nguyen DM, Chen GA, Schrump DS (2002) Modulation of p53, ErbB1, ErbB2, and Raf-1 expression in lung cancer cells by depsipeptide FR901228. *J Natl Cancer Inst* 94: 504–513

172 Fuino L, Bali P, Wittmann S, Donapaty S, Guo F, Yamaguchi H, Wang HG, Atadja P, Bhalla K (2003) Histone deacetylase inhibitor LAQ824 down-regulates Her-2 and sensitizes human breast cancer cells to trastuzumab, taxotere, gemcitabine, and epothilone B. *Mol Cancer Ther* 2: 971–984

173 Nimmanapalli R, Fuino L, Bali P, Gasparetto M, Glozak M, Tao J, Moscinski L, Smith C, Wu J, Jove R et al (2003) Histone deacetylase inhibitor LAQ824 both lowers expression and promotes proteasomal degradation of Bcr-Abl and induces apoptosis of imatinib mesylate-sensitive or -refractory chronic myelogenous leukemia-blast crisis cells. *Cancer Res* 63: 5126–5135

174 Sealy L, Chalkley R (1978) DNA associated with hyperacetylated histone is preferentially digested by DNase I. *Nucleic Acids Res* 5: 1863–1876

175 Huang H, Reed CP, Zhang JS, Shridhar V, Wang L, Smith DI (1999) Carboxypeptidase A3 (CPA3): a novel gene highly induced by histone deacetylase inhibitors during differentiation of prostate epithelial cancer cells. *Cancer Res* 59: 2981–2988

176 Medina V, Edmonds B, Young GP, James R, Appleton S, Zalewski PD (1997) Induction of caspase-3 protease activity and apoptosis by butyrate and trichostatin A (inhibitors of histone deacetylase): dependence on protein synthesis and synergy with a mitochondrial/cytochrome c-dependent pathway. *Cancer Res* 57: 3697–3707

177 Lee E, Furukubo T, Miyabe T, Yamauchi A, Kariya K (1996) Involvement of histone hyperacetylation in triggering DNA fragmentation of rat thymocytes undergoing apoptosis. *FEBS Lett* 395: 183–187

178 Bernhard D, Ausserlechner MJ, Tonko M, Loffler M, Hartmann BL, Csordas A, Kofler R (1999) Apoptosis induced by the histone deacetylase inhibitor sodium butyrate in human leukemic lymphoblasts. *FASEB J* 13: 1991–2001

179 Glick RD, Swendeman SL, Coffey DC, Rifkind RA, Marks PA, Richon VM, La Quaglia MP (1999) Hybrid polar histone deacetylase inhibitor induces apoptosis and CD95/CD95 ligand expression in human neuroblastoma. *Cancer Res* 59: 4392–4399
180 Qiu L, Kelso MJ, Hansen C, West ML, Fairlie DP, Parsons PG (1999) Anti-tumour activity *in vitro* and *in vivo* of selective differentiating agents containing hydroxamate. *Br J Cancer* 80: 1252–1258
181 Parsons PG, Hansen C, Fairlie DP, West ML, Danoy PA, Sturm RA, Dunn IS, Pedley J, Ablett EM (1997) Tumor selectivity and transcriptional activation by azelaic bishydroxamic acid in human melanocytic cells. *Biochem Pharmacol* 53: 1719–1724
182 Rajgolikar G, Chan KK, Wang HC (1998) Effects of a novel antitumor depsipeptide, FR901228, on human breast cancer cells. *Breast Cancer Res Treat* 51: 29–38
183 Byrd JC, Shinn C, Ravi R, Willis CR, Waselenko JK, Flinn IW, Dawson NA, Grever MR (1999) Depsipeptide (FR901228): a novel therapeutic agent with selective, *in vitro* activity against human B-cell chronic lymphocytic leukemia cells. *Blood* 94: 1401–1408
184 Gray SG, Yakovleva T, Hartmann W, Tally M, Bakalkin G, Ekstrom TJ (1999) IGF-II enhances trichostatin A-induced TGFbeta1 and p21(Waf1,Cip1, sdi1) expression in Hep3B cells. *Exp Cell Res* 253: 618–628
185 Koyama Y, Adachi M, Sekiya M, Takekawa M, Imai K (2000) Histone deacetylase inhibitors suppress IL-2-mediated gene expression prior to induction of apoptosis. *Blood* 96: 1490–1495
186 Futamura M, Monden Y, Okabe T, Fujita-Yoshigaki J, Yokoyama S, Nishimura S (1995) Trichostatin A inhibits both ras-induced neurite outgrowth of PC12 cells and morphological transformation of NIH3T3 cells. *Oncogene* 10: 1119–1123
187 Ruefli AA, Ausserlechner MJ, Bernhard D, Sutton VR, Tainton KM, Kofler R, Smyth MJ, Johnstone RW (2001) The histone deacetylase inhibitor and chemotherapeutic agent suberoylanilide hydroxamic acid (SAHA) induces a cell-death pathway characterized by cleavage of Bid and production of reactive oxygen species. *Proc Natl Acad Sci USA* 98: 10833–10838
188 Ruefli AA, Bernhard D, Tainton KM, Kofler R, Smyth MJ, Johnstone RW (2002) Suberoylanilide hydroxamic acid (SAHA) overcomes multidrug resistance and induces cell death in P-glycoprotein-expressing cells. *Int J Cancer* 99: 292–298
189 Rosato RR, Almenara JA, Grant S (2003) The histone deacetylase inhibitor MS-275 promotes differentiation or apoptosis in human leukemia cells through a process regulated by generation of reactive oxygen species and induction of p21CIP1/WAF1 1. *Cancer Res* 63: 3637–3645
190 Zhu WG, Lakshmanan RR, Beal MD, Otterson GA (2001) DNA methyltransferase inhibition enhances apoptosis induced by histone deacetylase inhibitors. *Cancer Res* 61: 1327–1333
191 Ng HH, Bird A (1999) DNA methylation and chromatin modification. *Curr Opin Genet Dev* 9: 158–163
192 Wade PA, Gegonne A, Jones PL, Ballestar E, Aubry F, Wolffe AP (1999) Mi-2 complex couples DNA methylation to chromatin remodelling and histone deacetylation. *Nat Genet* 23: 62–66
193 Cameron EE, Bachman KE, Myohanen S, Herman JG, Baylin SB (1999) Synergy of demethylation and histone deacetylase inhibition in the re-expression of genes silenced in cancer. *Nat Genet* 21: 103–107

194 Yang X, Ferguson AT, Nass SJ, Phillips DL, Butash KA, Wang SM, Herman JG, Davidson NE (2000) Transcriptional activation of estrogen receptor alpha in human breast cancer cells by histone deacetylase inhibition. *Cancer Res* 60: 6890–6894

195 Weiser TS, Guo ZS, Ohnmacht GA, Parkhurst ML, Tong-On P, Marincola FM, Fischette MR, Yu X, Chen GA, Hong JA et al (2001) Sequential 5-Aza-2 deoxycytidine-depsipeptide FR901228 treatment induces apoptosis preferentially in cancer cells and facilitates their recognition by cytolytic T lymphocytes specific for NY-ESO-1. *J Immunother* 24: 151–161

196 Kwon HJ, Kim MS, Kim MJ, Nakajima H, Kim KW (2002) Histone deacetylase inhibitor FK228 inhibits tumor angiogenesis. *Int J Cancer* 97: 290–296

197 Kim MS, Blake M, Baek JH, Kohlhagen G, Pommier Y, Carrier F (2003) Inhibition of histone deacetylase increases cytotoxicity to anticancer drugs targeting DNA. *Cancer Res* 63: 7291–7300

198 Yu C, Rahmani M, Almenara J, Subler M, Krystal G, Conrad D, Varticovski L, Dent P, Grant S (2003) Histone deacetylase inhibitors promote STI571-mediated apoptosis in STI571-sensitive and -resistant Bcr/Abl+ human myeloid leukemia cells. *Cancer Res* 63: 2118–2126

199 Jang ER, Lim SJ, Lee ES, Jeong G, Kim TY, Bang YJ, Lee JS (2004) The histone deacetylase inhibitor trichostatin A sensitizes estrogen receptor alpha-negative breast cancer cells to tamoxifen. *Oncogene* 23: 1724–1736

200 Aviram A, Zimrah Y, Shaklai M, Nudelman A, Rephaeli A (1994) Comparison between the effect of butyric acid and its prodrug pivaloyloxymethylbutyrate on histones hyperacetylation in an HL-60 leukemic cell line. *Int J Cancer* 56: 906–909

201 Ueda H, Manda T, Matsumoto S, Mukumoto S, Nishigaki F, Kawamura I, Shimomura K (1994) FR901228, a novel antitumor bicyclic depsipeptide produced by *Chromobacterium violaceum* No. 968. III. Antitumor activities on experimental tumors in mice. *J Antibiot (Tokyo)* 47: 315–323

202 Kosugi H, Ito M, Yamamoto Y, Towatari M, Ueda R, Saito H, Naoe T (2001) *In vivo* effects of a histone deacetylase inhibitor, FK228, on human acute promyelocytic leukemia in NOD / Shi-scid/scid mice. *Jpn J Cancer Res* 92: 529–536

203 Kim MS, Kwon HJ, Lee YM, Baek JH, Jang JE, Lee SW, Moon EJ, Kim HS, Lee SK, Chung HY et al (2001) Histone deacetylases induce angiogenesis by negative regulation of tumor suppressor genes. *Nat Med* 7: 437–443

204 Marks PA, Richon VM, Rifkind RA (2000) Histone deacetylase inhibitors: inducers of differentiation or apoptosis of transformed cells. *J Natl Cancer Inst* 92: 1210–1216

205 Cohen LA, Amin S, Marks PA, Rifkind RA, Desai D, Richon VM (1999) Chemoprevention of carcinogen-induced mammary tumorigenesis by the hybrid polar cytodifferentiation agent, suberanilohydroxamic acid (SAHA). *Anticancer Res* 19: 4999–5005

206 Komatsu Y, Tomizaki KY, Tsukamoto M, Kato T, Nishino N, Sato S, Yamori T, Tsuruo T, Furumai R, Yoshida M et al (2001) Cyclic hydroxamic-acid-containing peptide 31, a potent synthetic histone deacetylase inhibitor with antitumor activity. *Cancer Res* 61: 4459–4466

207 Thibault A, Cooper MR, Figg WD, Venzon DJ, Sartor AO, Tompkins AC, Weinberger MS, Headlee DJ, McCall NA, Samid D et al (1994) A phase I and pharmacokinetic study of intravenous phenylacetate in patients with cancer. *Cancer Res* 54: 1690–1694

208 Conley BA, Egorin MJ, Tait N, Rosen DM, Sausville EA, Dover G, Fram RJ, Van Echo DA (1998) Phase I study of the orally administered butyrate prodrug, tributyrin, in patients with solid tumors. *Clin Cancer Res* 4: 629–634

209 Gore SD, Carducci MA (2000) Modifying histones to tame cancer: clinical development of sodium phenylbutyrate and other histone deacetylase inhibitors. *Expert Opin Investig Drugs* 9: 2923–2934

210 Gilbert J, Baker SD, Bowling MK, Grochow L, Figg WD, Zabelina Y, Donehower RC, Carducci MA (2001) A phase I dose escalation and bioavailability study of oral sodium phenylbutyrate in patients with refractory solid tumor malignancies. *Clin Cancer Res* 7: 2292–2300

211 Novogrodsky A, Dvir A, Ravid A, Shkolnik T, Stenzel KH, Rubin AL, Zaizov R (1983) Effect of polar organic compounds on leukemic cells. Butyrate-induced partial remission of acute myelogenous leukemia in a child. *Cancer* 51: 9–14

212 Patnaik A, Rowinsky EK, Villalona MA, Hammond LA, Britten CD, Siu LL, Goetz A, Felton SA, Burton S, Valone FH et al (2002) A phase I study of pivaloyloxymethyl butyrate, a prodrug of the differentiating agent butyric acid, in patients with advanced solid malignancies. *Clin Cancer Res* 8: 2142–2148

213 Reid T, Valone F, Lipera W, Irwin D, Paroly W, Natale R, Sreedharan S, Keer H, Lum B, Scappaticci F et al (2004) Phase II trial of the histone deacetylase inhibitor pivaloyloxymethyl butyrate (Pivanex, AN-9) in advanced non-small cell lung cancer. *Lung Cancer* 45: 381–386

214 Gottlicher M, Minucci S, Zhu P, Kramer OH, Schimpf A, Giavara S, Sleeman JP, Lo Coco F, Nervi C, Pelicci PG et al (2001) Valproic acid defines a novel class of HDAC inhibitors inducing differentiation of transformed cells. *EMBO J* 20: 6969–6978

215 Vigushin DM (2002) FR-901228 Fujisawa/National Cancer Institute. *Curr Opin Investig Drugs* 3: 1396–1402

216 Chan KK, Bakhtiar R, Jiang C (1997) Depsipeptide (FR901228, NSC-630176) pharmacokinetics in the rat by LC/MS/MS. *Invest New Drugs* 15: 195–206

217 Sandor V, Bakke S, Robey RW, Kang MH, Blagosklonny MV, Bender J, Brooks R, Piekarz RL, Tucker E, Figg WD et al (2002) Phase I trial of the histone deacetylase inhibitor, depsipeptide (FR901228, NSC 630176), in patients with refractory neoplasms. *Clin Cancer Res* 8: 718–728

218 Prakash S, Foster BJ, Meyer M, Wozniak A, Heilbrun LK, Flaherty L, Zalupski M, Radulovic L, Valdivieso M, LoRusso PM (2001) Chronic oral administration of CI-994: a phase 1 study. *Invest New Drugs* 19: 1–11

219 Pauer LR, Olivares J, Cunningham C, Williams A, Grove W, Kraker A, Olson S, Nemunaitis J (2004) Phase I study of oral CI-994 in combination with carboplatin and paclitaxel in the treatment of patients with advanced solid tumors. *Cancer Invest* 22: 886–896

Progress in Drug Research, Vol. 63
(R. M. Schultz, Ed.)

Inhibitors of cyclin-dependent kinase modulators for cancer therapy

Adrian M. Senderowicz

Radiation Biology Branch
National Cancer Institute
National Institutes of Health
Bldg. 10, Room B3-B6, Bethesda
MD 20892, USA
<sendero@helix.nih.gov>

Key words

Cell cycle, molecular targets, cyclin-dependent kinases, flavopiridol, UCN-01, CYC202, BMS 387032, drug development.

Glossary of abbreviations

cdk, cyclin-dependent kinases; Rb, retinoblastoma; CAK, cdk-activating kinase; FU, fluorouracil; DLT, dose-limiting toxicity; MTD, maximal-tolerated dose; PKC, protein kinase C.

1 Brief overview of cell cycle regulation

Upon activation of mitogenic signaling cascades, cells commit to entry into a series of regulated steps allowing traverse of the cell cycle. Synthesis of DNA (genome duplication), also known as S phase, is followed by separation into two daughter cells (chromatid separation) or M phase. During the G_2 phase (the time between the S and M phases), cells can repair errors that occur during DNA duplication, preventing the propagation of these errors to daughter cells. In contrast, the G_1 phase, the time between the M and S phases, represents the period of commitment to cell cycle progression. In order for cells to continue cycling to the next phase, the prior phase has to be properly completed; otherwise, "fail safe" mechanisms, also known as "cell cycle checkpoints" are elicited [1].

The cell cycle machinery is governed by the cyclical activation of the cyclin-dependent kinases (cdk), serine-threonine kinases composed by the cdk catalytic subunit and cofactors such as cyclins and endogenous cdk inhibitors (CKI), such as $p21^{cip1/waf1}$. The main function of cdk is the phosphorylation of substrates required for cell cycle progression [2]. One crucial substrate of cdk is the gene product of the retinoblastoma gene (Rb), a tumor suppressor gene that is dysfunctional in the majority of human neoplasms due to "overactive" cdk [3, 4]. Thus, manipulation of cdk and cofactors is a potentially valuable strategy in cancer therapeutics [3, 4].

The fact that most tumors are aneuploid, reflecting abnormal sister chromatid separation has motivated increasing interest in the understanding of the mitotic checkpoints [5, 6]. There are at least two serine-threonine kinases relevant to mitotic checkpoints that are being targeted by small molecules: aurora and polo-like kinases [5, 7–10]. Depletion of several mitotic components (including aurora and polo-like kinases) by either small molecules, intracellular antibodies, dominant negative alleles or small interfering RNA (siRNA), promotes cell death in *in vitro* cancer models [8, 11–13]. This novel concept is being investigated intensely and several molecules are approaching phase I/II trials [14].

Another gene relevant to cell cycle regulation (and also to apoptosis) is p53, a tumor suppressor gene frequently inactivated in human cancer cells [15]. Transformed cells with inactivated p53 are unable to undergo apoptosis, which leads to growth imbalance and genomic instability [15]. Since the majority of tumor cells have lost the G_1 checkpoint (due to p53 mutations) but not the G_2 checkpoint, upon DNA damage they would arrest in G_2. Thus, the use of combination therapy of DNA-damaging agents (radiation or chemotherapy) and small molecules that selectively abrogate the G_2 checkpoint represents an attractive approach to cancer therapy. This approach could lead to tumor cell death due to accelerated mitosis and un-repaired DNA lesions, while sparing normal cells from some of the cytotoxic effects [4, 16, 17].

2 Cell cycle alterations in human neoplasms

In the last few years, it became clear that cyclins, cdk complexes, and other cell cycle regulators are mechanistically involved in the development of human tumors [18–20]. This is consistent with a large body of literature showing the importance of inactivation of the Rb pathway in tumor development [21]. The inactivation of Rb can be produced by direct mutation of the Rb protein, but this is a relatively rare event occurring only in retinoblastomas, osteosarcomas, and a minority of breast and some other tumors [22]. More frequent alterations of this pathway occur by functional inactivation of Rb by hyperphosphorylation. This is normally the result of elevated cdk activities caused by decrease in cdk endogenous inhibitor or by overexpression of cyclins and cdks. For example, several laboratories have reported that some tumors show loss of Rb or, alternatively, overexpression of cyclin D1 [23–25]. Similarly, in other tumors, loss of p16Ink4a and Rb are mutually exclusive [26, 27]. This observation led to the hypothesis that inactivation of the cyclin D/CDK/p16/pRb pathway can promote tumor development and that either loss of the suppressor activity of Rb or p16Ink4a, or overexpression of cyclin D1 can over-ride this checkpoint [22, 28]. Several reports have implicated D-type cyclins in neoplastic development, although limited information is available on the participation of its partner, cdk4, in these events. The involvement of cdk4 in the neoplastic process was suggested by the fact that cdk4 amplification and/or overexpression were detected in human glioblastomas, but in these tumors overexpression and/or amplification of D-type cyclins were not detected [29]. In addition, cdk4 mutations were identified in patients with familial melanoma [30] and, recently, amplification and overexpression of cdk4 were also detected in sporadic breast carcinomas [31], ovarian carcinomas [32], and sarcomas [33]. Taken together, proteins that govern cell cycle control are reasonable targets for cancer therapy [17, 34].

3 Manipulation of cdk activity for therapeutic purposes

Several strategies could be considered to modulate cdk activity. These strategies are divided into direct effects on the catalytic cdk subunit or indirect modulation of regulatory pathways that govern cdk activity [17, 34, 35]. Small molecular endogenous CKI (SCDKI) are compounds that directly target the catalytic cdk subunit. Most of these compounds modulate cdk activity by interacting specifically with the ATP-binding site of cdk [17, 34–37]. Examples of this class include flavopiridol, roscovitine, aminothiazole, UCN-01 (7-hydroxystaurosporine), BMS 387032, and alsterpaullone. The second class are compounds that modulate cdk activity by targeting the regulatory upstream pathways that govern cdk activity: by altering the expression and synthesis of the cdk/cyclin subunits or the cdk inhibitory proteins; by modulating the phosphorylation of cdk; by targeting cdk-activating kinase (CAK), cdc25, and wee1/myt1; or by manipulating the proteolytic machinery that regulates the catabolism of cdk/cyclin complexes or their regulators [3, 4, 35]. Examples for this class of compounds include perifosine and UCN-01, among others.

4 Small-molecule cdk modulators

As mentioned previously, cdk can be modulated by direct effects on the catalytic subunit and/or by disruption of upstream regulatory pathways. Several examples and mechanisms are described elsewhere [3, 4, 34–41].

5 Cdk modulators in clinical trials

5.1 Flavopiridol

5.1.1 Mechanism of antiproliferative effects

Flavopiridol (L86-8275 or HMR 1275) is a semisynthetic flavonoid derived from rohitukine, an indigenous plant from India. Initial studies with this flavonoid revealed clear evidence of G_1/S or G_2/M arrest, due to loss in cdk1 and cdk2 [42, 43]. Studies using purified cdk showed that the inhibition observed is reversible and competitively blocked by ATP, with a K_i of 41 nM [42–44]. Furthermore, the crystal structure of the complex of deschloroflavopiridol and cdk2 showed that flavopiridol binds to the ATP-binding pocket, with the benzopyran occupying the same region as the purine ring of ATP [45], confirming the earlier biochemical studies with flavopiridol [46]. Flavopiridol inhibits all cdk thus far examined (IC_{50} ~100 nM), but it inhibits cdk7 (CAK) less potently (IC_{50} ~300 nM) [46, 47].

In addition to directly inhibiting cdk, flavopiridol promotes a decrease in the level of cyclin D1, an oncogene that is overexpressed in many human neoplasias. Of note, neoplasms that overexpress cyclin D1 have a poor prognosis [48]. Depletion of cyclin D1 appears to lead to the loss of cdk activity [49]. Cyclin D1 decrease is caused by depletion of cyclin D1 mRNA and was associated with a specific decline in cyclin D1 promoter, measured by a luciferase reporter assay [49]. The transcriptional repression of cyclin D1 observed after treatment with flavopiridol is consistent with the effects of flavopiridol on yeast cells (see above) and underscores the conserved effect of flavopiridol on eukaryotic cyclin transcription [50]. In summary, flavopiridol can induce cell cycle arrest by at least three mechanisms: (1) direct inhibition of cdk activities by binding to the ATP-binding site; (2) prevention of the phosphorylation of cdk at threonine-160/161 by inhibition of cdk7/cyclin H [42, 44]; and (3) decrease in the amount of cyclin D1, an important cofactor for cdk4 and cdk6 activation (G_1/S arrest only).

In part, flavopiridol regulates transcription due to potent inhibition of P-TEFb (also known as cdk9/cyclin T), with a K_i of 3 nM, leading to inhibition of transcription by RNA polymerase II by blocking the transition into productive elongation. Interestingly, in contrast with all cdk tested so far, flavopiridol was not competitive with ATP in this reaction. P-TEFb is a required cellular cofactor for the human immunodeficiency virus (HIV-1) transactivator, Tat. Consistent with its ability to inhibit P-TEFb, flavopiridol blocked Tat transactivation of the viral promoter *in vitro*. Furthermore, flavopiridol blocked HIV-1 replication in both single-round and viral spread assays with an IC_{50} of less than 10 nM [51]. These actions of the drug led to the testing of flavopiridol through clinical trials for patients with HIV-related malignancies [52].

An important biochemical effect involved in the antiproliferative activity of flavopiridol is the induction of apoptotic cell death. Hematopoietic cell lines are often quite sensitive to flavopiridol-induced apoptotic cell death [53–57], but the mechanism(s) by which flavopiridol induces apoptosis have not yet been elucidated. Flavopiridol does not modulate topoisomerase I/II activity [56]. In certain hematopoietic cell lines, neither BCL-2/BAX nor p53 appeared to be affected [54, 58], whereas, in other systems, BCL-2 may be inhibited [55, 59]. It is still unclear whether the putative flavopiridol-induced inhibition of cdk activity is required for induction of apoptosis.

Clear evidence of cell cycle arrest along with apoptosis was observed in a panel of squamous head and neck cancer cell lines, including a cell line (HN30) that are refractory to several DNA-damaging agents, such as γ-irradiation and bleomycin [60]. Again, the apoptotic effect was independent of p53 status, and was associated with the depletion of cyclin D1 [60]. These findings have been corroborated in other preclinical models [49, 61–63].

Flavopiridol targets not only tumor cells but also angiogenesis pathways. Brusselbach et al. [64] incubated primary human umbilical vein endothelial cells (HUVEC) with flavopiridol and observed apoptotic cell death even in cells that were not cycling, leading to the notion that flavopiridol may have anti-angiogenic properties due to endothelial cytotoxicity. In other model systems, Kerr et al. [65] tested flavopiridol in an *in vivo* Matrigel model of angiogenesis, and found that flavopiridol decreased blood vessel formation, a surrogate marker for the anti-angiogenic effect of this compound. Furthermore, as mentioned earlier, Melillo et al. [66] demonstrated that, at low nanomolar concentrations, flavopiridol prevented the induction of vascular endothelial growth factor (VEGF) by hypoxic conditions in human monocytes due to decreased VEGF mRNA stability. Similar anti-angiogenic effects were observed in zebrafish *in vivo* models [67]. Thus, the antitumor activity of flavopiridol observed may be in part due to anti-angiogenic effects. Whether the various anti-angiogenic actions of flavopiridol result from its interaction with a cdk target or other targets requires further study.

The antitumor effect observed with flavopiridol can also be explained by activation of differentiation pathways. It became clear recently that cells become differentiated when exit of the cell cycle (G_0) and loss of cdk2 activity occur. Based on this information, Lee et al. [68] tested flavopiridol and roscovitine, both known cdk2 inhibitors, to determine if they induce a differentiated phenotype. For this purpose, NCI-H358 lung carcinoma cell lines were exposed to a cdk2 antisense construct, flavopiridol, or roscovitine. Clear evidence of mucinous differentiation along with loss in cdk2 activity was observed in this lung carcinoma model. Thus, it is plausible that the antitumor effect of flavopiridol in lung carcinoma models may be due to induction of differentiation, among others [68].

Several investigators determined that flavopiridol has synergistic effects with standard chemotherapeutic agents in several *in vitro* models. Synergistic effects were observed in A549 lung carcinoma cells when treatment with flavopiridol followed treatment with paclitaxel, cytarabine, topotecan, doxorubicin, or etoposide [69–72]. In contrast, a synergistic effect was observed with 5-fluorouracil (FU) only when cells were treated with flavopiridol for 24 h before the addition of 5-FU. Furthermore, synergistic effects with cisplatin were not schedule dependent [70]. However, Chien et al. [73] failed to demonstrate a synergistic effect between flavopiridol and cisplatin and/or γ-irradiation in bladder carcinoma models. One important issue to mention is that most of these studies were performed in *in vitro* models. Thus, confirmatory studies in *in vivo* animal models are needed.

Experiments using colorectal (Colo205) and prostate (LnCaP/DU-145) carcinoma xenograft models, in which flavopiridol was administered frequently over a protracted period, demonstrated that flavopiridol is cytostatic [74, 75]. These demonstrations led to human clinical trials of flavopiridol administered as a 72-h continuous infusion every 2 weeks [76] (see below). Subsequent studies in human leukemia/lymphoma xenografts demonstrated that flavopiridol administered intravenously as a bolus rendered animals tumor free, whereas flavopiridol administered as an infusion only delayed tumor growth [53]. Moreover, in HN-12 head and neck cancer xenografts flavopiridol administered intraperitoneally for 5 days demonstrated a substantial growth delay [60]. Again, apoptotic cell death and cyclin D1 depletion were observed in tissues from xenografts treated with flavopiridol [53]. Based on these results, a phase I trial of 1-h daily infusional flavopiridol every 3 weeks has been conducted at the NCI [77].

5.1.2 Clinical experience with flavopiridol

Two phase I clinical trials of flavopiridol administered as a 72-h continuous infusion every 2 weeks have been completed [76, 79]. In the NCI phase I trial (n = 76) of infusional flavopiridol, the dose-limiting toxicity (DLT) was secretory diarrhea with a maximal-tolerated dose (MTD) of 50 mg/m^2/day for 3 days. In the presence of anti-diarrheal prophylaxis (a combination of cholestyramine and loperamide), patients tolerated higher doses, defining a second MTD, 78 mg/m^2/day for 3 days. The DLT observed at the higher dose level was a substantial proinflammatory syndrome that is associated with induction of plasma IL-6 [76, 78]. Minor responses were observed in patients with non-Hodgkin's lymphoma, colon, and kidney cancer for more than 6 months. Moreover, one patient with refractory renal cancer achieved a partial response for more than 8 months [76]. Plasma concentrations of 300–500 nM flavopiridol, which inhibit cdk activity *in vitro*, were safely achieved during this trial [76].

In a complementary phase I trial also exploring the same schedule (72-h continuous infusion every 2 weeks), Thomas et al. [79] found that the DLT was diarrhea, corroborating the NCI experience. Moreover, plasma concentrations of 300–500 nM flavopiridol were also observed. Interestingly, there was one patient in this trial with refractory metastatic gastric cancer that progressed after a treatment regimen containing 5-FU. When treated with flavopiridol, this patient achieved a sustained complete response without any evidence of disease for more than 2 years after treatment was completed.

The first phase I trial of a daily 1-h infusion of flavopiridol was recently completed [77]. This schedule was based on antitumor results observed in leukemia/lymphoma and head and neck cancer xenografts treated with flavopiridol [53, 60]. A total of 55 patients were treated in this trial. The recommended phase II dose is 37.5 mg/m^2/day for 5 consecutive days. The DLT observed at 52.5 mg/m^2/day are nausea/vomiting, neutropenia, fatigue, and diarrhea [77]. Other side effects are local tumor pain and anorexia. To reach higher flavopiridol concentrations, the protocol was amended to administer flavopiridol for 3 days and then for 1 day only. With these protocol modifications, we were able to achieve concentrations (~4 µM) necessary to induce apoptosis in xenograft models [53, 60]. Of note, the half-life observed in this trial is much shorter (~3 h) than the infusional trial (~10 h). Thus, the high micromolar concentrations achieved in the 1-h infusional trial could be maintained only for short periods of time

Several phase II trials using the continuous infusion schedule (50 mg/m^2/day over 72 h) were recently conducted in several malignancies including melanoma, lung, kidney, and prostate cancer, and in patients with refractory head and neck cancer, chronic lymphocytic leukemia (CLL), and mantle cell lymphoma (MCL) among others. Unfortuntately, at this dose and schedule, flavopiridol monotherapy did not show significant antitumor activity [80–84].

Based on the interesting preclinical data in combination with cytotoxics and also based on the feasibility of flavopiridol administration as a short infusion, several phase I combination trials have been performed [85–88]. Activity was observed in patients with taxane-refractory disease. However, results of phase 3 trials with these combinations are needed before concluding that combinations are active in refractory cases.

5.2 UCN-01

5.2.1 Mechanism of antiproliferative activity

Staurosporine is a potent nonspecific protein and tyrosine kinase inhibitor, with a very low therapeutic index in animals [89]. Thus, efforts to find analogues of staurosporine have identified compounds specific for protein kinases. One staurosporine analogue, UCN-01, has potent activity against several protein kinase C (PKC) isoenzymes, particularly the Ca^{2+}-dependent PKC with an IC_{50} ~ 30 nM [90, 91]. In addition to its effects on PKC, UCN-01 has antiproliferative activity in several human tumor cell lines [91–93]. These effects appear not to be related to the effects of UCN-01 in PKC signaling [94].

Another interesting feature, again unrelated to PKC, is 'inappropriate activation' of cdk kinases in intact cells [94]. This phenomenon correlates with the G_2 abrogation checkpoint observed with this agent. Experimental evidence suggests that DNA damage leads to cell cycle arrest to allow DNA repair. In the presence of UCN-01, irradiated cells are unable to accumulate in the G_2 phase with subsequent early mitosis and the onset of apoptotic cell death [93]. The accelerated mitosis is due to activation of cdc2 kinase. These activations could be partially explained by the inactivation of wee1, the kinase that negatively regulates the G_2/M phase transition [95]. Moreover,

UCN-01 can have a direct effect on chk1, the protein kinase that regulates the G_2 checkpoint [96–98]. Thus, although UCN-01 at high concentrations can directly inhibit cdk *in vitro*, UCN-01 can modulate cellular 'upstream' regulators at much lower concentration, leading to inappropriate cdc2 activation. Studies from other groups suggest that not only is UCN-01 able to abrogate the G_2 checkpoint induced by DNA-damaging agents, it is also, in some circumstances, able to abrogate the DNA damage-induced S phase checkpoint [99, 100].

Another interesting property of UCN-01 is its ability to arrest cells in the G_1 phase of the cell cycle [91, 101–108]. When human epidermoid carcinoma A431 cells (mutated p53) or HN12 head and neck carcinoma cell lines are incubated with UCN-01, these cells were arrested in the G_1 phase with Rb hypophosphorylation and $p21^{waf1/p27kip1}$ accumulation [102, 106]. Chen et al. [103] suggested that Rb, but not p53, function is essential for UCN-01-mediated G_1 arrest. However, Shimizu et al. [107] demonstrated that lung carcinoma cell lines with either absent, mutant, or wild-type Rb exposed to UCN-01 displayed G_1 arrest and antiproliferative effects irrespective of Rb function. Thus, the exact role of Rb or p53 in the G_1 arrest induced by UCN-01 is still unknown. Further studies on the putative target(s) for UCN-01 in the G_1 phase arrest of cells are warranted.

Recently, Facchinetti et al. [104] demonstrated that the G_1/S arrest induced by UCN-01 is due to the transcriptional upregulation of p21. This effect is due to activation of the MAPK/ERK pathway, leading to p53-independent transactivation of p21. Further studies are needed to understand the mechanism by which UCN-01 activates MAPK.

As shown in several *in vitro* models, lack of functional p53 does not preclude the cell cycle arrest and cytotoxicity induced by this agent [91, 93, 94, 101–108]. Thus, a common feature observed in more than 50% of human neoplasias associated with poor outcome and refractoriness to standard chemotherapies [109, 110] may render tumor cells more sensitive to UCN-01.

A very exciting recent development is the discovery that UCN-01 can modulate the PI3 kinase/AKT survival pathway [111]. UCN-01 displays a potent inhibition *in vitro* of the pdk1 serine/threonine kinase, leading to dephosphorylation and inactivation of AKT [111]. Of note, induction of p21 is not due to inhibition of PDK1/AKT, but occurs by activation of MAPK [104]. Although this is an exciting novel feature of UCN-01, it is of utmost importance to demonstrate whether the antitumor effects of UCN-01 are mediated by this action. Moreover, demonstration that these effects also occur in *in vivo* settings is crucial.

As previously mentioned, synergistic effects of UCN-01 have been observed with many signal transduction and chemotherapeutic agents, including mitomycin C, 5-FU, carmustine, and camptothecin, among others [99, 100, 112–120]. Therefore, it is possible that combining UCN-01 with these or other agents could improve its therapeutic index. Moreover, UCN-01 has demonstrated synergistic effects with γ-irradiation [93, 121]. Clinical trials exploring these possibilities are currently being developed.

5.2.2 Clinical trials of UCN-01

In the first phase I trial of UCN-01, UCN-01 was initially administered as a 72-h continuous infusion every 2 weeks based on data from *in vitro* and xenograft preclinical models [122, 123]. However, it became apparent in the first few patients that the drug had an unexpectedly long half-life (~30 days). This half-life was 100 times longer than the half-life observed in preclinical models, most likely due to the avid binding of UCN-01 to α1-acid glycoprotein [124, 125]. Thus, the protocol was modified to administer UCN-01 every 4 weeks (one half-life) and, in subsequent courses, the duration of infusion was decreased by half (total 36 h). Thus, it was possible to reach similar peak plasma concentrations in subsequent courses with no evidence of drug accumulation. There was no evidence of myelotoxicity or gastrointestinal toxicity (prominent side effects observed in animal models), despite very high plasma concentrations achieved (35-50 μM) [122–125]. Major toxicities were nausea/vomiting (amenable to standard antiemetic treatments), symptomatic hyperglycemia associated with an insulin-resistance state (increase in insulin and c-peptide levels while receiving UCN-01), and pulmonary toxicity characterized by substantial hypoxemia without obvious radiological changes. The recommended phase II dose of UCN-01 given on a 72-h continuous infusion schedule was 42.5 mg/m^2/day [123]. One patient with refractory metastatic melanoma developed a partial response that lasted 8 months. Another patient with refractory anaplastic large-cell lymphoma that had failed multiple chemotherapeutic regimens including high-dose chemotherapy has no evidence of disease more than 4 years after the initiation of UCN-01. Moreover, a few patients with leiomyosarcoma, non-Hodgkin's lymphoma, and lung cancer demonstrated stable disease for 6 months [123, 126].

To estimate 'free UCN-01 concentrations' in body fluids, several methods were considered. Plasma ultracentrifugation and salivary determination of UCN-01 revealed similar results. At the recommended phase II dose (37.5 mg/m^2/day over 72 h), concentrations of 'free-salivary' UCN-01 (~100 nM) that may cause G_2 checkpoint abrogation can be achieved. As mentioned earlier, UCN-01 is a potent PKC inhibitor. To determine the putative signaling effects of UCN-01 in tissues, bone marrow aspirates and tumor cells were obtained from patients before and during the first cycle of UCN-01 administration. Western blot studies were performed in these samples against phosphorylated adducin, a cytoskeletal membrane protein and a specific substrate phosphorylated by PKC. A clear loss in phospho-adducin content in the post-treatment samples was observed in all tumor and bone marrow samples tested, leading to the conclusion that UCN-01 can modulate PKC activity in tissues from patients in this trial [122, 123].

Several groups have conducted shorter duration (3-h) infusional trials of UCN-01 [127, 128]. A recently published report by Dees et al. [128] presented the experience with 1-h (and then 3-h) infusions with UCN-01. A total of 24 patients participated in this trial. The study started as a 1-h infusion; however, it appeared too toxic. The MTD using the 3-h infusion was 95 mg/m^2 for the first course and 47.5 mg/m^2 over 3 h for second and subsequent courses. The DLT was hypotension. Other toxicities observed were similar to the 72-h infusion trial. However, in the 3-h infusion UCN-01 trial, CNS toxicities including seizures and change and mental status occurred. No objective responses were observed. Mean (SD) pharmacokinetic (PK) variable values in nine patients treated at 95 mg/m^2 over 3 h were volume of distribution at steady state, 14 (5.4) L; β half-life, 406 (151) h ; systemic clearance, 0.028 (0.017) L/h; C_{max}, 51 (16) μM; and area under the curve, 19,732 (12,195) μM/L h. When compared with the pharmacokinetics parameters of the 72-h infusional trial, the 3-h infusional trial has some similarities and differences. Unfortunately, based on the accelerated dose-escalation design [129], they were not able to have "robust" PK parameters. Despite these limitations, PK parameters are similar; it appears that, at the MTD, the 3-h trials demonstrated, as expected, a slightly higher peak plasma concentration than the 72 h. However, the area under the plasma concentration curve (AUC) in the former was slightly lower. In the 72-h infusion, antitumor activity was demonstrated in a patient with metastatic melanoma and in a patient with anaplastic Non-Hodgkin's lymphoma, while the 3-h infusion had no evidence of antitumor effects. Finally, evidence of "free" UCN-01 concentrations were demonstrated in the 72-h infusion trial by salivary UCN-01 concentration, by plasma centrifugation, by plasma G_2 checkpoint *ex vivo* assay, and by down-modulation of phospho-adducin, a known substrate of PKC. In contrast, the 3-h infusion showed salivary data in some patients at the MTD dose. In summary, it is still unknown what the best schedule to administer UCN-01 is.

Recently, a phase I combination study of 72-h infusion UCN-01 and 24-h weekly FU was reported [130]. Increasing doses of weekly 24-h infusion of FU were followed by UCN-01 dose of 135 mg/m^2 over 72 h in cycle 1, and 67.5 mg/m^2 over 36 h in subsequent cycles, based on the initial phase I trial [122, 123]. The authors were able to escalate FU up to 2600 mg/m^2 in combination with monthly UCN-01. The DLT included arrhythmia and syncope. Other toxicities included hyperglycemia, headache, and nausea and vomiting. Highest mean peak plasma concentration of UCN-01 (48.5 µM) was obtained in cohort 5 (1.265 mg/m^2 FU) of 48.5 µM. Of note, the lowest mean peak plasma UCN-01 concentration (17.6 µM) was observed in the highest FU dose administered (cohort 8, 2.600 mg/m^2) of 17.6 µM. The investigators proposed cohort 8 as the recommended phase II dose. Unfortunately, there were no objective responses.

A phase II trial of 3-h infusional UCN-01 in patients with progressive, metastatic renal cell carcinoma was recently reported [131]. Twenty-one patients were enrolled into this study and received 90 mg/m^2 over 3 h based on prior phase I trials using this schedule [127, 128]. Accrual was halted after failure to reach a predetermined efficacy requirement with seven patients remaining disease-progression free after 4 months. The median time to peak (TTP) for all patients was 2.67 months (range 0.4–7.6 months). There were no objective responses, and UCN-01 using this schedule was well tolerated [131].

6 Outstanding issues related to the modulation of cell cycle for cancer therapy

The role of cdk as targets for cancer therapy, especially with respect to cdk2 has been recently challenged [132–138]. Briefly, loss of cdk2 function in some colon carcinoma cell lines failed to arrest at the G_1/S entry [136]. Moreover, ablation of cdk2 and or cyclin E in mice demonstrated normal development with significant meiotic perturbations [132, 134–138]. The lack of significant somatic effects in these models may be explained by the redundancy of cdk [137]. To have significant antitumor activity, small-molecule cdk modulators may need to target more than one cdk to avoid the rescue by other redundant cdk.

7 Summary

Most human malignancies have an aberration in the Rb pathway due to 'cdk hyperactivation'. Several small-molecule cdk modulators are being discovered and tested in the clinic. The first ATP-competitive cdk inhibitors tested in clinical trials, flavopiridol and UCN-01, have shown promising results with evidence of antitumor activity and plasma concentrations sufficient to inhibit cdk-related functions. The best schedule to be administered, combination with standard chemotherapeutic agents, best tumor types to be targeted, and demonstration of cdk modulation from tumor samples from patients in these trials are important issues that need to be answered to advance these agents to the clinical arena.

References

1 Paulovich A, Toczyski D, Hartwell L (1997) When checkpoints fail. *Cell* 88: 315–321

2 Morgan DO (1997) Cyclin-dependent kinases: engines, clocks, and microprocessors. *Annu Rev Cell Dev Biol* 13: 261–291

3 Senderowicz AM (2003) Small-molecule cyclin-dependent kinase modulators. *Oncogene* 22: 6609–6620

4 Senderowicz AM (2003) Novel small molecule cyclin-dependent kinases modulators in human clinical trials. *Cancer Biol Ther* 2: S84–95

5 Bharadwaj R, Yu H (2004) The spindle checkpoint, aneuploidy, and cancer. *Oncogene* 23: 2016–2027

6 Lew DJ, Burke DJ (2003) The spindle assembly and spindle position checkpoints. *Annu Rev Genet* 37: 251–282

7 Chan GK, Yen TJ (2003) The mitotic checkpoint: a signaling pathway that allows a single unattached kinetochore to inhibit mitotic exit. *Prog Cell Cycle Res 5:* 431–439

8 Kops GJPL, Foltz DR, Cleveland DW (2004) Lethality to human cancer cells through massive chromosome loss by inhibition of the mitotic checkpoint. *Proc Natl Acad Sci USA* 101: 8699–8704

9 Meraldi P, Honda R, Nigg EA (2004) Aurora kinases link chromosome segregation and cell division to cancer susceptibility. *Curr Opin Genet Dev* 14: 29–36

10 Jiang Y, Zhang Y, Lees E, Seghezzi W (2003) AuroraA overexpression overrides the mitotic spindle checkpoint triggered by nocodazole, a microtubule destabilizer. *Oncogene* 22: 8293–8301

11 Harrington EA, Bebbington D, Moore J, Rasmussen RK, Ajose-Adeogun AO, Nakayama T, Graham JA, Demur C, Hercend T, Diu-Hercend A et al (2004) VX-680, a potent and selective small-molecule inhibitor of the Aurora kinases, suppresses tumor growth *in vivo*. *Nat Med* 10: 262–267
12 Hauf S, Cole RW, LaTerra S, Zimmer C, Schnapp G, Walter R, Heckel A, van Meel J, Rieder CL, Peters JM (2003) The small molecule Hesperadin reveals a role for Aurora B in correcting kinetochore-microtubule attachment and in maintaining the spindle assembly checkpoint. *J Cell Biol* 161: 281–294
13 Ditchfield C, Johnson VL, Tighe A, Ellston R, Haworth C, Johnson T, Mortlock A, Keen N, Taylor SS (2003) Aurora B couples chromosome alignment with anaphase by targeting BubR1, Mad2, and Cenp-E to kinetochores. *J Cell Biol* 161: 267–280
14 Sillje HH, Nigg EA (2003) Signal transduction. Capturing polo kinase. *Science* 299: 1190–1191
15 Vousden KH, Lu X (2002) Live or let die: the cell's response to p53. *Nat Rev Cancer* 2: 594–604
16 Kawabe T (2004) G2 checkpoint abrogators as anticancer drugs. *Mol Cancer Ther* 3: 513–519
17 Senderowicz AM (2004) Targeting cell cycle and apoptosis for the treatment of human malignancies. *Curr Opin Cell Biol* 16: 670–678
18 Motokura T, Bloom T, Kim HG, Juppner H, Ruderman JV, Kronenberg HM, Arnold A (1991) A novel cyclin encoded by a bcl1-linked candidate oncogene. *Nature* 350: 512–515
19 Weinberg RA (1992) The integration of molecular genetics into cancer management. *Cancer* 70: 1653–1658
20 Weinberg RA (1996) The molecular basis of carcinogenesis: understanding the cell cycle clock. *Cytokines Mol Ther* 2: 105–110
21 Hatakeyama M, Brill JA, Fink GR, Weinberg RA (1994) Collaboration of G1 cyclins in the functional inactivation of the retinoblastoma protein. *Genes Dev 8:* 1759–1771
22 Pines J (1995) Cyclins and cyclin-dependent kinases: a biochemical view. *Biochem J* 308: 697–711
23 Bartek J, Staskova Z, Draetta G, Lukas J (1993) Molecular pathology of the cell cycle in human cancer cells. *Stem Cells* 11 Suppl 1: 51–58
24 Lukas J, Aagaard L, Strauss M, Bartek J (1995) Oncogenic aberrations of p16INK4/CDKN2 and cyclin D1 cooperate to deregulate G1 control. *Cancer Res* 55*:* 4818–4823
25 Bartek J, Bartkova J, Lukas J (1996) The retinoblastoma protein pathway and the restriction point. *Curr Opin Cell Biol* 8: 805–814
26 Aagaard L, Lukas J, Bartkova J, Kjerulff AA, Strauss M, Bartek J (1995) Aberrations of p16Ink4 and retinoblastoma tumour-suppressor genes occur in distinct sub-sets of human cancer cell lines. *Int J Cancer* 61: 115–120
27 Lukas J, Bartkova J, Bartek J (1996) Convergence of mitogenic signalling cascades from diverse classes of receptors at the cyclin D-cyclin-dependent kinase-pRb-controlled G1 checkpoint. *Mol Cell Biol* 16: 6917–6925
28 Sherr C J (2000) Cell cycle control and cancer. *Harvey Lect* 96: 73–92
29 Sonoda Y, Yoshimoto T, Sekiya T (1995) Homozygous deletion of the MTS1/p16 and MTS2/p15 genes and amplification of the CDK4 gene in glioma. *Oncogene* 11: 2145–2149

30 Wolfel T, Hauer M, Schneider J, Serrano M, Wolfel C, Klehmann-Hieb E, De Plaen E, Hankeln T, Meyer zum Buschenfelde KH, Beach D (1995) A p16INK4a-insensitive CDK4 mutant targeted by cytolytic T lymphocytes in a human melanoma. *Science* 269: 1281–1284
31 An HX, Beckmann MW, Reifenberger G, Bender HG, Niederacher D (1999) Gene amplification and overexpression of CDK4 in sporadic breast carcinomas is associated with high tumor cell proliferation. *Am J Pathol* 154: 113–118
32 Masciullo V, Scambia G, Marone M, Giannitelli C, Ferrandina G, Bellacosa A, Benedetti Panici P, Mancuso S (1997) Altered expression of cyclin D1 and CDK4 genes in ovarian carcinomas. *Int J Cancer* 74: 390–395
33 Kanoe H, Nakayama T, Murakami H, Hosaka T, Yamamoto H, Nakashima Y, Tsuboyama T, Nakamura T, Sasaki MS, Toguchida J (1998) Amplification of the CDK4 gene in sarcomas: tumor specificity and relationship with the RB gene mutation. *Anticancer Res* 18: 2317–2321
34 Meijer L (2000) Cyclin-dependent kinases inhibitors as potential anticancer, antineurodegenerative, antiviral and antiparasitic agents. *Drug Resist Updat* 3: 83–88
35 Senderowicz AM, Sausville EA (2000) Preclinical and clinical development of cyclin-dependent kinase modulators. *J Natl Cancer Inst* 92: 376–387
36 Zaharevitz DW, Gussio R, Leost M, Senderowicz AM, Lahusen T, Kunick C, Meijer L, Sausville EA (1999) Discovery and initial characterization of the paullones, a novel class of small-molecule inhibitors of cyclin-dependent kinases. *Cancer Res* 59: 2566–2569
37 De Azevedo WF, Leclerc S, Meijer L, Havlicek L, Strnad M, Kim SH (1997) Inhibition of cyclin-dependent kinases by purine analogues: crystal structure of human cdk2 complexed with roscovitine. *Eur J Biochem* 243: 518–526
38 Meijer L, Borgne A, Mulner O, Chong JP, Blow JJ, Inagaki N, Inagaki M, Delcros JG, Moulinoux JP (1997) Biochemical and cellular effects of roscovitine, a potent and selective inhibitor of the cyclin-dependent kinases cdc2, cdk2 and cdk5. *Eur J Biochem* 243: 527–536
39 Misra RN, Xiao HY, Kim KS, Lu S, Han WC, Barbosa SA, Hunt JT, Rawlins DB, Shan W, Ahmed SZ et al (2004) N-(cycloalkylamino)acyl-2-aminothiazole inhibitors of cyclin-dependent kinase 2. N-[5-[[[5-(1,1-dimethylethyl)-2-oxazolyl]methyl]thio]-2-thiazolyl]-4-piperidinecarboxamide (BMS-387032), a highly efficacious and selective antitumor agent. *J Med Chem* 47: 1719–1728
40 Mettey Y, Gompel M, Thomas V, Garnier M, Leost M, Ceballos-Picot I, Noble M, Endicott J, Vierfond JM, Meijer L (2003) Aloisines, a new family of CDK/GSK-3 inhibitors. SAR study, crystal structure in complex with CDK2, enzyme selectivity, and cellular effects. *J Med Chem* 46: 222–236
41 Ortega MA, Montoya ME, Zarranz B, Jaso A, Aldana I, Leclerc S, Meijer L, Monge A (2002) Pyrazolo[3,4-b]quinoxalines. A new class of cyclin-dependent kinases inhibitors. *Bioorg Med Chem* 10: 2177–2184
42 Worland PJ, Kaur G, Stetler-Stevenson M, Sebers S, Sartor O, Sausville EA (1993) Alteration of the phosphorylation state of p34cdc2 kinase by the flavone L86-8275 in breast carcinoma cells. Correlation with decreased H1 kinase activity. *Biochem Pharmacol* 46: 1831–1840
43 Kaur G, Stetler-Stevenson M, Sebers S, Worland P, Sedlacek H, Myers C, Czech J, Naik R, Sausville E (1992) Growth inhibition with reversible cell cycle arrest of carcinoma cells by flavone L86-8275. *J Natl Cancer Inst* 84: 1736–1740

44 Carlson BA, Dubay MM, Sausville EA, Brizuela L, Worland PJ (1996) Flavopiridol induces G1 arrest with inhibition of cyclin-dependent kinase (CDK) 2 and CDK4 in human breast carcinoma cells. *Cancer Res* 56: 2973–2978
45 De Azevedo WF Jr, Mueller-Dieckmann HJ, Schulze-Gahmen U, Worland PJ, Sausville E, Kim SH (1996) Structural basis for specificity and potency of a flavonoid inhibitor of human CDK2, a cell cycle kinase. *Proc Natl Acad Sci USA* 93: 2735–2740
46 Losiewicz MD, Carlson BA, Kaur G, Sausville EA, Worland PJ (1994) Potent inhibition of CDC2 kinase activity by the flavonoid L86-8275. *Biochem Biophys Res Commun* 201: 589–595
47 Carlson B, Pearlstein R, Naik R, Sedlacek H, Sausville E, Worland P (1996) Inhibition of CDK2, CDK4 and CDK7 by flavopiridol and structural analogs. *Proc Am Assoc Cancer Res* 1996: 424
48 Fredersdorf S, Burns J, Milne AM, Packham G, Fallis L, Gillett CE, Royds JA, Peston D, Hall PA, Hanby AM et al (1997) High level expression of p27(kip1) and cyclin D1 in some human breast cancer cells: inverse correlation between the expression of p27(kip1) and degree of malignancy in human breast and colorectal cancers. *Proc Natl Acad Sci USA* 94: 6380–6385
49 Carlson B, Lahusen T, Singh S, Loaiza-Perez A, Worland PJ, Pestell R, Albanese C, Sausville EA, Senderowicz AM (1999) Down-regulation of cyclin D1 by transcriptional repression in MCF-7 human breast carcinoma cells induced by flavopiridol. *Cancer Res* 59: 4634–4641
50 Gray NS, Wodicka L, Thunnissen AM, Norman TC, Kwon S, Espinoza FH, Morgan DO, Barnes G, LeClerc S, Meijer L *et al* (1998) Exploiting chemical libraries, structure, and genomics in the search for kinase inhibitors. *Science* 281: 533–538
51 Chao SH, Fujinaga K, Marion JE, Taube R, Sausville EA, Senderowicz AM, Peterlin BM, Price DH (2000) Flavopiridol inhibits P-TEFb and blocks HIV-1 replication. *J Biol Chem* 275: 28345–28348
52 Wright J, Blatner GL, Cheson BD (1998) Clinical trials referral resource. Clinical trials of flavopiridol. *Oncology (Huntingt)* 12: 1014–1023
53 Arguello F, Alexander M, Sterry J, Tudor G, Smith E, Kalavar N, Greene J, Koss W, Morgan D, Stinson S *et al* (1998) Flavopiridol induces apoptosis of normal lymphoid cells, causes immunosuppresion, and has potent antitumor activity *in vivo* against human and leukemia xenografts. *Blood* 91: 2482–2490
54 Byrd JC, Shinn C, Waselenko JK, Fuchs EJ, Lehman TA, Nguyen PL, Flinn IW, Diehl LF, Sausville E, Grever MR (1998) Flavopiridol induces apoptosis in chronic lymphocytic leukemia cells via activation of caspase-3 without evidence of bcl-2 modulation or dependence on functional p53. *Blood* 92: 3804–3816
55 Konig A, Schwartz GK, Mohammad RM, Al-Katib A, Gabrilove JL (1997) The novel cyclin-dependent kinase inhibitor flavopiridol downregulates Bcl-2 and induces growth arrest and apoptosis in chronic B-cell leukemia lines. *Blood* 90: 4307–4312
56 Parker B, Kaur G, Nieves-Neira W, Taimi M, Kolhagen G, Shimizu T, Pommier Y, Sausville E, Senderowicz AM (1998) Early induction of Apoptosis in hematopoietic cell lines after exposure to flavopiridol. *Blood* 91: 458–465
57 Decker RH, Dai Y, Grant S (2001) The cyclin-dependent kinase inhibitor flavopiridol induces apoptosis in human leukemia cells (U937) through the mitochondrial rather than the receptor-mediated pathway. *Cell Death Differ* 8: 715–724

58 Parker BW, Kaur G, Nieves-Neira W, Taimi M, Kohlhagen G, Shimizu T, Losiewicz MD, Pommier Y, Sausville EA, Senderowicz AM (1998) Early induction of apoptosis in hematopoietic cell lines after exposure to flavopiridol. *Blood* 91: 458–465

59 Kitada S, Zapata JM, Andreeff M, Reed JC (2000) Protein kinase inhibitors flavopiridol and 7-hydroxy-staurosporine down-regulate antiapoptosis proteins in B-cell chronic lymphocytic leukemia. *Blood* 96: 393–397

60 Patel V, Senderowicz AM, Pinto D, Igishi T, Raffeld M, Quintanilla-Martinez L, Ensley JF, Sausville EA, Gutkind JS (1998) Flavopiridol, a novel cyclin-dependent kinase inhibitor, suppresses the growth of head and neck squamous cell carcinomas by inducing apoptosis. *J Clin Invest* 102: 1674–1681

61 Guedez L, Quintanilla-Martinez L, Lahusen T, Davies T, Singh SS, Barotto N, Vistica D, Raffeld M, Sausville EA, Senderowicz AM (1999) Flavopiridol-induced apoptosis is associated with a decrease in cyclin D1 in mantle lymphoma cell lines. *Proc Am Assoc Cancer Res* 1999: 3413

62 Schrump DS, Matthews W, Chen GA, Mixon A, Altorki NK (1998) Flavopiridol mediates cell cycle arrest and apoptosis in esophageal cancer cells. *Clin Cancer Res* 4: 2885–2890

63 Wu K, Wang C, D'Amico M, Lee RJ, Albanese C, Pestell RG, Mani S (2002) Flavopiridol and trastuzumab synergistically inhibit proliferation of breast cancer cells: association with selective cooperative inhibition of cyclin D1-dependent kinase and Akt signaling pathways. *Mol Cancer Ther* 1: 695–706

64 Brusselbach S, Nettelbeck DM, Sedlacek HH, Muller R (1998) Cell cycle-independent induction of apoptosis by the anti-tumor drug Flavopiridol in endothelial cells. *Int J Cancer* 77: 146–152

65 Kerr JS, Wexler RS, Mousa SA, Robinson CS, Wexler EJ, Mohamed S, Voss ME, Devenny JJ, Czerniak PM, Gudzelak A Jr, Slee AM (1999) Novel small molecule alpha v integrin antagonists: comparative anti-cancer efficacy with known angiogenesis inhibitors. *Anticancer Res* 19: 959–968

66 Melillo G, Sausville EA, Cloud K, Lahusen T, Varesio L, Senderowicz AM (1999) Flavopiridol, a protein kinase inhibitor, down-regulates hypoxic induction of vascular endothelial growth factor expression in human monocytes. *Cancer Res* 59: 5433–5437

67 Parng C, Seng WL, Semino C, McGrath P (2002) Zebrafish: a preclinical model for drug screening. *Assay Drug Dev Technol* 1: 41–48

68 Lee HR, Chang TH, Tebalt MJ 3rd, Senderowicz AM, Szabo E (1999) Induction of differentiation accompanies inhibition of Cdk2 in a non-small cell lung cancer cell line. *Int J Oncol* 15: 161–166

69 Schwartz G, Farsi K, Maslak P, Kelsen D, Spriggs D (1997) Potentiation of apoptosis by flavopiridol in mitomycin-C-treated gastric and breast cancer cells. *Clin Cancer Res* 3: 1467–1472

70 Bible KC, Kaufmann SH (1997) Cytotoxic synergy between flavopiridol (NSC 649890, L86-8275) and various antineoplastic agents: the importance of sequence of administration. *Cancer Res* 57: 3375–3380

71 Yu C, Krystal G, Dent P, Grant S (2002) Flavopiridol potentiates STI571-induced mitochondrial damage and apoptosis in BCR-ABL-positive human leukemia cells. *Clin Cancer Res* 8: 2976–2984

72 Dai Y, Rahmani M, Pei XY, Dent P, Grant S (2004) Bortezomib and Flavopiridol interact synergistically to induce apoptosis in chronic myeloid leukemia cells resistant

to imatinib mesylate through both Bcr/Abl-dependent and -independent mechanisms. *Blood* 104: 509–518
73 Chien M, Astumian M, Liebowitz D, Rinker-Schaeffer C, Stadler WM (1999) *In vitro* evaluation of flavopiridol, a novel cell cycle inhibitor, in bladder cancer. *Cancer Chemother Pharmacol* 44: 81–87
74 Sedlacek HH, Czech J, Naik R, Kaur G, Worland P, Losiewicz M, Parker B, Carlson B, Smith A, Senderowicz A, Sausville E (1996) Flavopiridol (L86-8275, NSC-649890), a new kinase inhibitor for tumor therapy. *Int J Oncol* 9: 1143–1168
75 Drees M, Dengler W, Roth T, Labonte H, Mayo J, Malspeis L, Grever M, Sausville E, Fiebig H (1997) Flavopiridol (L86-8275): Selective antitumor activity *in vitro* and activity *in vivo* for prostate carcinoma cells. *Clin Cancer Res* 32: 273–279
76 Senderowicz AM, Headlee D, Stinson SF, Lush RM, Kalil N, Villalba L, Hill K, Steinberg SM, Figg WD, Tompkins A, Arbuck SG, Sausville EA (1998) Phase I trial of continuous infusion flavopiridol, a novel cyclin- dependent kinase inhibitor, in patients with refractory neoplasms. *J Clin Oncol* 16: 2986–2999
77 Tan AR, Headlee D, Messmann R, Sausville EA, Arbuck SG, Murgo AJ, Melillo G, Zhai S, Figg WD, Swain SM et al (2002) Phase I clinical and pharmacokinetic study of flavopiridol administered as a daily 1-hour infusion in patients with advanced neoplasms. *J Clin Oncol* 20: 4074–4082
78 Messmann RA, Ullmann CD, Lahusen T, Kalehua A, Wasfy J, Melillo G, Ding I, Headlee D, Figg WD, Sausville EA et al (2003) Flavopiridol-related proinflammatory syndrome is associated with induction of interleukin-6. *Clin Cancer Res* 9: 562–570
79 Thomas JP, Tutsch KD, Cleary JF, Bailey HH, Arzoomanian R, Alberti D, Simon K, Feierabend C, Binger K, Marnocha R et al (2002) Phase I clinical and pharmacokinetic trial of the cyclin-dependent kinase inhibitor flavopiridol. *Cancer Chemother Pharmacol* 50: 465–472
80 Stadler WM, Vogelzang NJ, Amato R, Sosman J, Taber D, Liebowitz D, Vokes EE (2000) Flavopiridol, a novel cyclin-dependent kinase inhibitor, in metastatic renal cancer: a University of Chicago Phase II Consortium study. *J Clin Oncol* 18: 371–375
81 Schwartz GK, Ilson D, Saltz L, O'Reilly E, Tong W, Maslak P, Werner J, Perkins P, Stoltz M, Kelsen D (2001) Phase II study of the cyclin-dependent kinase inhibitor flavopiridol administered to patients with advanced gastric carcinoma. *J Clin Oncol* 19: 1985–1992
82 Shapiro GI, Supko JG, Patterson A, Lynch C, Lucca J, Zacarola PF, Muzikansky A, Wright JJ, Lynch TJ Jr, Rollins BJ (2001) A phase ii trial of the cyclin-dependent kinase inhibitor flavopiridol in patients with previously untreated stage IV non-small cell lung cancer. *Clin Cancer Res* 7: 1590–1599
83 Aklilu M, Kindler HL, Donehower RC, Mani S, Vokes EE (2003) Phase II study of flavopiridol in patients with advanced colorectal cancer. *Ann Oncol* 14: 1270–1273
84 Liu G, Gandara DR, Lara PN Jr, Raghavan D, Doroshow JH, Twardowski P, Kantoff P, Oh W, Kim K, Wilding G (2004) A Phase II trial of flavopiridol (NSC #649890) in patients with previously untreated metastatic androgen-independent prostate cancer. *Clin Cancer Res* 10: 924–928
85 Bible K, Lensing J, Nelson S, Atherton P, Sloan J, Erlichman C (2003) A phase 1 trial of flavopiridol combined with 5-fluorouracil (5-FU) and leucovorin (CF) in patients with advanced malignancies. *Proc Am Soc Clin Oncol* 2003: 129

86 Schwartz GK, O'Reilly E, Ilson D, Saltz L, Sharma S, Tong W, Maslak P, Stoltz M, Eden L, Perkins P *et al* (2002) Phase I study of the cyclin-dependent kinase inhibitor flavopiridol in combination with paclitaxel in patients with advanced solid tumors. *J Clin Oncol* 20: 2157–2170

87 Gries J, Kasimis B, Schwarzenberger P, Shapiro G, Fidias P, Rodrigues L, Cogswell J, Bukowski R (2002) Phase I study of flavopiridol (HMR1275) in combination with paclitaxel and carboplatin in non-small cell lung cancer (NCSLC) patients. *Eur J Cancer* 38: S49–S50

88 Tan AR, Yang X, Berman A, Zhai S, Sparreboom A, Parr AL, Chow C, Brahim JS, Steinberg SM, Figg WD et al (2004) Phase I trial of the cyclin-dependent kinase inhibitor flavopiridol in combination with docetaxel in patients with metastatic breast cancer. *Clin Cancer Res* 10: 5038–5047

89 Tamaoki T (1991) Use and specificity of staurosporine, UCN-01, and calphostin C as protein kinase inhibitors. *Methods Enzymol* 201: 340–347

90 Takahashi I, Kobayashi E, Asano K, Yoshida M, Nakano H (1987) UCN-01, a selective inhibitor of protein kinase C from *Streptomyces*. *J Antibiot (Tokyo)* 40: 1782–1784

91 Seynaeve CM, Stetler-Stevenson M, Sebers S, Kaur G, Sausville EA, Worland PJ (1993) Cell cycle arrest and growth inhibition by the protein kinase antagonist UCN-01 in human breast carcinoma cells. *Cancer Res* 53: 2081–2086

92 Akinaga S, Gomi K, Morimoto M, Tamaoki T, Okabe M (1991) Antitumor activity of UCN-01, a selective inhibitor of protein kinase C, in murine and human tumor models. *Cancer Res* 51: 4888–4892

93 Wang Q, Fan S, Eastman A, Worland PJ, Sausville EA, O'Connor P (1996) UCN-01: a potent abrogator of G2 checkpoint function in cancer cells with disrupted p53. *J Natl Cancer Inst* 88: 956–965

94 Wang Q, Worland PJ, Clark JL, Carlson BA, Sausville EA (1995) Apoptosis in 7-hydroxystaurosporine-treated T lymphoblasts correlates with activation of cyclin-dependent kinases 1 and 2. *Cell Growth Differ* 6: 927–936

95 Yu L, Orlandi L, Wang P, Orr MS, Senderowicz AM, Sausville EA, Silvestrini R, Watanabe N, Piwnica-Worms H, O'Connor PM (1998) UCN-01 abrogates G2 arrest through a Cdc2-dependent pathway that is associated with inactivation of the Wee1Hu kinase and activation of the Cdc25C phosphatase. *J Biol Chem* 273: 33455–33464

96 Sarkaria JN, Busby EC, Tibbetts RS, Roos P, Taya Y, Karnitz LM, Abraham RT (1999) Inhibition of ATM and ATR kinase activities by the radiosensitizing agent, caffeine. *Cancer Res* 59: 4375–4382

97 Graves PR, Yu L, Schwarz JK, Gales J, Sausville EA, O'Connor PM, Piwnica-Worms H (2000) The Chk1 protein kinase and the Cdc25C regulatory pathways are targets of the anticancer agent UCN-01. *J Biol Chem* 275: 5600–5605

98 Busby EC, Leistritz DF, Abraham RT, Karnitz LM, Sarkaria JN (2000) The radiosensitizing agent 7-hydroxystaurosporine (UCN-01) inhibits the DNA damage checkpoint kinase hChk1. *Cancer Res* 60: 2108–2112

99 Shao RG, Cao CX, Shimizu T, O'Connor PM, Kohn KW, Pommier Y (1997) Abrogation of an S-phase checkpoint and potentiation of camptothecin cytotoxicity by 7-hydroxystaurosporine (UCN-01) in human cancer cell lines, possibly influenced by p53 function. *Cancer Res* 57: 4029–4035

100 Bunch RT, Eastman A (1996) Enhancement of cisplatin-induced cytotoxicity by 7-hydroxystaurosporine (UCN-01), a new G2-checkpoint inhibitor. *Clin Cancer Res* 2: 791–797

101 Akinaga S, Nomura K, Gomi K, Okabe M (1994) Effect of UCN-01, a selective inhibitor of protein kinase C, on the cell-cycle distribution of human epidermoid carcinoma, A431 cells. *Cancer Chemother Pharmacol* 33: 273–280

102 Akiyama T, Sugiyama K, Shimizu M, Tamaoki T, Akinaga S (1999) G1-checkpoint function including a cyclin-dependent kinase 2 regulatory pathway as potential determinant of 7-hydroxystaurosporine (UCN-01)-induced apoptosis and G1-phase accumulation. *Jpn J Cancer Res* 90: 1364–1372

103 Chen X, Lowe M, Keyomarsi, K (1999) UCN-01-mediated G1 arrest in normal but not tumor breast cells is pRb-dependent and p53-independent. *Oncogene* 18: 5691–5702

104 Facchinetti MM, De Siervi A, Toskos D, Senderowicz AM (2004) UCN-01-induced cell cycle arrest requires the transcriptional induction of p21(waf1/cip1) by activation of mitogen-activated protein/extracellular signal-regulated kinase kinase/extracellular signal-regulated kinase pathway. *Cancer Res* 64: 3629–3637

105 Kawakami K, Futami H, Takahara J, Yamaguchi K (1996) UCN-01, 7-hydroxyl-staurosporine, inhibits kinase activity of cyclin-dependent kinases and reduces the phosphorylation of the retinoblastoma susceptibility gene product in A549 human lung cancer cell line. *Biochem Biophys Res Commun* 219: 778–783

106 Patel V, Lahusen T, Leethanakul C, Igishi T, Kremer M, Quintanilla-Martinez L, Ensley JF, Sausville EA, Gutkind JS, Senderowicz AM (2002) Antitumor activity of UCN-01 in carcinomas of the head and neck is associated with altered expression of cyclin D3 and p27(KIP1). *Clin Cancer Res* 8: 3549–3560

107 Shimizu E, Zhao MR, Nakanishi H, Yamamoto A, Yoshida S, Takada M, Ogura T, Sone S (1996) Differing effects of staurosporine and UCN-01 on RB protein phosphorylation and expression of lung cancer cell lines. *Oncology* 53: 494–504

108 Usuda J, Saijo N, Fukuoka K, Fukumoto H, Kuh HJ, Nakamura T, Koh Y, Suzuki T, Koizumi F, Tamura T, Kato H, Nishio K (2000) Molecular determinants of UCN-01-induced growth inhibition in human lung cancer cells. *Int J Cancer* 85: 275–280

109 Marchetti A, Buttitta F, Merlo G, Diella F, Pellegrini S, Pepe S, Macchiarini P, Chella A, Angeletti CA, Callahan R et al (1993) p53 alterations in non-small cell lung cancers correlate with metastatic involvement of hilar and mediastinal lymph nodes. *Cancer Res* 53: 2846–2851

110 Lowe SW, Bodis S, Bardeesy N, McClatchey A, Remington L, Ruley HE, Fisher DE, Jacks T, Pelletier J, Housman DE (1994) Apoptosis and the prognostic significance of p53 mutation. *Cold Spring Harb Symp Quant Biol* 59: 419–426

111 Sato S, Fujita N, Tsuruo T (2002) Interference with PDK1-Akt survival signaling pathway by UCN-01 (7-hydroxystaurosporine). *Oncogene* 21: 1727–1738

112 Tsuchida E, Tsuchida M, Urano M (1997) Synergistic cytotoxicity between a protein kinase C inhibitor, UCN-01, and monoclonal antibody to the epidermal growth factor receptor on MDA-468 cells. *Cancer Biother Radiopharm* 12: 117–121

113 Sugiyama K, Shimizu M, Akiyama T, Tamaoki T, Yamaguchi K, Takahashi R, Eastman A, Akinaga S (2000) UCN-01 selectively enhances mitomycin C cytotoxicity in p53 defective cells which is mediated through S and/or G(2) checkpoint abrogation. *Int J Cancer* 85: 703–709

114 Pollack IF, Kawecki S, Lazo JS (1996) Blocking of glioma proliferation *in vitro* and *in vivo* and potentiating the effects of BCNU and cisplatin: UCN-01, a selective protein kinase C inhibitor. *J Neurosurg* 84: 1024–1032

115 Jones CB, Clements MK, Redkar A, Daoud SS (2000) UCN-01 and camptothecin induce DNA double-strand breaks in p53 mutant tumor cells, but not in normal or p53 negative epithelial cells. *Int J Oncol* 17: 1043–1051

116 Husain A, Yan XJ, Rosales N, Aghajanian C, Schwartz GK, Spriggs DR (1997) UCN-01 in ovary cancer cells: effective as a single agent and in combination with cis-diamminedichloroplatinum(II)independent of p53 status. *Clin Cancer Res* 3: 2089–2097

117 Hsueh CT, Kelsen D, Schwartz GK (1998) UCN-01 suppresses thymidylate synthase gene expression and enhances 5-fluorouracil-induced apoptosis in a sequence-dependent manner. *Clin Cancer Res* 4: 2201–2206

118 Akinaga S, Nomura K, Gomi K, Okabe M (1993) Enhancement of antitumor activity of mitomycin C *in vitro* and *in vivo* by UCN-01, a selective inhibitor of protein kinase C. *Cancer Chemother Pharmacol* 32: 183–189

119 Hahn M, Li W, Yu C, Rahmani M, Dent P, Grant S (2005) Rapamycin and UCN-01 synergistically induce apoptosis in human leukemia cells through a process that is regulated by the Raf-1/MEK/ERK, Akt, and JNK signal transduction pathways. *Mol Cancer Ther* 4: 457–470

120 Dasmahapatra GP, Didolkar P, Alley MC, Ghosh S, Sausville EA, Roy KK (2004) *In vitro* combination treatment with perifosine and UCN-01 demonstrates synergism against prostate (PC-3) and lung (A549) epithelial adenocarcinoma cell lines. *Clin Cancer Res* 10: 5242–5252

121 Tsuchida E, Urano M (1997) The effect of UCN-01 (7-hydroxystaurosporine), a potent inhibitor of protein kinase C, on fractionated radiotherapy or daily chemotherapy of a murine fibrosarcoma. *Int J Radiat Oncol Biol Phys* 39: 1153–1161

122 Senderowicz AM, Headlee D, Lush R, Bauer K, Figg W, Murgo AS, Arbuck S, Inoue K, Kobashi S, Kuwabara T, Sausville E (1999) Phase I trial of infusional UCN-01, a novel protein kinase inhibitor, in patients with refractory neoplasms. *Proc Am Soc Clin Oncol* 1999: 3111

123 Sausville EA, Arbuck SG, Messmann R, Headlee D, Bauer KS, Lush RM, Murgo A, Figg WD, Lahusen T, Jaken S et al (2001) Phase I trial of 72-hour continuous infusion UCN-01 in patients with refractory neoplasms. *J Clin Oncol* 19: 2319–2333

124 Fuse E, Tanii H, Kurata N, Kobayashi H, Shimada Y, Tamura T, Sasaki Y, Tanigawara Y, Lush RD, Headlee D et al (1998) Unpredicted clinical pharmacology of UCN-01 caused by specific binding to human alpha1-acid glycoprotein. *Cancer Res* 58: 3248–3253

125 Sparreboom A, Chen H, Acharya MR, Senderowicz AM, Messmann RA, Kuwabara T, Venzon DJ, Murgo AJ, Headlee D, Sausville EA et al (2004) Effects of alpha1-acid glycoprotein on the clinical pharmacokinetics of 7-hydroxystaurosporine. *Clin Cancer Res* 10: 6840–6846

126 Wilson WH, Sorbara L, Figg WD, Mont EK, Sausville E, Warren KE, Balis FM, Bauer K, Raffeld M, Senderowicz AM et al (2000) Modulation of clinical drug resistance in a B cell lymphoma patient by the protein kinase inhibitor 7-hydroxystaurosporine: presentation of a novel therapeutic paradigm. *Clin Cancer Res* 6: 415–421

127 Tamura T, Sasaki Y, Minami H, Fujii H, Ito K, Igarashi T, Kamiya Y, Kurata T, Ohtsu T, Onozawa Y et al (1999) Phase I study of UCN-01 by 3-hour infusion. *Proc Am Soc Clin Oncol* 1999: 159

128 Dees EC, Baker SD, O'Reilly S, Rudek MA, Davidson SB, Aylesworth C, Elza-Brown K, Carducci MA, Donehower RC (2005) A phase I and pharmacokinetic study of short infusions of UCN-01 in patients with refractory solid tumors. *Clin Cancer Res* 11: 664–671
129 Simon R, Freidlin B, Rubinstein L, Arbuck SG, Collins J, Christian MC (1997) Accelerated titration designs for phase I clinical trials in oncology. *J Natl Cancer Inst* 89: 1138–1147
130 Kortmansky J, Shah MA, Kaubisch A, Weyerbacher A, Yi S, Tong W, Sowers R, Gonen M, O'Reilly E, Kemeny N, Ilson DI et al (2005) Phase I trial of the cyclin-dependent kinase inhibitor and protein kinase C inhibitor 7-hydroxystaurosporine in combination with Fluorouracil in patients with advanced solid tumors. *J Clin Oncol* 23: 1875–1884
131 Rini BI, Weinberg V, Shaw V, Scott J, Bok R, Park JW, Small EJ (2004) Time to disease progression to evaluate a novel protein kinase C inhibitor, UCN-01, in renal cell carcinoma. *Cancer* 101: 90–95
132 Mendez J (2003) Cell proliferation without cyclin E-CDK2. *Cell* 114: 398–399
133 Geng Y, Yu Q, Sicinska E, Das M, Schneider JE, Bhattacharya S, Rideout WM, Bronson RT, Gardner H, Sicinski P (2003) Cyclin E ablation in the mouse. *Cell* 114: 431–443
134 Ortega S, Prieto I, Odajima J, Martin A, Dubus P, Sotillo R, Barbero JL, Malumbres M, Barbacid M (2003) Cyclin-dependent kinase 2 is essential for meiosis but not for mitotic cell division in mice. *Nat Genet* 35: 25–31
135 Lents NH, Baldassare JJ (2004) CDK2 and cyclin E knockout mice: lessons from breast cancer. *Trends Endocrinol Metab* 15: 1–3
136 Tetsu O, McCormick F (2003) Proliferation of cancer cells despite CDK2 inhibition. *Cancer Cell* 3: 233–245
137 Sherr CJ, Roberts JM (2004) Living with or without cyclins and cyclin-dependent kinases. *Genes Dev* 18: 2699–2711
138 Berthet C, Aleem E, Coppola V, Tessarollo L, Kaldis P (2003) Cdk2 knockout mice are viable. *Curr Biol* 13: 1775–1785

Progress in Drug Research, Vol. 63
(R. M. Schultz, Ed.)

Targeting cyclo-oxygenase-2 for cancer prevention and treatment

Stephen T. Gately

RND Pharmaceuticals, Inc.
853 N. Quentin Road, Suite 195
Palatine, IL 60067, USA
<SGATELY@RNDPHARM.COM>

Key words

Angiogenesis, celecoxib, lumiracoxib, non-steroidal anti-inflammatory drug, rofecoxib.

1 Introduction

More than 30 years ago the mechanism of action for aspirin and aspirin-like drugs was established as the inhibition of prostaglandin (PG) H_2 synthase [1]. Twenty years later at least two cyclooxygenase (COX) isoforms were identified [2], and more recently a third isoform, COX-3 has been described [3]. The development of therapeutic agents that target the cyclooxygenases has a record of being almost continuous [4]. Many of the early drugs developed were non-selective; they inhibited both COX-1 and COX-2. Other compounds, including meloxicam, etodolac, and nimesulide had an improved gastrointestinal safety profile and appeared to be more selective for COX-2 [4, 5].

In 1990, data on DuP697, an effective anti-inflammatory agent with reduced ulcerogenic properties was reported [6]. This improved safety profile was considered to be related to the novel, non-acidic, chemical structure of the compound. Additional experimental molecules, NS398, flosulide and CGP28238 were generated also exhibiting an improved gastrointestinal safety profile [4]. With the discovery of COX-2, the improved gastrointestinal safety was soon related to selectivity of these molecules for the COX-2 isozyme. The chemical structures of DuP697 and NS398 were central for industrial chemists in the design of new COX-2 selective inhibitors, and now four COX-2 selective agents have gained regulatory approval. Celecoxib (Celebrex®) is indicated for the treatment of osteoarthritis and adult rheumatoid arthritis, and the second generation selective inhibitor valdecoxib (Bextra®) is indicated for acute and chronic treatment of the signs and symptoms of adult rheumatoid arthritis and osteoarthritis, as well as the relief of pain associated with primary dysmenorrhea. The U.S. Food and Drug Administration (FDA) later approved celecoxib as an oral adjunct for usual care for patients with familial adenomatous polyposis (FAP), a rare hereditary disease that, left untreated, leads to the development of colorectal cancer. This approval in the cancer prevention setting has led to numerous clinical studies of COX-2 selective inhibitors in the oncology setting.

Rofecoxib (Vioxx®) was approved in the U.S. in 1999 for the relief of the signs and symptoms of osteoarthritis and adult rheumatoid arthritis, management of acute pain in adults, primary dysmenorrhea and acute treatment of migraine attacks with or without aura in adults. It was also approved for the relief of the signs and symptoms of the most common forms of juvenile rheumatoid arthritis in children. The second generation selective inhibitor etoricoxib (Arcoxia™) was approved by the European regulatory authority, and has been launched in 38 countries worldwide in Europe, Latin America and the Asia-Pacific region.

Rofecoxib has now been withdrawn from the market following interim analysis of the data from the Adenomatous Polyp Prevention on Vioxx (APPROVe) study, designed to determine the effect of rofecoxib on benign sporadic colonic adenomas [7]. There was a significant increase in the incidence of serious thromboembolic adverse events in the group receiving 25 mg rofecoxib per day as compared with the placebo group [7]. Blood pressure was elevated in patients in the rofecoxib group, and the incidence of myocardial infarction and thrombotic stroke in the two groups began to diverge progressively after 1 year or more of treatment [7]. Meta-analyses of randomized controlled trials of rofecoxib also identified evidence for the adverse cardiovascular effects of rofecoxib [8].

In November 2004, the valdecoxib label had to be revised to include a black-box warning regarding serious skin reactions, and a contraindication for use in patients who have undergone bypass surgery [9]. A letter to the editor in the New England Journal of Medicine later recommended that clinicians stop prescribing valdecoxib except in extraordinary circumstances until better cardiovascular safety data were available [9].

In mid-December 2004, Pfizer announced that celecoxib more than doubled the risk of heart attack in patients from a large cancer-prevention trial sponsored by the National Cancer Institute. The Adenoma Prevention with Celecoxib (APC) trial found that patients taking 400 mg and 800 mg celecoxib daily had an approximately 2.5-fold increase in their risk of experiencing a major fatal or non-fatal cardiovascular event compared to those patients taking placebo.

In a separate long-term study, the Prevention of Spontaneous Adenomatous Polyps (PreSAP) trial, no increased cardiovascular risk was found for patients taking 400 mg celecoxib daily compared with those taking placebo. These findings were based on an identical analysis to that used to assess cardiovascular risk in the APC trial, and were conducted by the same independent safety review board.

Additionally, data have recently been reported suggesting that the adverse cardiovascular effects of these agents may be limited to rofecoxib [10]. In a case-control study, the adjusted odds ratio for myocardial infarction (MI) among celecoxib and rofecoxib users was analyzed, and demonstrated a statistically significant difference in the odds of non-fatal MI. This difference was not due to an increased risk of MI among rofecoxib users, but rather was due to lower odds of MI among celecoxib users [10]. Notwithstanding these data, randomized trials will be needed to fully understand the adverse cardiovascular effects for this class of agents.

It remains to be determined if the increased cardiovascular toxicity is related to the entire class of COX-2 selective inhibitors, or whether it is related to the chemical structure of some of these inhibitors [11]. The mechanism proposed for the increased cardiovascular toxicity for selective COX-2 inhibitors is the inhibition of PGI_2 formation without coincidental inhibition of thromboxane A_2 (TxA_2) that is formed by the unrestrained action of COX-1 from platelets [12]; TxA_2 is a potent vasoconstrictor and platelet agonist [12]. Additionally, inhibition of PGE_2 and PGI_2 within the kidney could lead to sodium and water retention, with resultant blood pressure elevations [13].

The toxicity could be related to the chemical structures of the COX-2 selective inhibitors. The approved drugs belong to the diarylheterocycle class of compounds that contain a sulfur moiety (Tab. 1). In contrast, lumiracoxib is an analogue of diclofenac (Tab. 1) that has the highest degree of COX-2 selectivity (Tab. 2) [14]. Results of the Therapeutic Arthritis Research and Gastrointestinal Event Trial (TARGET) found the incidence of MI did not differ between lumiracoxib and either ibuprofen or naproxen, irrespective of aspirin use [15]. This finding could suggest that molecules not based on the diarylheterocycle structure may not be associated with increased cardiovascular risk.

The observation of increased cardiovascular toxicity may not have negative implications for the use of this class of agents in the treatment of patients with cancer; therapies for cancer treatment are often associated with cardiovascular toxicity [16]. The targeted therapy bevacizumab (Avastin™) is associated with increased rate of hypertension, and a 1–2% increased risk of gastrointestinal perforations and cardiovascular events [17]. In the face of

Table 1.

First Generation	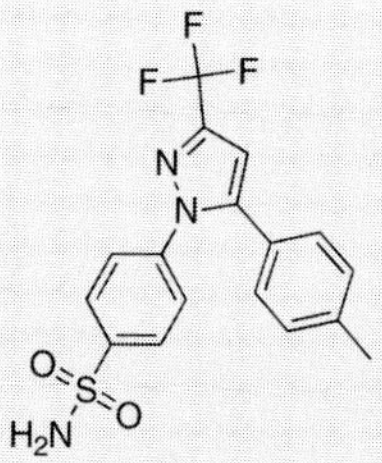 **Celecoxib**	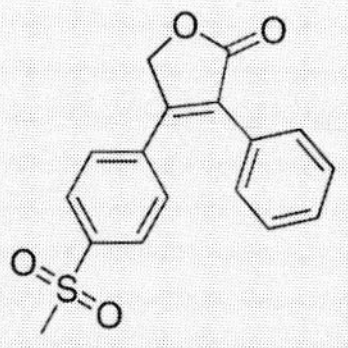 **Rofecoxib**
Second Generation	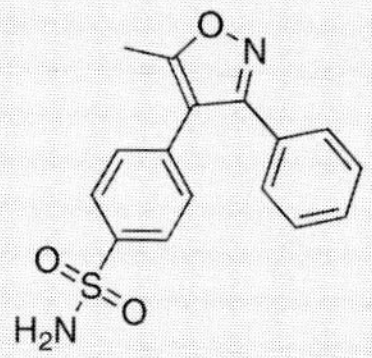 **Valdecoxib**	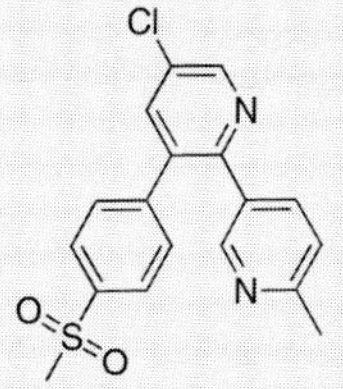 **Etoricoxib**
Second Generation Different Chemical Structure	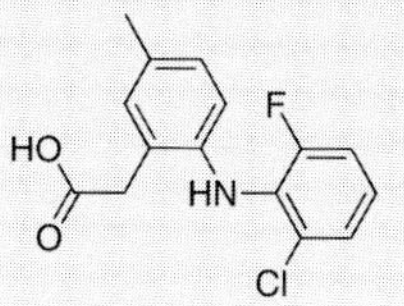 **Lumiracoxib**	

Table 2.

	Inhibitor	Ratio COX-2/COX-1
↑	Lumiracoxib	700
	Etoricoxib	344
Increasing	Rofecoxib	272
COX-2	Valdecoxib	61
Selectivity	Celecoxib	30

these data, bevacizumab was approved for use in combination with intravenous 5-fluorouracil-based chemotherapy as a first-line treatment for patients with metastatic cancer of the colon or rectum [17]. This suggests that regulators and physicians may accept agents with cardiovascular toxicities for use in patients with life-threatening conditions.

2 Cyclooxygenase-1 and 2

The major COX isozymes (COX-1 and COX-2) are the rate-limiting enzymes for the production of prostaglandins and thromboxanes from free arachidonic acid [18, 19]. COX-1 is constitutively expressed and is responsible for normal kidney and platelet function as well as the maintenance of the gastrointestinal mucosa [18]. In contrast, the COX-2 enzyme is induced by a variety of stimuli, including oncogenes, growth factors, tumor promoters, and chemotherapy via RAS and protein kinase C-mediated signaling [20, 21].

3 Cycloxygenase-2

Increased amounts of COX-2 are commonly detected in premalignant and malignant tissues [20]. Transcription factors including AP-1, CREB/NF-IL-6, NF-κB, NFAT, PEA3, PPARγ response elements, and Ets sites have all been identified as stimulators of COX-2 transcription [20, 21]. Wild-type p53 and the adenomatous polyposis coli gene can inhibit COX-2 transcription [22, 23], demonstrating that a balance between oncogenes and tumor suppressor genes regulates the expression of COX-2 in tumors.

Post-transcriptional mechanisms have also been shown to be involved in the elevated levels of COX-2 found in tumors. The 3′-untranslated domain of the COX-2 mRNA contains AU-rich elements (AREs) that are the sites for interaction with a variety of ARE-binding factors [21]. These binding factors, which include HuR, tristetraprolin, and AUF, influence the fate of COX-2 mRNA by controlling degradation, stabilization, or translation of COX-2 mRNA [24]. Variation in the amount or activity of these ARE-binding factors can therefore dramatically impact COX-2 levels in tumors.

Importantly, standard cancer treatments appear to increase the level of COX-2 in tumors. Paclitaxel and docetaxel stimulate COX-2 transcription via an AP-1-dependent mechanism [25, 26]. Taxane treatment also enhances the stability of the COX-2 mRNA [25, 26]. Ionizing radiation has also been shown to induce COX-2 expression [27, 28], again supporting that therapeutic interventions can be responsible, in part, for the elevated levels of COX-2 found in tumors.

4 Cellular expression of COX-2

Elevated expression of COX-2 in cancer has been localized to the neoplastic epithelium [29], within the microvasculature [30] and to stromal cells [31]. These data show that multiple cell types in the tumor microenvironment contribute to the elevated COX-2 expression. Overexpression of COX-2 by these different cell types leads to the increased production of the prostanoids, PGE_2, $PGF_{2\alpha}$, PGD_2, TxA_2 and PGI_2. The prostanoids mediate their effects by binding to G protein-coupled receptors that contain a series of transmembrane domains [20]. PGE_2 is the most abundant prostanoid detected in epithelial malignancies [20]. PGE_2, is known to promote colon carcinoma growth and invasion [32], and was found to be a potent inducer of the angiogenic switch during mammary cancer progression [33]. Elevated PGE_2 also demonstrates potent immunosuppressive effects [34–36], stimulates TCF-β-catenin-mediated transcription leading to expression of cyclin D1 and c-myc [37], activates cAMP/protein kinase A [38], and transactivates the epidermal growth factor (EGF) receptor [39]. PGE_2 was also shown to be a mediator of vascular endothelial growth factor (VEGF)- and basic fibroblast growth factor (bFGF)-induced CXCR4-dependent angiogenesis; these angiogenic effects of PGE_2 require CXCR4 expression [40]. PGE_2 has also been shown to induce the expression of aromatase, resulting in the increased synthesis of estrogen [41–43]

5 Non-clinical evidence supporting targeting COX-2 in cancer management

Numerous genetic and pharmacological non-clinical studies have focused on targeting COX-2 to determine the therapeutic or preventive benefit in cancer.

5.1 Genetic studies

The significant contribution of COX-2 in cancer promotion was demonstrated experimentally in an animal model of human familial adenomatous polyposis [44]. Mice, genetically predisposed for polyp formation by a targeted truncation deletion in the adenomatous polyposis coli protein tumor suppressor gene, were crossed with COX-2 knockout mice [44]. The tumor burden of the double-mutant offspring was significantly reduced by the genetic knockout of COX-2; furthermore, the reduction in polyp formation was equal to that achieved by treating the polyp-forming mice with a selective COX-2 inhibitor [44]. Additionally, it was shown that fibroblasts obtained from COX-2 knockout mice demonstrated a 94% reduction in levels of the angiogenic protein VEGF when compared to wild-type fibroblasts [31]. Pharmacological exposure of wild-type fibroblasts to a selective COX-2 inhibitor also resulted in a 92% reduction in VEGF production [31]. Tumors grown in COX-2 knockout mice demonstrated decreased expression of VEGF mRNA, as well as a 30% decrease in vascular density compared to COX-2 wild-type mice [31].

Mice engineered to overexpress human COX-2 in mammary glands were reported to develop focal mammary gland hyperplasia, dysplasia, and transformation of tissue into metastatic tumors [33, 45]. A similar finding was also observed in mice that were engineered to overexpress COX-2 in basal keratinocytes, where mice developed epidermal hyperplasia as well as dysplastic features [46]. COX-2 overexpression in the basal keratinocytes led to elevated levels of epidermal PGE_2, $PGF_{2\alpha}$, and 15-deoxy-$\delta^{12,14}$-PGJ_2, that sensitized the skin for genotoxic carcinogens [47].

5.2 Pharmacological studies

There have been numerous non-clinical studies using a variety of pharmacological inhibitors of COX-2 that have confirmed that this isozyme is an important therapeutic target [20]. The growth inhibitory mechanism of a selective COX-2 inhibitor was evaluated in an *in vivo* oncogenic mouse model of spontaneous breast cancer [48]. The oncogenic mice carried the polyoma middle T antigen driven by the mouse mammary tumor virus promoter and developed primary adenocarcinomas of the breast. Oral administration of celecoxib caused a significant reduction in mammary tumor burden associated with increased tumor cell apoptosis and decreased proliferation *in vivo* [48].

Celecoxib and sulindac were also evaluated in a transgenic mouse prostate (TRAMP) model that resembles many features of human prostate cancer [49]. These compounds caused significant reductions in prostatic intraepithelial neoplasia lesions, and reduced levels of androgen receptor, VEGF, NF-κB, p65, Bcl-2 and AKT [49].

Celecoxib treatment was found to reduce both Sp1 DNA binding activity and transactivating activity [50]. This decreased activity correlated with reduced Sp1 protein and its phosphorylation [50]. In an animal model of orthotopic pancreatic cancer, celecoxib treatment inhibited tumor growth and metastasis via inhibition of angiogenesis, a finding that was correlated with decreased Sp1 activity and VEGF expression [50].

The combination of COX-2 selective inhibitors with ionizing radiation has demonstrated that selective COX-2 inhibitors can act synergistically with radiotherapy to improve tumor debulking and control in preclinical models [51, 52]. The mechanism for the observed synergy between celecoxib and radiotherapy results from the inhibition of COX-2-derived PGE_2, a factor shown to be essential for the tumor growth and associated vasculature [53].

6 Application of COX-2 selective inhibitors in cancer

Based on the numerous compelling non-clinical studies, it is clear that agents that selectively target COX-2 should be evaluated in human clinical studies. Three distinct applications of COX-2 inhibitors could be envisioned in the cancer setting. The most straightforward is in anti-tumor therapy, where a COX-2 inhibitor is used, with or without chemotherapeutic agents or ionizing radiation, to directly treat the tumor burden. A second application is in the adjuvant setting, where a COX-2 inhibitor could be used, with or without other drugs, to eradicate or control occult micro-metastases following surgery or radiation. The third setting consists of prevention of cancer, and includes primary prevention (prevention of first occurrence of a cancer) and secondary prevention (prevention of recurrence of a cancer). While primary prevention is desirable, demonstrating it in a clinical setting is difficult for a variety of reasons including: (1) defining the target population; (2) clinical trial length; (3) trial size; and (4) trial cost. It is, therefore, most likely that these agents will be used in secondary prevention studies; however, with growing safety concerns, these agents may be exclusively evaluated in the cancer treatment setting.

Most cancers presenting at a late stage are poorly managed, and even early-stage patients suffer a high recurrence rate. Current therapies are generally limited by their toxicities, and are inappropriate for chronic administration. Therefore, a COX-2 selective inhibitor having a generally well-tolerated safety profile could have potential in the management of patients with cancer.

7 COX-2 selective inhibitors and cancer prevention

Retrospective analyses suggest a 40–50 % reduction in the relative risk of developing colon cancer in persons taking aspirin or other NSAIDs on a regular basis [54–56]. In a double-blind, placebo-controlled study, celecoxib was tested in patients with familial adenomatis polyposis (FAP) [57]. In this trial, treatment with celecoxib (100 or 400 mg twice daily) or placebo was carried out for 6 months. The study found that 6 months of twice-daily treatment with 400 mg celecoxib led to a significant reduction in the number of colorectal polyps [57]. The outcomes from this trial resulted in the U.S. Food and Drug Administration approving celecoxib as an adjunctive therapy for the management of polyps in patients with FAP. A similar study using another COX-2 selective drug, rofecoxib, found that once-daily treatment with 25 mg rofecoxib, significantly decreased the number and size of rectal polyps in FAP patients [58].

At the time of this writing, there are 14 oncology prevention-related clinical trials ongoing (www.clinicaltrials.gov) involving regimens that include celecoxib alone or in combination with other agents. The studies target patients with: FAP, oral leukoplakia, head and neck dysplasia, sporadic adenomatous colorectal polyps, basal cell and squamous cell carcinoma of the skin, stage I non-small cell lung cancer (NSCLC), breast cancer *in situ*, lobular breast carcinoma *in situ*, stage I adenocarcinoma of the colon, monoclonal gammopathy of undetermined significance, cervical cancer, high-grade squamous intraepithelial lesion, and early-stage noninvasive carcinoma of the bladder.

8 COX-2 and cancer therapy

Large quantities of prostanoids are detected in human and animal tumors compared with normal adjacent tissues [21, 59]. In addition, many immunohistochemical studies have examined the expression of COX-1 and COX-2 in tumor tissues from various cancers [55, 60]. COX-1 is ubiquitously expressed in both normal and neoplastic regions in all tissues, and appeared to be particularly expressed in the stroma, including fibroblasts, smooth muscle cells and the vasculature. Moderate to intense COX-2 expression was consistently observed in the inflammatory cells, neoplastic cells, and blood vessels in epithelial-derived human cancers, again supporting a role for COX-2 in the formation and/or maintenance of human tumors [60].

Selective COX-2 inhibitors are being evaluated alone and in combination with chemotherapy and radiation for a variety of human cancers [61–63]. Reviews of ongoing and planned clinical trials can be found for: colorectal [54]; breast [64]; upper aerodigestive [65]; genitourinary [66]; and lung [67, 68] cancers.

It is too early to know if these studies will demonstrate a role for targeting COX-2 in human cancers; however, a recent uncontrolled phase II study suggests preliminary activity [69]. Twenty-nine patients with stages IB–IIIA NSCLC were treated with two preoperative cycles of paclitaxel and carboplatin, as well as daily celecoxib, 400 mg b.i.d. followed by surgical resection. The study end points were toxicity, response rate, and the measurement of intratumoral levels of PGE_2. The overall clinical response rate was 65% (48% with partial response; 17% with complete response) [69]. The comparison with previously reported response rates suggests that the addition of a COX-2 selective inhibitor may enhance the response to preoperative paclitaxel and carboplatin in patients with NSCLC. The study also demonstrated that treatment with celecoxib 400 mg twice daily was sufficient to normalize the increase in PGE_2 levels found in NSCLC patients after treatment with paclitaxel and carboplatin [69].

9 Future directions

The growing volume of non-clinical and clinical data strongly supports the study of COX-2 selective agents in the prevention and treatment of cancer. There are, however, outstanding issues that will need to be addressed.

9.1 Selectivity

The current COX-2 inhibitors were designed to be highly selective for COX-2, and were thought not to interact with other protein targets [70]. Recent data demonstrate that these agents are active against COX-independent targets [71]. In addition, higher concentrations of NSAIDs or COX-2 selective agents can inhibit the growth of cells that do not express COX-2 [72]. In addition, celecoxib derivatives lacking COX-2 inhibitory activity were found to be effective anti-cancer growth inhibitory and apoptotic agents [73–76]. Taken together these data suggest that both COX-dependent and -independent effects could account for the potent anticancer activity of the COX-2 selective agents.

9.2 Cellular target

The precise cellular target for the COX-2 selective agents remains unknown. Certainly tumor cells have elevated levels of COX-2; however, the COX-2 selective drugs are also potent inhibitors of angiogenesis [77]. COX-2 mediates angiogenesis through multiple mechanisms, including: (a) increasing VEGF production; (b) generating proangiogenic eicosanoid products (TxA_2, PGI_2, PGE_2) that directly stimulate endothelial cell sprouting, migration and tube formation; (c) enhancing vascular endothelial cell survival by upregulation of the anti-apoptotic proteins Bcl-2 and activation of the PI3K-Akt pathway; (d) upregulating matrix metalloproteinases required for vascular invasion; (e) promoting angiogenic functions of the $\alpha v\beta 3$ integrin; (f) activating the EGF receptor to cause downstream angiogenic events; and (g) decreasing production of the endogenous angiogenesis inhibitor IL-12 [77]. It has also been shown that stromal expression of COX-2 is essential for tumor growth and angiogenesis [31]. These data suggest that the effects of COX-2 selective agents may be directly targeting tumor cells, and/or the indirect targeting of angiogenesis as well as the multiple other cell types found in the tumor microenvironment.

9.3 Anti-cancer dose

The dose for celecoxib that is being evaluated in current phase II and III trials is the approved dose for patients with FAP, 400 mg b.i.d. There have been no phase I single agent dose-escalation trials conducted with celecoxib to determine if the 400 mg b.i.d. dose is the most efficacious dose for cancer treatment alone or in combination with 'standard of care' therapies. It is clear from the study by Altorki et al. [69] in patients with NSCLC that the 400 mg b.i.d. dose was sufficient to normalize the increase in PGE_2 levels found in NSCLC patients after treatment with paclitaxel and carboplatin. It is unclear if there would be an improvement if activity if these compounds were tested at higher concentrations that appear to be associated with COX-independent activities of the molecules.

9.4 Safety

The recent voluntary withdrawal of rofecoxib from the market and the discontinuation of large colorectal prevention trials evaluating celecoxib, due to cardiovascular complications, would suggest that the safety of COX-2 selective drugs needs to be more closely monitored in ongoing prevention and treatment trials. Larger cooperative group, placebo-controlled studies that include selective COX-2 inhibitors will certainly provide much needed safety data in the oncology therapeutic arena. Importantly, the National Institutes of Health announced that early data from a study evaluating naproxen and celecoxib for Alzheimer's disease prevention revealed an apparent increase in cardiovascular events among patients receiving naproxen (NIH Press release, 23 December 2004). If these data are confirmed, it would suggest that naproxen would be a poor comparator for cardiovascular safety assessments of COX-2 selective agents.

Alternatively, the evaluation of COX-2 selective drugs derived from nonselective NSAIDs could provide important opportunities if the cardiovascular complications are in some manner related to the diarylheterocycle chemistry of the compounds. Lumiracoxib (Prexige) is an analogue of diclofenac [78] with the greatest degree of selectivity towards COX-2 [14, 70]. Lumiracoxib is currently awaiting U.S. approval for the indications of osteoarthritis and acute pain, pending the submission of the final report of the ongoing TARGET trial. Additionally, a series of indomethacin amide derivatives were generated that were shown to be highly selective COX-2 inhibitors [79]. These derivatives of older NSAIDs may be more appropriate in the cancer treatment setting as they have been shown to target key anti-cancer pathways including: activation of peroxisome proliferator-activated receptor γ, cyclin-D1, NF-κB, β-catenin, Akt, NAG-1 [80].

In summary, the use of COX-2 selective inhibitors still represents a viable therapeutic option alone, and in combination with established therapeutics, not only for the treatment of existing disease, but as an alternative for individuals at high risk of developing cancer, or in individuals at high risk of disease relapse.

References

1 Vane JR (1971) Inhibition of prostaglandin synthesis as a mechanism of action for aspirin-like drugs. *Nat New Biol* 231: 232–235

2 Fu JY, Masferrer JL, Seibert K, Raz A, Needleman P (1990) The induction and suppression of prostaglandin H2 synthase (cyclooxygenase) in human monocytes. *J Biol Chem* 265: 16737–16740

3 Simmons DL, Botting RM, Robertson PM, Madsen ML, Vane JR (1999) Induction of an acetaminophen-sensitive cyclooxygenase with reduced sensitivity to nonsteroid antiinflammatory drugs. *Proc Natl Acad Sci USA* 96: 3275–3280

4 Flower RJ (2003) The development of COX2 inhibitors. *Nat Rev Drug Discov* 2: 179–191
5 Warner TD, Giuliano F, Vojnovic I, Bukasa A, Mitchell JA, Vane JR (1999) Nonsteroid drug selectivities for cyclo-oxygenase-1 rather than cyclo-oxygenase-2 are associated with human gastrointestinal toxicity: a full *in vitro* analysis. *Proc Natl Acad Sci USA* 96: 7563–7568
6 Gans KR, Galbraith W, Roman RJ, Haber SB, Kerr JS, Schmidt WK, Smith C, Hewes WE, Ackerman NR (1990) Anti-inflammatory and safety profile of DuP 697, a novel orally effective prostaglandin synthesis inhibitor. *J Pharmacol Exp Ther* 254: 180–187
7 Fitzgerald GA (2004) Coxibs and cardiovascular disease. *N Engl J Med* 351: 1709–1711
8 Juni P, Nartey L, Reichenbach S, Sterchi R, Dieppe PA, Egger M (2004) Risk of cardiovascular events and rofecoxib: cumulative meta-analysis. *Lancet* 364: 2021–2029
9 Ray WA, Griffen MR, Stein CM (2004) Cardiovascular toxicity of valdecoxib. *N Engl J Med* 351: 2767
10 Kimmel SE, Berlin JA, Reilly M, Jaskowlak J, Kishel L, Chittams J, Strom BL (2005) Patients exposed to rofecoxib and celecoxib have different odds of nonfatal myocardial infarction. *Ann Intern Med* 142: 157–164
11 Davies NM, Jamali F (2004) COX-2 selective inhibitors cardiac toxicity: getting to the heart of the matter. *J Pharm Pharm Sci* 7: 332–336
12 Cheng Y, Austin SC, Rocca B, Koller BH, Coffman TM, Grosser T, Lawson JA, FitzGerald GA (2002) Role of prostacyclin in the cardiovascular response to thromboxane A2. *Science* 296: 539–541
13 Krum H, Liew D, Aw J, Haas S (2004) Cardiovascular effects of selective cyclooxygenase-2 inhibitors. *Expert Rev Cardiovasc Ther* 2: 265–270
14 Brune K, Hinz B (2004) Selective cyclooxygenase-2 inhibitors: similarities and differences. *Scand J Rheumatol* 33: 1–6
15 Farkouh ME, Kirshner H, Harrington RA, Ruland S, Verheugt FW, Schnitzer TJ, Burmester GR, Mysler E, Hochberg MC, Doherty M et al (2004) Comparison of lumiracoxib with naproxen and ibuprofen in the Therapeutic Arthritis Research and Gastrointestinal Event Trial (TARGET), cardiovascular outcomes: randomised controlled trial. *Lancet* 364: 675–684
16 Schimmel KJ, Richel DJ, van den Brink RB, Guchelaar HJ (2004) Cardiotoxicity of cytotoxic drugs. *Cancer Treat Rev* 30: 181–191
17 Hurwitz H (2004) Integrating the anti-VEGF-A humanized monoclonal antibody bevacizumab with chemotherapy in advanced colorectal cancer. *Clin Colorectal Cancer* 4 Suppl 2: S62–S68
18 Dannenberg AJ, Subbaramaiah K (2003) Targeting cyclooxygenase-2 in human neoplasia: rationale and promise. *Cancer Cell* 4: 431–436
19 Herschman HR (1996) Prostaglandin synthase 2. *Biochim Biophys Acta* 1299: 125–140
20 Subbaramaiah K, Dannenberg AJ (2003) Cyclooxygenase 2: a molecular target for cancer prevention and treatment. *Trends Pharmacol Sci* 24: 96–102
21 Simmons DL, Botting RM, Hla T (2004) Cyclooxygenase isozymes: the biology of prostaglandin synthesis and inhibition. *Pharmacol Rev* 56: 387–437
22 Subbaramaiah K, Altorki N, Chung WJ, Mestre JR, Sampat A, Dannenberg AJ (1999) Inhibition of cyclooxygenase-2 gene expression by p53. *J Biol Chem* 274: 10911–10915

23 Araki Y, Okamura S, Hussain SP, Nagashima M, He P, Shiseki M, Miura K, Harris CC (2003) Regulation of cyclooxygenase-2 expression by the Wnt and ras pathways. *Cancer Res* 63: 728–734

24 Dixon DA (2004) Dysregulated post-transcriptional control of COX-2 gene expression in cancer. *Curr Pharm Des* 10: 635–646

25 Subbaramaiah K, Hart JC, Norton L, Dannenberg AJ (2000) Microtubule-interfering agents stimulate the transcription of cyclooxygenase-2. Evidence for involvement of ERK1/2 AND p38 mitogen-activated protein kinase pathways. *J Biol Chem* 275: 14838–14845

26 Subbaramaiah K, Marmo TP, Dixon DA, Dannenberg, AJ (2003) Regulation of cyclooxgenase-2 mRNA stability by taxanes: evidence for involvement of p38, MAPKAPK-2, and HuR. *J Biol Chem* 278: 37637–37647

27 Fukuda K, Sakakura C, Miyagawa K, Kuriu Y, Kin S, Nakase Y, Hagiwara A, Mitsufuji S, Okazaki Y, Hayashizaki Y et al (2004) Differential gene expression profiles of radioresistant oesophageal cancer cell lines established by continuous fractionated irradiation. *Br J Cancer* 91: 1543–1550

28 Tessner TG, Muhale F, Schloemann S, Cohn SM, Morrison AR, Stenson WF (2004) Ionizing radiation up-regulates cyclooxygenase-2 in I407 cells through p38 mitogen-activated protein kinase. *Carcinogenesis* 25: 37–45

29 Tsujii M, Kawano S, Tsuji S, Sawaoka H, Hori M, DuBois RN (1998) Cyclooxygenase regulates angiogenesis induced by colon cancer cells. *Cell* 93: 705–716

30 Masferrer JL, Leahy KM, Koki AT, Zweifel BS, Settle SL, Woerner BM, Edwards DA, Flickinger AG, Moore RJ, Seibert K (2000) Antiangiogenic and antitumor activities of cyclooxygenase-2 inhibitors. *Cancer Res* 60: 1306–1311

31 Williams CS, Tsujii M, Reese J, Dey SK, DuBois RN (2000) Host cyclooxygenase-2 modulates carcinoma growth. *J Clin Invest* 105: 1589–1594

32 Wang D, Wang H, Shi Q, Katkuri S, Walhi W, Desvergne B, Das SK, Dey SK, DuBois RN (2004) Prostaglandin E(2) promotes colorectal adenoma growth via transactivation of the nuclear peroxisome proliferator-activated receptor delta. *Cancer Cell* 6: 285–295

33 Chang SH, Liu CH, Conway R, Han DK, Nithipatikom K, Trifan OC, Lane TF, Hla T (2004) Role of prostaglandin E2-dependent angiogenic switch in cyclooxygenase 2-induced breast cancer progression. *Proc Natl Acad Sci USA* 101: 591–596

34 Akasaki Y, Liu G, Chung NH, Ehtesham M, Black KL, Yu JS (2004) Induction of a $CD4^+$ T regulatory type 1 response by cyclooxygenase-2-overexpressing glioma. *J Immunol* 173: 4352–4359

35 Pockaj BA, Basu GD, Pathangey LB, Gray RJ, Hernandez JL, Gendler SJ, Mukherjee P (2004) Reduced T-cell and dendritic cell function is related to cyclooxygenase-2 overexpression and prostaglandin E2 secretion in patients with breast cancer. *Ann Surg Oncol* 11: 328–339

36 Holla VR, Wang D, Brown JR, Mann JR, Katkuri S, Dubois RN (2004) Prostaglandin E2 regulates the complement inhibitor CD55/decay accelerating factor in colorectal cancer. *J Biol Chem* 280: 476–483

37 Fujino H, Vielhauer GA, Regan JW (2004) Prostaglandin E2 selectively antagonizes prostaglandin F2alpha-stimulated T-cell factor/beta-catenin signaling pathway by the FPB prostanoid receptor. *J Biol Chem* 279: 43386–43391

38 Shao J, Evers BM, Sheng H (2004) Prostaglandin E2 synergistically enhances receptor tyrosine kinase-dependent signaling system in colon cancer cells. *J Biol Chem* 279: 14287–14293

39 Buchanan FG, Wang D, Bargiacchi F, DuBois RN (2003) Prostaglandin E2 regulates cell migration via the intracellular activation of the epidermal growth factor receptor. *J Biol Chem* 278: 35451–35457

40 Salcedo R, Zhang X, Young HA, Michael N, Wasserman K, Ma WH, Martins-Green M, Murphy WJ, Oppenheim JJ (2003) Angiogenic effects of prostaglandin E2 are mediated by up-regulation of CXCR4 on human microvascular endothelial cells. *Blood* 102: 1966–1977

41 Goss PE, Strasser-Weippl K (2004) Prevention strategies with aromatase inhibitors. *Clin Cancer Res* 10: 372S–379S

42 Richards JA, Brueggemeier RW (2003) Prostaglandin E2 regulates aromatase activity and expression in human adipose stromal cells via two distinct receptor subtypes. *J Clin Endocrinol Metab* 88: 2810–2816

43 Brueggemeier RW, Richards JA, Petrel TA (2003) Aromatase and cyclooxygenases: enzymes in breast cancer. *J Steroid Biochem Mol Biol* 86: 501–507

44 Oshima M, Dinchuk JE, Kargman SL, Oshima H, Hancock B, Kwong E, Trzaskos JM, Evans JF, Taketo MM (1996) Suppression of intestinal polyposis in Apc delta716 knockout mice by inhibition of cyclooxygenase 2 (COX-2). *Cell* 87: 803–809

45 Liu CH, Chang SH, Narko K, Trifan OC, Wu MT, Smith E, Haudenschild C, Lane TF, Hla T (2001) Overexpression of cyclooxygenase-2 is sufficient to induce tumorigenesis in transgenic mice. *J Biol Chem* 276: 18563–18569

46 Neufang G, Furstenberger G, Heidt M, Marks F, Muller-Decker K (2001) Abnormal differentiation of epidermis in transgenic mice constitutively expressing cyclooxygenase-2 in skin. *Proc Natl Acad Sci USA* 98: 7629–7634

47 Muller-Decker K, Neufang G, Berger I, Neumann M, Marks F, Furstenberger G (2002) Transgenic cyclooxygenase-2 overexpression sensitizes mouse skin for carcinogenesis. *Proc Natl Acad Sci USA* 99: 12483–12488

48 Basu GD, Pathangey LB, Tinder TL, Lagioia M, Gendler SJ, Mukherjee P (2004) Cyclooxygenase-2 inhibitor induces apoptosis in breast cancer cells in an *in vivo* model of spontaneous metastatic breast cancer. *Mol Cancer Res* 2: 632–642

49 Narayanan BA, Narayanan NK, Pittman B, Reddy BS (2004) Regression of mouse prostatic intraepithelial neoplasia by nonsteroidal anti-inflammatory drugs in the transgenic adenocarcinoma mouse prostate model. *Clin Cancer Res* 10: 7727–7737

50 Wei D, Wang L, He Y, Xiong HQ, Abbruzzese JL, Xie K (2004) Celecoxib inhibits vascular endothelial growth factor expression in and reduces angiogenesis and metastasis of human pancreatic cancer via suppression of Sp1 transcription factor activity. *Cancer Res* 64: 2030–2038

51 Kishi K, Petersen S, Petersen C, Hunter N, Mason K, Masferrer JL, Tofilon PJ, Milas L (2000) Preferential enhancement of tumor radioresponse by a cyclooxygenase-2 inhibitor. *Cancer Res* 60: 1326–1331

52 Petersen C, Petersen S, Milas L, Lang FF, Tofilon PJ (2000) Enhancement of intrinsic tumor cell radiosensitivity induced by a selective cyclooxygenase-2 inhibitor. *Clin Cancer Res* 6: 2513–2520

53 Davis TW, O'Neal JM, Pagel MD, Zweifel BS, Mehta PP, Heuvelman DM, Masferrer JL (2004) Synergy between celecoxib and radiotherapy results from inhibition of cy-

clooxygenase-2-derived prostaglandin E2, a survival factor for tumor and associated vasculature. *Cancer Res* 64: 279–285
54 Koehne CH, Dubois RN (2004) COX-2 inhibition and colorectal cancer. *Semin Oncol* 31: 12–21
55 Thun MJ, Henley SJ, Patrono C (2002) Nonsteroidal anti-inflammatory drugs as anticancer agents: mechanistic, pharmacologic, and clinical issues. *J Natl Cancer Inst* 94: 252–266
56 Rao CV, Reddy BS (2004) NSAIDs and chemoprevention. *Curr Cancer Drug Targets* 4: 29–42
57 Steinbach G, Lynch PM., Phillips RK, Wallace MH, Hawk E, Gordon GB, Wakabayashi N, Saunders B, Shen Y, Fujimura T, Su LK, Levin B (2000) The effect of celecoxib, a cyclooxygenase-2 inhibitor, in familial adenomatous polyposis. *N Engl J Med* 342: 1946–1952
58 Higuchi T, Iwama T, Yoshinaga K, Toyooka M, Taketo MM, Sugihara K (2003) A randomized, double-blind, placebo-controlled trial of the effects of rofecoxib, a selective cyclooxygenase-2 inhibitor, on rectal polyps in familial adenomatous polyposis patients. *Clin Cancer Res* 9: 4756–4760
59 Levine L (1981) Arachidonic acid transformation and tumor production. *Adv Cancer Res* 35: 49–79
60 Koki A, Khan NK, Woerner BM, Dannenberg AJ, Olson L, Seibert K, Edwards D, Hardy M, Isakson P, Masferrer JL (2002) Cyclooxygenase-2 in human pathological disease. *Adv Exp Med Biol* 507: 177–184
61 Gasparini G, Longo R, Sarmiento R, Morabito A (2003) Inhibitors of cyclo-oxygenase 2: a new class of anticancer agents? *Lancet Oncol* 4: 605–615
62 Karamouzis MV, Papavassiliou AG (2004) COX-2 inhibition in cancer therapeutics: a field of controversy or a magic bullet? *Expert Opin Investig Drugs* 13: 359–372
63 Evans JF, Kargman SL (2004) Cancer and cyclooxygenase-2 (COX-2) inhibition. *Curr Pharm Des* 10: 627–634
64 Arun B, Goss P (2004) The role of COX-2 inhibition in breast cancer treatment and prevention. *Semin Oncol* 31: 22–29
65 Altorki NK, Subbaramaiah K, Dannenberg AJ (2004) COX-2 inhibition in upper aerodigestive tract tumors. *Semin Oncol* 31: 30–36
66 Sabichi AL, Lippman SM (2004) COX-2 inhibitors and other nonsteroidal anti-inflammatory drugs in genitourinary cancer. *Semin Oncol* 31: 36–44
67 Sandler AB, Dubinett SM (2004) COX-2 inhibition and lung cancer. *Semin Oncol* 31: 45–52
68 Riedl K, Krysan K, Pold M, Dalwadi H, Heuze-Vourc'h N, Dohadwala M, Liu M, Cui X, Figlin R, Mao JT et al (2004) Multifaceted roles of cyclooxygenase-2 in lung cancer. *Drug Resist Updat* 7: 169–184
69 Altorki NK, Keresztes RS, Port JL, Libby DM, Korst RJ, Flieder DB, Ferrara CA, Yankelevitz DF, Subbaramaiah K, Pasmantier MW et al (2003) Celecoxib, a selective cyclo-oxygenase-2 inhibitor, enhances the response to preoperative paclitaxel and carboplatin in early-stage non-small-cell lung cancer. *J Clin Oncol 21*: 2645–2650
70 FitzGerald GA (2003) COX-2 and beyond: Approaches to prostaglandin inhibition in human disease. *Nat Rev Drug Discov* 2: 879–890
71 Weber A, Casini A, Heine A, Kuhn D, Supuran CT, Scozzafava A, Klebe G (2004) Unexpected nanomolar inhibition of carbonic anhydrase by COX-2-selective cele-

coxib: new pharmacological opportunities due to related binding site recognition. *J Med Chem* 47: 550–557
72 Zhang X, Morham SG, Langenbach R, Young DA (1999) Malignant transformation and antineoplastic actions of nonsteroidal antiinflammatory drugs (NSAIDs) on cyclooxygenase-null embryo fibroblasts. *J Exp Med* 190: 451–459
73 Ding H, Han C, Zhu J, Chen CS, D'Ambrosio SM (2005) Celecoxib derivatives induce apoptosis via the disruption of mitochondrial membrane potential and activation of caspase 9. *Int J Cancer* 113: 803–810
74 Johnson AJ, Smith LL, Zhu J, Heerema NA, Jefferson S, Mone A, Grever M, Chen CS, Byrd JC (2004) A novel celecoxib derivative, OSU03012, induces cytotoxicity in primary CLL cells and transformed B-cell lymphoma via a caspase and Bcl-2 independent mechanism. *Blood* 105: 2504–2509
75 Zhu J, Huang JW, Tseng PH, Yang YT, Fowble J, Shiau CW, Shaw YJ, Kulp SK, Chen CS (2004) From the cyclooxygenase-2 inhibitor celecoxib to a novel class of 3-phosphoinositide-dependent protein kinase-1 inhibitors. *Cancer Res* 64: 4309–4318
76 Kulp SK, Yang YT, Hung CC, Chen KF, Lai JP, Tseng PH, Fowble JW, Ward PJ, Chen CS (2004) 3-Phosphoinositide-dependent protein kinase-1/Akt signaling represents a major cyclooxygenase-2-independent target for celecoxib in prostate cancer cells. *Cancer Res* 64: 1444–1451
77 Gately S, Li WW (2004) Multiple roles of COX-2 in tumor angiogenesis: a target for antiangiogenic therapy. *Semin Oncol* 31: 2–11
78 Lyseng-Williamson KA, Curran MP (2004) Lumiracoxib. *Drugs* 64: 2237–2246
79 Kalgutkar AS, Marnett AB, Crews BC, Remmel RP, Marnett LJ (2000) Ester and amide derivatives of the nonsteroidal antiinflammatory drug, indomethacin, as selective cyclooxygenase-2 inhibitors. *J Med Chem* 43: 2860–2870
80 Hull MA, Gardner SH, Hawcroft G (2003) Activity of the non-steroidal anti-inflammatory drug indomethacin against colorectal cancer. *Cancer Treat Rev* 29: 309–320

Progress in Drug Research, Vol. 63
(R. M. Schultz, Ed.)

Antisense approaches in drug discovery and development

Elizabeth Rayburn[1],
Wei Wang[1], Ruiwen Zhang[1,2,3]
and Hui Wang[1,2]

[1]Department of Pharmacology
and Toxicology
Division of Clinical Pharmacology
University of Alabama at
Birmingham, VH 112, Box 600
1670 University Blvd.
Birmingham, AL 35294–0019, USA
<hui.wang@ccc.uab.edu>

[2]Comprehensive Cancer Center
University of Alabama at
Birmingham, Birmingham
Alabama, USA

[3]Gene Therapy Center
University of Alabama at
Birmingham, Birmingham
Alabama, USA

Glossary of abbreviations

AR, androgen receptor; aPTT, activated partial thromboplastin time; cGLP, current Good Labortory Practices; CeNA, cyclohexene nucleic acid; CMV, cytomegalovirus; ds/ssRNA, double/single stranded RNA; GPCRs, G protein-coupled receptors; MBO, mixed backbone oligo; MDM2, mouse double minute 2; MOE, methoxyethyl; PKA, cAMP-dependent protein kinase (protein kinase A); PKC, protein kinase C; pRb, hypophosphorylated retinoblastoma (Rb); PS, phosphorothioate; RNAi, RNA interference; SCID, severe combined immunodeficient; siRNA/shRNA, short interfering/short hairpin RNA; SNP, single nucleotide polymorphism; TNF-α, tumor necrosis factor alpha; VEGF(R), vascular endothelial growth factor (receptor); XIAP, X-chromosome linked inhibitor-of-apoptosis.

1 Introduction

Modern cancer therapy relies on better understanding of cancer biology and cancer genetics. The majority of human cancers are derived from single somatic cells that undergo a series of genetic and epigenetic changes, leading to alterations in gene activity, loss of control of proliferation, and development of cancer phenotypes, including the disregard of signals to differentiate and to stop proliferating, the capacity for sustained proliferation, a loss of apoptosis, and increased invasion and angiogenesis [1]. In the last two decades, progress has been made in identifying, cloning, sequencing and characterizing pathogenic genes important to cancer development, leading to the development of genetic-based therapy. Genetic therapy can be summarized into two general approaches: the first, termed gene therapy, is the introduction of a vector that is capable of inserting a gene of interest into the genetic code to restore normal function or correct an abnormal function; the second, termed RNA-based therapy, includes antisense technology, and delivers RNA silencing molecules that can hybridize with and specifically inhibit the expression of pathogenic genes to target cells.

Generally speaking, antisense nucleic acids (DNA, RNA, and DNA/RNA chimeras) are single-stranded oligonucleotides (oligos) that are complementary to the sequence of a target RNA or DNA. This concept was first introduced by Zamecnik and his colleagues over 25 years ago [2]. In fact, antisense RNA is a naturally occurring means of regulation of gene expression in living cells, including plants, animals and humans [3]. However, the early groundbreaking work did not generate much interest until the late 1980s. After a major breakthrough in automated oligo synthesis, and better understanding of gene regulation in living cells, antisense techniques have developed rapidly. Among the many potential applications, antisense technology as an RNA silencing approach will have utility in the following four areas:

a Identification of gene function: The function of a gene of interest can be investigated by specifically blocking gene expression, with or without knowing the protein encoded by the gene.
b Identification of novel targets for therapy: With high specificity and affinity, RNA silencing approaches target specific molecular targets for the treatment of various diseases such as cancer, cardiovascular diseases and infectious diseases. This serves to validate the therapeutic targeting of these molecules, not only by antisense techniques, but also by providing a basis for designing other specific, rational inhibitors.
c Applications in pharmacogenetics and pharmacogenomics: Recent technological advances have moved oligo arrays into the realm of standard laboratory technology. RNA silencing approaches aid in the identification of novel genes responsible for variations in response to drug treatment and/or toxicity, which facilitates the development of individualized medicine.
d Development of novel therapeutic agents: Antisense oligos and ribozymes identified in gene function target validation studies can often be developed as therapeutic agents. These agents can be administered alone or in combination with conventional therapies, including anti-viral drugs, antibodies, chemotherapy or radiation therapy. Compared with conventional therapy, this approach provides higher specificity and efficacy, and lower toxicity.

Many published studies suggest the potential use of antisense oligos in the treatment of various human diseases such as cancer, genetic disorders, viral infections, hypertension, and other cardiovascular diseases [4–12]. The first antisense drug, Vitravene, has been approved for the treatment of patients with cytomegalovirus-induced retinitis [10]. Several other antisense oligos have entered phases I–III clinical trials as anticancer agents (Tab. 1), and many more are in preclinical development (Tab. 2).

Table 1.
Antisense anti-cancer drugs in clinical trials since 1995.

Name of drug	Target	Chemical modification(s)	Phase	Company	Ref.
Affinitak/ ISIS3521/ Aprinocarsen	PKC-alpha	PS	II/III	Lilly/ISIS	[58]
Oblimersen, G3139	Bcl-2	PS	II/III	Aventis/Genta	[24]
ISIS 2503	H-ras	PS	II	ISIS	[62, 63]
GTI-2040	RR R2 subunit	PS	II	Lorus Therapeutics	[144]
GTI-2501	RR R1 subunit	PS	II	Lorus Therapeutics	[145]
GEM-231	PKA	MBO (PS/2′-O-Me)	II	Hybridon	[146]
MG98	DNA methyl-transferase	MBO (PS/2′-O-Me)	II	MethyGene/ MGI Pharma/ British Biotech	[147]
Oncomyc-NG/ AVI 4126	c-myc	Morpholino	II	AVI BioPharma	[148, 149]
AVI 4557	Cyp3A4	Phosphoro-diamidate Morpholino	II (oral)	AVI BioPharma	[150]
AP12009	TGF-B2	PS	II	Antisense Pharma	[151]
ISIS 5132	c-raf	PS	I/II	ISIS	[152]
LErafAON	c-raf	PS (liposome)	I/II	NeoPharm	[153, 154]
OGX-011	Clusterin	MBO (PS/2′-O-Me)	I/II	Oncogenix/ ISIS	[155]
LR-3001	c-myb	PS	I	Lynx Therapeutics/ Inex/Temple Univ.	[156]
OL(1)p53/ EL-625	p53	PS	I	Lynx Therapeutics/ Elos Inc.	[157, 158]
GEM 640/ AEG 35156	XIAP	MBO (PS/2′-O-Me)	pre-clinical/I	Hybridon/Aegera Therapeutics	[159]
ISIS 23722	Survivin	MOE gapmer	pre-clinical/I	Lilly/ISIS	[160]

Table 2.
Pre-clinical targeting of proteins by antisense oligonucleotides since 2000.

Target	Function of protein	Cancer	Modifications	*In vivo* model	Corporate affiliation	Combination	Reference
Androgen receptor	Cell signaling/ proliferation	Prostate	Phosphoro-diamidate morpholino	Prostate xenograft	Novartis		[161]
ATP synthase subunit E	Energy transport/ cell signaling	Hepatocellular carcinoma		n/a			[162]
Bcl-xL	Apoptosis	Colon, various	PS, MOE, LNA Gapmer			Oxaliplatin, radiation	[163, 164]
c-FLIP	Apoptosis	Prostate					[165]
CSF-1	Growth factor/ immune regulation			Breast xenograft			[166]
cyp3A2	Drug metabolism		Phosphoro-diamidate morpholino		Avi BioPharma		[150]
DNA-dependent protein kinase	DNA repair	NSCLC				Wortmannin, radiation	[167]
EGFR	Growth factor	SCC, NSCLC	Morpholino		Hybridon	Docetaxel	[168, 169]
Egr-1	Transcription factor/growth factor	Prostate		TRAMP			[170]
GLUT5	Facilitated transport	Breast					[171]
Ferritin	Iron storage	Breast					[172]
FGFR/bFGF	Growth factor			Orthotoptic germ cell tumor			[173]

Table 2 (continued).

Target	Function of protein	Cancer	Modifications	In vivo model	Corporate affiliation	Combination	Reference
Glucosyl-ceramide synthase	Lipid synthesis/ drug resistance	Breast		Mouse melanoma		Doxorubicin	[174, 175]
Glucosyl-transferase	Lipid synthesis	Glioma					[176]
HER-2	Oncogene/ signaling	Head and neck, breast, ovarian		Breast xenograft		Various chemotherapy agents	[177, 178]
Hif-1-alpha	Stress response	Glioblastoma					[179]
hTERT	DNA synthesis/ regulation	Hepatoma					[180]
HUS1	DNA repair/ cell cycle control	Lung				Cisplatin	[181]
KGFR	Growth factor/ motility	Breast					[182]
Ki-67	Proliferation	Renal cell carcinoma	PS	Orthotopic RCC model			[183]
k-ras	Signaling/ proliferation	Pancreatic, colon					[184, 185]
Ku70	Apoptosis/ DNA repair	Colon					[186]
Ku86	DNA synthesis/ repair	Glioma	2′-MOE/PS			Radiation, various chemo-therapeutic agents	[187]

Table 2 (continued).

Target	Function of protein	Cancer	Modifications	In vivo model	Corporate affiliation	Combination	Reference
Laminin-8	Structural component/ angiogenesis	Glioma	Morpholino				[188]
Mcl-1	Apoptosis	Melanoma		Melanoma xenograft		Dacarbazine	[189]
MDM2	Oncogene/cell cycle regulation	Various	MBO	Various xenografts	Hybridon (GEM 240)	Various, radiation	[139]
MDR1	Drug resistance	Brain, HUV-ECC cells				Doxorubicin	[190]
MMP-9	Matrix degradation	Prostate	Phosphoro-diamidate morpholino		Avi BioPharma		[191]
MRP1	Drug resistance	Glioma	PS			Etoposide	[192]
n-myc	Cell signaling	Neuro-blastoma	Peptide nucleic acid				[193]
p21	Cell cycle regulation	Breast		Mouse mammary carcinoma			[194]
PKC-eta	Cell signaling/ oncogenesis	Lung adeno-carcinoma				Vincristine, paclitaxel	[195]
RelA	Cell signaling/ inflammation	Ovarian				TNF-alpha, paclitaxel	[196]
Ribosomal protein P2	Protein synthesis	Pancreatic					[197]

Table 2 (continued).

Target	Function of protein	Cancer	Modifications	In vivo model	Corporate affiliation	Combination	Reference
RNA polymerase II	Protein synthesis	Pancreatic, prostate	PS, locked nucleic acid	Panc and prostate xenografts			[198, 199]
Survivin (also see clinical trials in Table 2)	Apoptosis	Non-Hodgkin's lymphoma		Lymphoma xenograft		Rituximab	[113]
Telomerase	DNA synthesis and regulation	Cervical	Thiophos-phoro-amidate		Geron		[24]
TGF-alpha	Signaling	Prostate				Taxol	[200]
Thrombo-modulin	Regulate coagulation	Lung adeno-carcinoma					[201]
Thymidylate synthase	Drug metabo-lism/nucleotide synthesis	Various				5-fluorode-oxyuridine	[202]
Type 1 insulin-like growth factor receptor	Cell signaling/ proliferation	Breast, prostate	PS	Breast xenograft			[203, 204]
Urokinase-plasminogen activator receptor	Matrix degradation/ cell motility	Melanoma	PS	Melanoma xenograft			[205]
VEGF	Angiogenesis	HNSCC, renal cell carcinoma	MBO		Hybridon/ VasGene		[94, 95]

2 Antisense drug design

In theory, the concept and rationale of antisense therapy is simple: antisense oligos specifically bind to and interact with their complementary target RNA and thereby block gene expression, resulting in therapeutic effects in a sequence-dependent manner. However, it has now been realized that antisense oligos exert their biological effects on target genes through several distinct mechanisms, including both antisense and non-antisense mechanisms in target and non-target cells or tissues [13–19].

2.1 Antisense mechanisms

Although it has been known for nearly 30 years that antisense oligos can decrease expression of a target gene product, the exact mechanisms of action are still being sorted out. The oligos may produce their effect by multiple mechanisms. These include the inhibition of transcription by forming triplexes with DNA, inhibiting pre-mRNA processing, inhibiting the transport of the mRNA to the cytoplasm, blocking translation of the mRNA, or by causing enzymatic degradation of the mRNA. Oligos can also interact directly with a protein to inhibit its function, although this is not considered an "antisense" effect. The most important mechanisms of action are translation arrest and degradation by RNase H enzyme. An overview of the five main mechanisms of action can be seen in Figure 1.

Two members of the RNase H family, RNase H1 and RNase H2, are expressed in human tissues. The RNase H family has several members of varying sizes, but all function as endonucleases and require divalent cations for catalysis. RNase H is activated by the presence of DNA/RNA hybrids, making the DNA oligos which bind to mRNA effective RNase H activators. Upon recognition of the hybrid, RNase H degrades the RNA, leaving the DNA untouched, but preventing the translation of the target mRNA. A recent report identified human RNase 1 as the major enzyme responsible for the antisense effects of the oligos. The same report also identified several new human RNase H enzymes that may contribute to the effects [20].

Many of the natural (phosphodiester) and modified oligos are capable of activating RNase H; however, some of the chemical modifications make the oligo unable to activate the enzyme. These oligos rely on the other mechanisms of action to achieve their antisense effect. Translation arrest is the

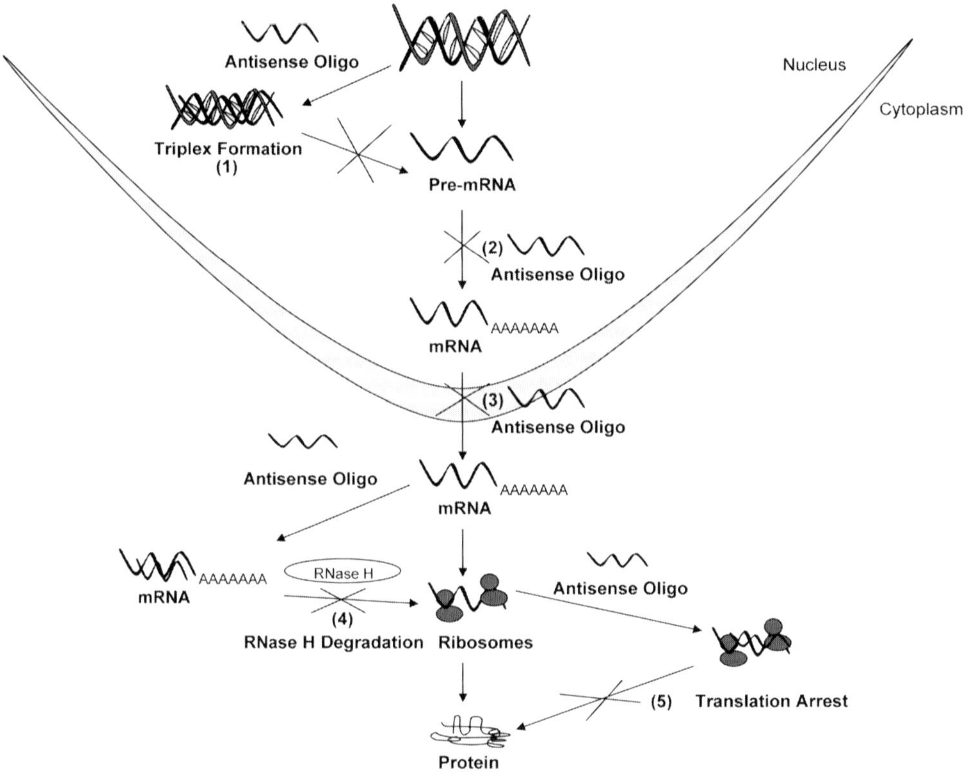

Figure 1.
Major mechanisms of action of antisense oligos. 1. Triplex formation with DNA. 2. Interference with pre-mRNA processing. 3. Interference with nuclear export of mRNA. 4. Degradation of mRNA by RNase H. 5. Translation arrest.

dominant mechanism for non enzyme-mediated antisense effects, although it may be less effective for preventing expression of a gene product. However, by interfering with translation, it may be possible to influence the proteins produced. This is especially useful for preventing the synthesis of truncated splice variants, and could perhaps alleviate the cause of several diseases. These mechanisms will be discussed in later sections relating to specific oligos.

2.2 Antisense chemistry

As a result of more than 20 years of investigations, considerable changes have been made to antisense oligos to enhance their specificity, increase their

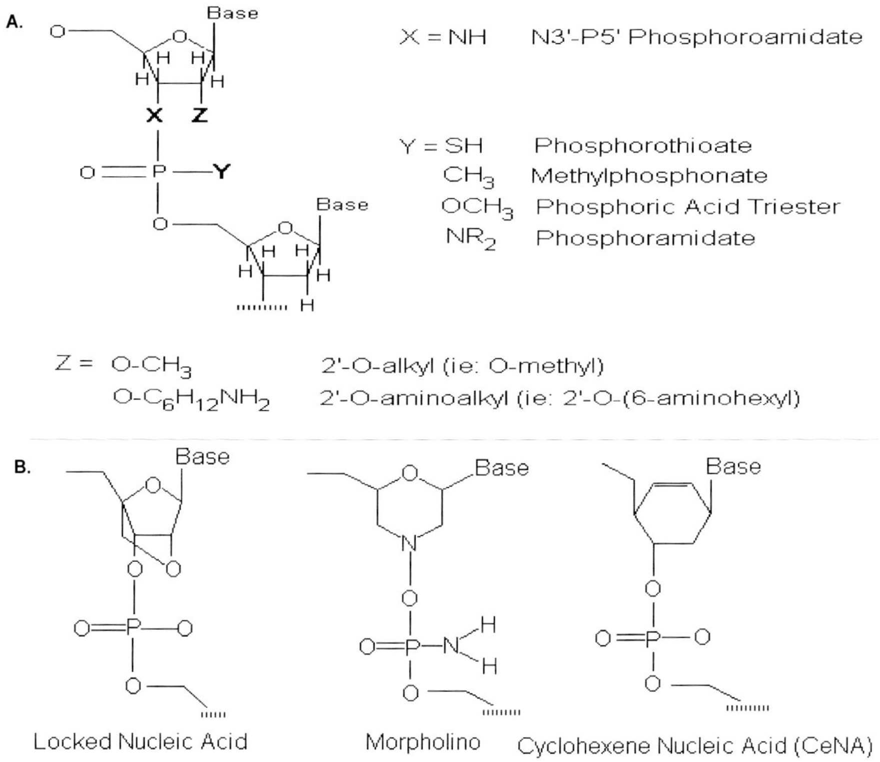

Figure 2.
Examples of chemical modifications made to improve antisense oligos. A. Substitutions made to the 2′ and 3′ positions and the non-bonding oxygen to enhance binding efficiency, decrease enzymatic degradation, and decrease immune system stimulation. B. Example modifications made to create "third generation" antisense oligos.

stability and increase their efficiency. Derived from the earliest phosphodiester-linked oligos, there are now a variety of more advanced antisense molecules. Some of the modifications made to the basic chemical structure can be seen in Figure 2. The first generation phosphodiester oligonucleotides were rapidly degraded by cellular nucleases, but were easily administered both *in vitro* and *in vivo*. Unfortunately, the short half-life of the oligos rendered them unable to achieve a sufficient antisense response. One of the most important developments in antisense chemistry was the incorporation of phosphorothioate (PS) backbones; that is, a non-bridging oxygen of the phosphodiester bond between nucleotides was replaced by sulfur. This allowed the oligos to avoid degradative nucleases, increasing the half-life of the oligos to hours or days, in comparison to the minutes of the phosphodiester oligos. PS oligos are capable of acting by both translation arrest and activation of RNase H. The phosphorothioate oligos have gained in popularity, and most of the antisense oligos being used in clinical trials, including the only FDA-approved antisense drug, Vitravene, have PS linkages. A wide variety of other modifications have been made, including substitution of the non-bridging oxygen with an amino-alkyl or a methyl group (phosphoroamidate or methylphosphonate) [21].

Unfortunately, there were some problems associated with the PS-modified oligos, including nonspecific toxicity. These problems will be discussed in-depth later in this chapter, but the next generation of oligos resolved some of these problems by making modifications to the 2′ position of the ribose ring. The -*O*-methyl and -*O*-methoxyethyl substitutions for the hydrogen at the 2′ position make the oligos less toxic than their DNA counterparts, but unfortunately also make the oligos unable to activate RNase H. It appears that these modified oligos can still exert antisense effects when designed properly, and 2′-methoxy and -methoxyethyl oligos are being used to prevent expression of a variety of molecules, including Clusterin, which was recently targeted in phase I clinical trials using a methoxyethyl oligo [4, 22].

Alternatively, avoiding the activation of RNase H is a necessity for altering incorrect splicing. This mechanism of oligo action could prove to be useful. There are an estimated 30000 genes in the human genome, and many genes are already known to have variant and aberrant splicing products. For example, as of 2004, more than 40 splicing variants of mdm2 have been found [23]. If other genes have a similar number of variant proteins, there are likely to be hundreds of thousands, if not millions, of splice variants resulting in different protein products. Some of these are responsible for disease states. The activation of RNase H by an antisense oligo targeting a variant would cause destruction of the mRNA without resolving the disease state. The disease phenotype would likely persist because the necessary full-length protein would not be produced. On the other hand, causing translation arrest can enable the translation of a correct, full-length mRNA when damaging splice variants would otherwise be produced. Thus, while the antisense effect may still be possible for these modified oligos, if RNase H is not activated, the oligos can also act in a different manner when necessary. An excellent example is the use of a 2′-*O*-methyl oligoribonucleotide to target a mutated intron in the β-globin gene which causes β-thalassemia. The oligo does not activate RNase H, but does cause translation arrest. This allows the full-length gene to be translated, the entire protein to be produced, and the mutation to be corrected [24].

In general, however, activation of RNase H is necessary for efficient antisense effects. For this reason, RNA oligos have generally been rejected for use. To allow for the modifications to DNA oligos to be made to decrease toxicity, and still allow for the activation of RNase H, a new technology was developed. The "gapmer" oligos consist of fully PS-modified backbones, and have nucleosides with only PS modifications alternating with those with both PS and 2′-*O*-methyl modifications. These alterations result in a change in conformation that helps prevent degradation by nucleases, while still maintaining a sufficient region for RNase H activation. Other modified oligos known as mixed backbone oligos (MBOs) have a short central stretch of DNA flanked by 2′-*O*-methoxyethyl modified ribonucleosides on both the 3′ and 5′ ends [25]. These oligos may also be more specific than traditional PS-modified oligos, because the shorter stretch of DNA may decrease the overlap with non-targeted sequences. MBOs have been used in preclinical and clinical trials, and have shown promising results. In our laboratory, we have been evaluating an MBO targeting the mdm2 oncogene, and have seen efficient knockdown and anti-cancer effects [26, 27].

Still other, more dramatic, modifications have been made. These include conversion of the ribose sugar to a hexose (for cyclohexene nucleic acids, CeNA), or double substitution to make morpholino phosphoroamidate nucleic acids (a six-membered morpholino ring is substituted for the ribose sugar, and nitrogen is substituted for one of the non-bridging oxygens in the backbone) or locked nucleic acids (where the 2′ position contains an oxygen atom, bonded by a methylene bridge to the 4′ position, resulting in stabilization of the conformation). Chimeric locked nucleic acid/DNA oligos are more stable, more efficient, and have a nearly 10°C higher melting temperature than traditional DNA-only oligos or the newer MBOs [21, 24]. There are a few morpholino-modified oligos being used in preclinical and clinical trials. For example, one oligo is being used to treat β-thalassemia, for the same reasons as the 2′-*O*-methyl was used [24]. Like the second generation oligos, these "third generation" oligos do not activate RNase H.

Another strategy similar to antisense in is RNA interference (RNAi). Like the modified oligos, RNAi molecules do not activate RNase H. However,

RNAi molecules do activate another nuclease complex, involving RNase III, to achieve their effects [28]. Like antisense strategies, RNAi activates specific enzymes to result in the cleavage of target mRNA, resulting in the downregulation of gene product expression. This alternative gene suppression strategy will be discussed in more detail in a later section of this chapter.

As mentioned earlier, nearly all of the antisense oligos being used in clinical trials are the phosphorothioate-modified oligos. Unfortunately, delivery of PS oligos still poses problems. While they are water soluble and resistant to nucleases, PS oligos are not easily taken up by the cell. To increase cellular uptake of PS oligos, a number of novel delivery systems have been evaluated.

2.3 Target validation

Although there are now several antisense drugs being used clinically and developed for future clinical use, antisense oligos have been useful in the past for validating therapeutic targets and will continue to prove valuable for this purpose, and for deducing the functions of specific gene products.

In vitro, antisense oligos are effective for knocking down expression of a variety of genes, allowing their effects in cells to be elucidated. Usually this involves evaluating the cells for a specific phenotype or simply examining the proliferation of the cells. For other knockdown studies, especially those related to development of potential anti-neoplastic agents, apoptosis and invasiveness are evaluated. From these types of studies, it can be determined whether a gene plays a role in the disease state, or in the resistance to traditional therapies.

In our laboratory, we have been evaluating mdm2 as a potential anti-cancer target for several years. We have been examining the effects of knocking down MDM2, and have seen that our antisense oligo prevents cancer cell proliferation and increases apoptosis *in vitro* [26]. Thus, MDM2 is a viable target for cancer therapy. Following our *in vitro* work, we proceeded to *in vivo* studies, which confirmed the anti-neoplastic effect of targeting MDM2. There are many similar reports about validating the targeting of a wide variety of other genes for therapeutic potential for cancer, cardiovascular diseases, infectious diseases and genetic disorders. Of the 30000 genes in the human genome, only about 500 are being targeted by current therapies [29]. This is less than 2% of the potential targets. Antisense strategies present a useful technology for knocking down expression of other genes for target validation.

2.4 Antisense delivery

In vitro uptake of antisense oligos has been accomplished using a variety of systems. In our laboratory, we typically use cationic liposomes (Lipofectin™ or Cytofectin™) to increase cellular uptake of the oligo. Lipids facilitate delivery into cells, apparently by an endocytic pathway. Other groups have used physical methods (e.g., electroporation), cyanoacrylate "nanoparticles," polycationic polymers, poly-(L-lysine) derivatives, basic or pore-forming peptides, and amphotericin B derivatives [30]. Some of these delivery systems can be targeted to specific receptors (especially the poly-lysine derivatives and basic peptides).

Other groups have used dendrimers (large, highly branched structures capable of interacting with a variety of molecules), and have seen an increase in cytosolic delivery. The dendrimers bind less tightly to serum proteins, and can be delivered *in vitro* even in media containing 30% serum [31]. Microparticles, similar to the nanoparticles, have also been investigated *in vitro*. These are made of biodegradable polymers, and slowly release the oligo as the polymer is degraded. This is useful for possible sustained release of the antisense oligos, and would facilitate *in vivo* delivery [31]. Different physical methods, in addition to electroporation, have been suggested, such as shockwaves, pressure-mediated delivery and ultrasound. Additionally, one research group suggests that using double-stranded oligo complexes may increase cellular uptake and make the antisense oligo more effective. These oligos would be made of one stable antisense oligo (with a chemically modified backbone) and one easily degraded oligodeoxynucleotide, and would be administered using Lipofectamine 2000™. The investigators saw that their oligo targeting MDR1 resulted in more efficient knockdown of the target, even in the presence of serum [32].

As a general rule, the longer an oligo sequence is, the more difficult it is to deliver it into a cell. Thus, most oligos being used now are fewer than 30 nucleotides in length. In addition to the structural modifications, the nucleotide sequence of the oligo can also make a difference in cellular uptake.

To date, most preclinical and clinical trials have not used any of these systems for delivery. Most oligos are delivered "naked" in a saline solution. Unfortunately, oligos, particularly PS-modified oligos, bind to proteins in the blood. This may increase their stability and allow them to be released over a longer period of time from complexes formed with cellular or plasma proteins, but the actual concentration of drug entering the cell may be less than 2% of the administered dose [31]. Other modifications made to oligos [e.g., methylphosphonate or peptide nucleic acids (PNA)] reduce cellular uptake even more. As a result, in some cases, delivery has also been evaluated using the same systems used *in vitro*. Lipids, poly (L-lysine) derivatives and nanoparticles have been used in mice, and sometimes have resulted in increased uptake and stability of the oligos. However, there was also often a concurrent increase in toxicity.

Other delivery systems also exist. One of these is cyclodextrins. These oligosaccharides have a central cavity that can accommodate the antisense oligo. Cyclodextrins are water soluble, and may decrease toxicity, while enhancing the bioavailability of the oligo [31]. More recently, long-term knockdown of expression has been investigated using various viral vector systems [33].

3 Preclinical evaluation of antisense drugs

As mentioned above, the concept of antisense therapy is simple and rational: to inhibit gene expression at the mRNA level in a sequence-specific manner. In the last decade, there have been numerous reports demonstrating the capacity of antisense oligos, especially PS oligos and their analogs, to block gene expression of host genes and foreign pathogenic genes, in various *in vitro* and *in vivo* disease models. However, the underlying mechanisms are still not fully understood, and the optimal specificity and efficacy have yet to be realized, especially in the clinical setting.

3.1 Proof of principle

Perhaps the most important aspect of pharmacological evaluation of antisense oligos is the target effectiveness and specificity of these agents. These agents are usually tested at both *in vitro* and *in vivo* levels. In the early days of antisense development, the biological activity of a given oligo was assayed in a cell-free, *in vitro* system using a high concentration of oligo, often resulting in false-positive reports. *In vitro*, cell-based assays have been routinely employed to establish the basis for further investigation of test oligos. Although there is some variability in cellular uptake, depending on cell type, drug concentration, cell culture conditions, and the delivery system, many oligos can cross the cell membrane and be distributed to the cytosol in sufficient quantities to exert the desired effect. To increase cellular uptake *in vitro*, several means of delivery, such as liposomes, are now routinely used to avoid the need for extremely high concentrations of the oligo. In the development of antisense antitumor agents, various assays have been used to demonstrate *in vitro* antitumor activity. Western blot analysis and Northern blot analysis are used to evaluate the effects of the test oligo on protein expression and mRNA expression and stability. Assays to determine cell viability, proliferation and apoptosis are used to illustrate antitumor activity of test oligos. However, these assays may produce false-positive and false-negative results. For example, some lipids used to increase oligo uptake are themselves cytotoxic. Therefore, proper controls (e.g., negative, positive, and mismatch controls) are needed. Dose-, time-, and sequence-dependent responses are better evidence for antisense effects, and are necessary to establish a basis for further *in vivo* evaluation of the test oligo.

Strong evidence showing *in vivo* activity for antisense oligos is critical during the development stages, but it is more difficult to produce convincing, reproducible results in animal models. In the development of antisense antitumor oligos, murine models are used most frequently. In fact, most antitumor oligos that have entered clinical trials have been tested in nude mouse xenograft models. In these models, human cancer cell lines are transplanted into nude mice or SCID mice. The endpoints for efficacy can be tumor size, survival, molecular markers, and/or histopathological observations. Three types of test models can be used, depending on the molecular target and the treatment schedule. First, the effect of the oligo on tumor onset and formation can be determined using an *ex vivo* protocol in which cells are treated with the oligo prior to implantation of the tumor, or an *in vivo* treatment protocol in which oligo treatment begins immediately after cancer cell implantation. The tumor formation rate and growth inhibition can be major endpoints in these models. Second, the inhibitory effects of the oligo on tumor growth can be assayed using an *in vivo* treatment protocol in which oligo treatment begins in the early stage of tumor growth, usually when the tumor size reaches 50–100 mg. In these models, tumor growth inhibition and molecular/pathology markers are the major endpoints. Third, the antitumor activity of oligos can also be tested in late stage tumors using a protocol in which oligo treatment begins usually when the tumor size reaches

500–1000 mg depending on tumor type. In these models, tumor growth inhibition and survival can be major endpoints.

It is crucial to establish dose-response relationships in *in vivo* models. Proper controls (e.g., untreated, vehicle, mismatch oligo controls) should be included. *In vivo* evidence for a block of specific gene expression is also desirable. The *in vivo* antitumor activity of a given antisense oligo is not necessarily the result of an antisense mechanism, and may be associated with nonspecific activity and/or sequence-specific non-antisense activity.

3.2 *In vitro* and *in vivo* biological activity

As mentioned earlier, endpoints of *in vitro* studies are usually the survival, proliferation and invasiveness of cells, but also can include neoangiogenesis and anchorage-independent growth analyses. Quantification of these anticancer endpoints has been achieved by viable cell counts (Trypan blue staining), Annexin V-FITC conjugation, MTT or BrdU assays, invasion through matrigel, or growth in soft agar. Other groups have looked at the capacity of antisense oligos to enhance the effects of traditional chemotherapeutic drugs and/or radiation.

Antisense oligos can influence all of these endpoints. Our oligo targeting MDM2 increases apoptosis, arrests cells in G_1, and makes cells sensitive to several chemotherapeutic drugs and gamma irradiation. The effects of the oligo obviously depend on its target gene, and the anticancer effects of the MDM2 oligo are related to both its p53-dependent and -independent interactions with other molecules. There are theoretically as many potential therapeutic targets as there are molecules involved in cancer initiation, growth and metastasis.

3.2.1 *In vitro* toxicity and nonspecific effects

There are some genes that cannot be knocked out without permanently harming cells. These effects are sequence specific, and sometimes give new information about gene function. There are also sometimes unintended knockdowns of expression when there is an overlap in nucleotide sequence with a non-targeted gene.

In cell culture, the antisense oligos generally do not have toxic nonspecific effects. The delivery system (e.g., Lipofectin™) is sometimes responsible for cell death and cell cycle arrest, but aside from sequence-specific targeted effects and sequence-specific non-targeted effects, the oligos are relatively non-cytotoxic at the doses used.

3.2.2 *In vitro* pharmacology of antisense oligos

The concentration of the oligo used depends on the oligo and cell line being employed, but efficacy is achieved at concentrations covering a wide range (nanomolar to millimolar). These concentrations are derived from dose-dependence studies, and are generally kept as low as possible so that the concentration more closely resembles a pharmacologically relevant dose. Knockdown of protein expression can last for hours to days, depending on the target gene, the cell line and the oligo used. Proteins with a long half-life make evaluation of knockdown by Western blots difficult. It may be necessary to treat cells with antisense oligos for several days to see an effect at the protein level. On the other hand, changes in the mRNA level can usually be seen within 24 h of treatment.

3.2.3 *In vivo* biological activity

In various animal models (mouse, rat and non-human primate), antisense oligos are effective for knocking down expression of genes. Most studies are done in mouse models because the mouse genome is well characterized. BLAST searches can be performed to avoid homology with other mouse genes when designing the oligos, decreasing the possibility of knocking down untargeted genes. Many cancer studies are accomplished using xenograft mouse models. This facilitates observation of tumor growth, and allows human-targeted oligos to be used against the tumor. In numerous studies of various types of cancer, antisense oligos decrease tumor growth, increase sensitivity to therapy, and sometimes completely eradicate tumors. As a general rule, the endpoint of *in vivo* mouse studies are tumor size, tumor growth rate, response to chemotherapy or radiation, and survival of the animals. To evaluate the toxicity of the oligo, body weight is usually recorded throughout the experiment, and after animals are sacrificed, certain tissues (e.g., spleen, kidneys and liver) are often examined for specific or systemic toxicity (e.g., immune system stimulation).

Although most antisense oligos are tested *in vivo* as monotherapy, combination treatment with antisense oligos and conventional chemotherapeutic agents has also been investigated. There have been a number of preclinical studies demonstrating that downregulation of specific gene products with antisense oligos sensitizes cancer cells to chemotherapeutic agents, resulting in an additive or synergistic anticancer activity. These antisense targets include MDM2, the epidermal growth factor receptor, cAMP-dependent protein kinase, c-myc, PKC, and Bcl-2 among others (Tab. 2). These antisense oligos increase the therapeutic effects of chemotherapeutic agents such as paclitaxel, 5-fluorouracil, cisplatin, carboplatin, taxotere, camptothecin, irinotecan, leucovorin, gemcitabine, doxorubicin, adriamycin, and dacarbazine. However, the mechanisms responsible for such additive or synergistic effects are not fully understood. The synergy between the two classes of agents may result from interactions at several stages, such as cell cycle arrest, induction of apoptosis, induction of immune response and production of cytokines. Although most studies showed that the additive or synergistic effects are sequence specific, recent studies have demonstrated that antisense oligos can also potentiate the antitumor activity of irinotecan in a sequence-independent manner [34–36]. Presumably, this occurs through an interaction at the pharmacokinetic and/or metabolic level to increase the conversion to the active metabolite [36].

3.3 Pharmacology and drug delivery, toxicology

As mentioned, there is always a possibility for sequence-specific, but unintended, knockdown resulting in toxicity. This can usually be avoided by careful selection of the oligo sequence. *In vivo* work typically follows *in vitro* target validation studies, and although many antisense oligos are effective *in vitro*, and may achieve the desired knockdown, they also often produce unforeseen side effects in animals. For example, both PS modifications and CpG sequences contained within many of the oligos used in the past contribute to their nonspecific toxicity because they stimulate the immune system. Although the immune stimulation by even high doses of PS oligo is not (usually) life-threatening, the doses of oligo used to achieve an antisense effect could potentially be if the oligos contain CpG sequences. Several of the oligos in clinical trials contain CpG sequence motifs, including G3139 (Genasense), which was recently in phase III clinical trials. The toxicity profile of these drugs has still been acceptable so far, but inclusion of CpG motifs is now avoided in new oligo designs.

Another potential source of toxicity of the PS oligos relates to their polyanionic properties, which are responsible for the propensity of the oligos for binding to proteins. Particularly when administered i.v., PS oligos bind to serum proteins, including thrombin, which leads to a decrease in coagulation and a prolongation of the activated partial thromboplastin time (aPTT) [37]. This side effect is not life-threatening at up to 15 mg/kg doses used for 2 weeks (three times/week) [37], but some of the newer modifications avoid this coagulopathy.

The efficiency of the knockdown depends on the nucleotide sequence, backbone modifications, dose, administration route, target tissue/location and the target gene. As would be expected, delivering oligos to the brain is more difficult than to other tissues, while delivery to blood cells is more easily achieved. With some of the receptor-targeted structural modifications, it may eventually be possible to target oligos to specific cell types.

PS-modified oligos, as well as other modified oligos, are usually administered by i.v. or i.p. routes, while some special formulations have been made allowing other types of administration. For example, ISIS 104838, a 2′-*O*-methyl oligo targeting TNF-α being used in phase II trials for rheumatoid arthritis and psoriasis, has been formulated in a sodium caprate pellet for oral delivery [38]. Other groups have been investigating the possibility of respiratory administration of oligos [39, 40].

Regardless of the route of administration, the oligos are distributed rapidly to tissues, including tumors. When administered i.v., PS-modified oligos are eliminated from the plasma, and are distributed to highly perfused organs, usually within an hour of administration [15]. The same general tissue distribution occurs for i.p. and s.c. administration of the oligos. Following metabolism in the liver, most of the oligo metabolites are excreted in the urine (75%) and feces (5–10%) within 90 days [41].

4 Clinical evaluation of antisense drug

4.1 *In vivo* efficacy: Proof of principle

Compared with preclinical studies, far fewer clinical studies of oligos have been reported (Tab. 1). Most clinically tested antisense antitumor oligos are PS modified, and have an acceptable safety profile and initial antitumor efficacy. In addition, several antisense oligos and chemotherapeutic agent combination treatments are under clinical evaluation [42].

In most published phase I trials, antisense oligos were well tolerated. Side effects include thrombocytopenia, prolongation of aPTT, and slight elevation in liver enzymes. No appreciable liver or renal toxicity has been reported. Pharmacokinetic studies have been accomplished in patients, and indicate a short plasma distribution half-life and prolonged elimination half-life [43]. Urinary excretion represents the major pathway of excretion, with mainly degraded products being observed. Limited phase II and III trials have been reported. Although there have been few clinical trials, the oligos do specifically inhibit the expression of targeted genes, and can mediate an antitumor response.

4.2 *In vivo* biological activity

There are more than 20 antisense oligos currently being tested in human clinical trials [12]. Since 1995, at least 17 antisense oligos have been (or are still being) evaluated for use as cancer therapy. Unfortunately, although an antisense drug was approved for use against CMV, no antisense oligo has yet received FDA approval for use for cancer. This is partly due to the fact that many of the oligos that have been evaluated were not as advanced as the oligos being designed today. Many of the antisense oligos contained CpG sequences or sequence homology to other genes that resulted in toxicity. Additionally, newer oligos, such as the MBOs, avoid nuclease degradation, but do not activate the immune system like the completely PS-modified oligos.

4.3 Pharmacology and toxicology

Thorough toxicity studies are a key component of antisense drug development. A number of PS-modified oligos have been studied extensively for their safety profiles in several species, including mice, rats, monkeys, and humans. As mentioned earlier, the dose-dependent side effects in rats and mice included thrombocytopenia, splenomegaly, and elevation of liver transaminases [44, 45]. Histopathological changes include mononuclear cell infiltration into tissues such as liver, kidney, and spleen, and reticuloendothelial cell and lymphoid cell hyperplasia. The severity of side effects is dependent on the dose, frequency, and duration of the administration of oligos. In general, the toxicity profiles are similar for PS oligos of various lengths and base compositions, with the exception of the presence of certain sequence motifs, such as CpG-dinucleotides [44, 46] and poly-G motifs [47], which contribute to the severity of toxicity.

Preclinical toxicity studies are used to guide a starting dose and dose escalation scheme of clinical trials, and are expected to be conducted in accordance with current Good Laboratory Practices (cGLP). To support clinical phase I trials, animal toxicity studies using two animal species are usually conducted in one rodent species and one non-rodent species. For antisense oligos, non-human primates are often used. In addition, special toxicity studies have been suggested to determine cardiotoxicity, hepatotoxicity, and immunotoxicity. Interested readers are directed to a published review for details [48].

5 Examples of antisense anticancer drugs under development

5.1 Bcl-2

Perhaps the best known anti-cancer antisense oligo is G3139 (Oblimersen, Genasense), which targets Bcl-2. Bcl-2 is an anti-apoptotic oncoprotein, which is associated with an aggressive clinical course, poor survival, and increased resistance to chemotherapy and radiation therapy in patients with B-cell cancers (chronic lymphocytic leukemia, multiple myeloma and non-Hodgkin's lymphoma) [49]. G3139 showed great promise in mice for the treatment of B-cell cancers, melanoma and solid tumors [50, 51]. It also decreased the resistance of purified multiple myeloma cells from patients to dexamethasone and doxorubicin [52]. It was found, by use of a different anti-Bcl-2 oligo, that reducing Bcl-2 levels decreased the resistance of multiple myeloma cells to dexamethasone, paclitaxel and p53 gene therapy [53].

G3139 has been used in phase II/III clinical trials for CLL, multiple myeloma, malignant melanoma, non-small cell and small-cell lung cancers and prostate cancer. Preliminary data from a large international randomized trial in melanoma showed a trend toward increased survival and improved response rates and response duration when oblimersen was added to dacarbazine [4]. Although oblimersen showed promise, the largest and most recent clinical trial of the drug did not show substantial improvement in the survival of patients with melanoma. These disappointing results led to a negative review of a recent NDA application. However, the drug is still being evaluated for other types of cancer and in different combination therapies. For example, combination with docetaxel was evaluated in phase I studies, and it is being used as a first-line salvage therapy in patients who relapsed or were refractory after one chemotherapy regimen [54]. The future of G3139 is uncertain, but the drug may still be useful for certain kinds of cancers.

5.2 PKC

The protein kinase C family is composed of at least ten serine-threonine kinases that are involved in the signal transduction controlling proliferation and apoptosis. The PKCs, particularly PKC-α, are involved in cancer initiation and progression. PKC-α is also responsible for the tumorigenicity of phorbol esters. An early study using antisense oligos to knockdown PKC-α expression resulted in efficient knockdown of the protein in A549 cells, and confirmed the role of the protein in the action of phorbol esters [55]. The same research group used their oligo (which is now known as Aprinocarsen, Affinitak or ISIS 3521) in mice, and saw that it caused dose-dependent and sequence-dependent knockdown of protein expression. After a single dose, a 64% decrease in protein expression was noted [56]. The investigators later combined the oligo with cisplatin, mitomycin-C, vinblastine, estracyt or adriamycin in nude mouse xenograft models, and saw superadditive effects from all of the combinations [57].

Following this preclinical work, Aprinocarsen entered clinical trials. It has been used for CNS malignancies, non-small-cell lung cancer, lymphomas, and ovarian, colorectal, breast and prostate carcinomas [58]. Some encouraging results were seen in non-Hodgkin's lymphoma patients, but the single agent was not effective for the treatment of other cancers, although it showed better effects when combined with chemotherapeutic agents [59]. Currently, a phase III study is underway evaluating the combination of Aprinocarsen and gemcitabine [4].

5.3 H-ras

Ras is a membrane-associated G-protein that mediates receptor tyrosine kinase activation of downstream proteins. There are three different ras protooncogenes, and there are oncogenic mutations in ras in about 30% of human cancers. Mutations to one of the ras proteins, H-ras, are common in bladder, kidney and thyroid carcinomas [60]. Like other proteins involved in cell signaling, H-ras has been targeted by antisense oligos. Preclinically, an anti-H-ras oligo decreased expression by about 90%, and prevented the formation of foci in transformed mouse cells. An anti-H-ras oligo also decreased the growth of xenograft tumors in nude mice when the cells were pre-treated with the oligo. In mice implanted with bladder xenograft tumors, treatment for 31 days with the oligo resulted in an 80% inhibition of tumor growth [61].

Based on these types of preclinical studies, clinical studies of an H-ras antisense oligo, ISIS 2503, were performed. These included phase I studies of the oligo as a single agent and in combination with gemcitabine, and phase II studies in pancreatic, metastatic breast, and non-small-cell lung cancer alone and in combination with gemcitabine [60, 62, 63]. These studies gave some promising results, particularly with pancreatic cancer. Phase III studies are likely to begin soon.

5.4 PKA

cAMP-dependent protein kinase (PKA) is involved in various cellular functions such as cell proliferation, gene induction, and metabolism [64], and its regulatory subunits have been suggested as a drug target for cancer and other diseases [65]. PKA is composed of two catalytic (C) and two regulatory (R) subunits and has type I and type II isozymes, with different R subunits, termed RI and RII, interacting with an identical C subunit [64]. Thus far, four isoforms of R subunits RIα, RIβ, RIIα, and RIIβ have been identified. The RI- and RII-regulatory subunits of PKA have opposing roles in cell growth and differentiation, with RI being growth stimulatory and RII being growth inhibitory [65]. Increased expression of the RIα subunit of PKA occurs during chemical or viral carcinogenesis and correlates with cell proliferation and neoplastic growth [65]. The RIα subunit of PKA is overexpressed in a variety of human tumor tissues and cell lines, including those from lung [66], breast [67], ovaries [68], and colon [69]. Furthermore, overexpression of the RIα subunit of PKA correlates with malignancy and poor prognosis in cancer patients [66–68]. More recently, studies have suggested that extracellular PKA activity may serve as a diagnostic and prognostic marker for cancer [69]. In addition, the RIα subunit is associated with multidrug resistance and decreased tumor sensitivity to chemotherapeutic agents [71–73]. Therefore, the RIα subunit of PKA is a potential target for human cancer therapy, with several selective type I PKA inhibitors being tested both in preclinical and clinical settings [65–78]. Examples of PKA RI inhibitors include 8-Cl-cAMP [74] and antisense oligos [75–78].

Selectively downregulating the expression of the RIα subunit of PKA using unmodified and PS oligos inhibits growth and differentiation of various cancer cell lines, and results in antitumor activity in tumor xenograft models [75]. While the PS oligo is selective, specific, and potent in inhibiting tumor growth, repeated administration caused side effects in mice, thereby limiting its therapeutic utility. In contrast, a novel MBO, composed of a modified PS oligo that has four 2′-*O*-methylribonucleotides substituted for deoxynucleosides at both the 3 -end and 5′-ends, provided improvements in the safety profile compared to PS oligos [76–78]. Our previous studies demonstrated that these MBOs are bioavailable following oral administration [79]. Following extensive preclinical studies by various routes of administration, a novel MBO targeted to the RIα subunit of PKA entered a clinical phase I study [78], and is presently being evaluated in phase II trials in patients with solid tumors. In addition, one of the major applications of anti-PKA oligos is to improve the therapeutic effectiveness of conventional cancer therapies, including DNA damaging agents and radiation. We and others have demonstrated that the MBO enhanced the therapeutic effectiveness of several clinically used chemotherapeutic agents including cisplatin and Taxol.

5.5 XIAP

Apoptosis plays an important role in various biological processes, such as cell turnover, development, metamorphosis and maintenance of homeostasis. Abnormalities in apoptosis are involved in carcinogenesis, chemotherapy, radiation therapy, and drug resistance. Upon being activated, apoptosis-inducing pathways eventually converge to activate caspases, which are cysteine proteases, leading to the cleavage of important cellular substrates, including poly(ADP-ribose) polymerase and the laminins.

The activities of caspases are negatively regulated by the inhibitor-of-apoptosis (IAP) family of proteins, among which X-chromosome-linked IAP (XIAP) is the most notable and the most potent [80]. The human XIAP gene is located on chromosome Xq25 [81] and encodes a 54-kDa protein that has three BIR (baculovirus inhibition of apoptosis repeat) motifs. The XIAP protein binds to and inhibits caspase-9 through its BIR3 domain and caspases-3 and -7 through its linker-BIR2 domain [82]. It also interferes with the BAX/cytochrome c cell death pathway [83]. XIAP promotes caspase-3 degradation through the proteasome by facilitating its ubiquitination via a ubiquitin E3 ligase activity in a RING finger domain located near its C terminus [84]. Overexpression of XIAP inhibits cellular apoptosis induced by a variety of stimuli, including TNF-α, Fas, serum or growth factor withdrawal, ischemia, chemotherapy and irradiation [85]. XIAP is present at basal levels in normal adult tissues, but it is up-regulated in many types of human tumors [86]. In acute myeloid leukemia patients, higher XIAP protein levels may indicate a poor prognosis [87]. In renal cell carcinomas, XIAP expression correlates with tumor stages, with the highest levels being present in poorly differentiated cancers [88, 89]. Moreover, its overexpression correlates with the resistance of cancer cells to chemotherapy and irradiation [86]. Cancer cells with deleted XIAP show remarkable sensitivity to TRAIL (TNF-related apoptosis-inducing ligand), suggesting that XIAP is a nonredundant modulator of TRAIL-induced apoptosis [90].

Preliminary studies have shown antitumor and chemosensitization effects from treatment with XIAP-specific antisense oligos and short interfering RNA (siRNA) molecules [85, 91–93]. Stable expression of short-hairpin RNAs (shRNAs) directed against XIAP resulted in the generation of three MDA-MB-231 cell lines (XIAP shRNA cells) with reductions in XIAP mRNA and protein levels by more than 85% relative to the expression levels seen in cells stably transfected with the U6 RNA polymerase III promoter alone (U6 cells). This RNAi approach dramatically sensitized the cells to killing by TRAIL [92]. Loss of XIAP also sensitized the cells to taxanes, but had no additional effects on the efficiency of carboplatin- and doxorubicin-mediated cell killing. The increased sensitivity of the XIAP shRNA cells to TRAIL and taxanes correlated with enhanced caspase cleavage and activation, including caspase-8, and robust processing of poly(ADP-ribose) polymerase and BID compared to U6 cells. The effects observed upon stable RNAi with respect to TRAIL sensitization were also achieved following the downregulation of XIAP in Panc-1 cells treated with a second-generation, mixed-backbone antisense oligo, AEG 35156/GEM640 [92, 93].

5.6 VEGF

Vascular endothelial growth factor (VEGF) expression is related to the growth rate of tumors, vascularity of tumors, and tumor metastasis [94]. VEGF is thus an attractive therapeutic target for cancer. One group used an anti-VEGF oligo to treat Caki-1 (renal cell carcinoma) cells. The antisense oligo reduced expression of VEGF, and led to a decrease in proliferation and migration of co-cultured endothelial cells. Cells pre-treated with the oligo generated half as many vessels in nude mice as untreated cells. Mice with Caki-1 xenografts receiving the oligo showed a decreased tumor growth rate [94]. Another group evaluating an anti-VEGF oligo saw that the oligo decreased VEGF expression in a human head and neck squamous cell carcinoma (HNSCC) cell line, and decreased growth of HNSCC xenografts in nude mice [95]. Dual targeting of VEGF and VEGF signaling has also been explored. For example, the same group that was studying the Caki-1 cells later examined a combination of antisense-mediated VEGF knockdown with a small molecule inhibitor of VEFG/bFGF receptor tyrosine kinase function. Both agents led to inhibition of tumor growth, and the combination had a greater effect than either agent alone. Another group targeted the VEGF receptor, Flk-1. Treatment with a chimeric oligo reduced Flk-1 expression and phosphorlyation, and inhibited VEGF activities [96]. A combination of Flk-1 and VEGF antisense oligos may lead to a more dramatic decrease in VEGF activity. There have not yet been any clinical trials using an antisense oligo against VEGF, but oligos targeting the protein will likely be used clinically in the near future.

5.7 β-catenin

Mutations to the Wnt/β-catenin pathway are responsible for a large proportion of colon cancers, and also likely play a role in the tumorigenesis of other tissues. β-catenin interacts with a variety of proteins, including Wnt and E-cadherin, and nuclear β-catenin interacts with Tcf/LEF transcription factors, resulting in an increase in c-Myc and cyclin D1, among other downstream genes [97, 98]. Thus, because of its interactions and its involvement in cancer initiation and progression, β-catenin is another attractive target for antisense therapy.

Antisense oligos against β-catenin have been used in colon carcinoma, esophageal carcinoma, leukemia and lymphoma cell lines. The oligos decreased β-catenin expression in a dose-dependent manner, and decreased Tcf transcription. In colon cancer cell lines treated with a β-catenin antisense oligo, there was a decrease in cell proliferation, invasiveness and anchorage-independent growth [99, 100]. In a study with colon cancer xenografts, the oligo decreased tumor growth and brought about complete tumor regression in 60% of animals [100]. Esophageal carcinoma cell lines were also affected by the antisense oligo. The oligo decreased mRNA expression by about 50%, increased apoptosis, and decreased cell proliferation by about 80% [101]. An antisense oligo did not seem to affect the viability of leukemia or lymphoma cell lines, but did decrease the amount of aggregation [102]. There may also be a link between VEGF and β-catenin. When an antisense oligo was used to knockdown expression of β-catenin, there was also a more than 50% reduction in VEGF-A expression [103]. Thus, an anti-β-catenin oligo may also help control tumor angiogenesis.

5.8 Survivin

Survivin, which plays important roles in the inhibition of apoptosis and regulation of cell division, was initially identified through hybridization screening of a human genomic library with the cDNA of the effector cell protease receptor-1 [104]. The human survivin gene is located on chromosome 17q25, and encodes the smallest member of the IAP family at only 16.5 kDa [105]. The survivin protein has only one BIR domain. Overexpression of survivin prevents cellular apoptosis induced by a variety of stimuli [105]; transgenic mice expressing survivin in the skin show impaired UVB-induced apoptosis [106]. In a variety of tumor models, downregulation of survivin through techniques involving antisense oligos, ribozymes or RNAi leads to suppression of tumor growth [105]. Although the mechanisms mediating its inhibitory effects remain to be elucidated, there is evidence that survivin blocks apoptosis through p21Waf1 [107]. It may also bind to and inhibit the activities of caspases-3, -7, and -9 [108]. Another mechanism could involve regulation of the subcellular location of apoptosis-inducing factor (AIF) [109].

Survivin is present in high levels in a variety of human malignancies, including carcinomas of lung, breast, colon, stomach, esophagus, liver, pancreas, uterus, ovaries, and in Hodgkin's- and non-Hodgkin's lymphomas, neuroblastoma, various leukemias, sarcoma, and melanoma [105]. Considerable retrospective evidence indicates that survivin levels correlate negatively with clinical prognosis and survival, and positively with aggressiveness, recurrence, and resistance to the therapy [105]. Survivin, transfected into rat tumor cells, inhibits apoptosis; it also promotes tumorigenesis of these cells when they are transplanted into SCID mice [110].

The potential of survivin as a target for cancer therapy is also suggested by evidence derived from use of an antisense molecule to downregulate survivin expression in leukemic HL60 cells. Accompanying survivin inhibition, there is cell cycle arrest at the G_2/M phase, followed by apoptosis [111]. In xenograft models of human gastric carcinoma, non-Hodgkin's lymphoma, thymic lymphoma, and lung cancer, antisense oligos have antitumor and radiosensitization effects [112–116]. Based on preclinical results, antisense molecules targeting survivin are under development for clinical use [108].

5.9 MDM2

The MDM2 protein contains a p53-binding domain at the N terminus, a nuclear localization signal, a central acidic domain and three C-terminal zinc-finger motifs [117]. MDM2 acts as a negative regulator of p53. The expression of MDM2 is induced by p53, and MDM2 binds to p53 with high affinity and inhibits its transcriptional activity. Via an E3 ligase activity in its RING finger domain, MDM2 is able to facilitate the ubiquitination of p53, accelerating its degradation by the proteasome. p53 regulates the cell cycle, maintains the genomic integrity of cells, and controls the cellular response to DNA damage [118–125]. DNA damaging treatments, including γ-irradiation and chemotherapeutic drugs, increase p53 levels, leading to G_1 arrest or apoptosis [126]. Modulating p53-mediated cell cycle arrest and/or apoptosis may lead to the sensitization of tumor cells to DNA damaging chemotherapeutic agents and radiation therapy [126, 127]. Thus, because it both inhibits the ability of p53 to induce cell cycle arrest and apoptosis, and decreases the stability of the p53 protein, MDM2 overexpression confers tumorigenicity to cells. Many published studies suggest that overexpression of MDM2 is associated with inactivation of wild-type p53 [128–130]. Many cancer therapeutic agents exert their cytotoxic effects through activation of wild-type p53. However, the activation of p53 by DNA damage from chemotherapy and radiation treatment may be limited in cancers with MDM2 expression, especially those with MDM2 overexpression.

The MDM2 gene is amplified in a number of human tumors, including human cancers of breast, colon, esophagus, bladder, prostate, liver, pancreas, and kidney, as well as lymphoma, leukemia, and other tumors such as soft tissue sarcoma, melanoma, glioma, and peripheral nerve sheath tumors (reviewed in [128–131]). Further, MDM2 amplification and/or overexpression have been implicated as a prognostic factor in cancer patients [128–130], and MDM2 overexpression is associated with aspects of advanced disease, such as invasive tumors, high grade/late stage tumors, recurrence, and metastasis [128–130]. Inactivation of the MDM2/p53 negative feed-back loop may increase the magnitude of p53 activation following DNA damaging treatment, thus enhancing the therapeutic effectiveness of DNA damaging drugs and radiation therapy and improving the prognosis for patients.

The MDM2 oncoprotein has other, p53-independent, activities. MDM2 binds to and interacts with pRB, E2F1, the ribosomal protein L5, and RNA [128–130]. The biological consequences of these activities are not clear, but may be associated with the transformational properties of MDM2. In addition, MDM2 may inhibit p21 [131]. In a transgenic mouse model, overexpression of MDM2 predisposes mice to spontaneous tumor formation in both the presence and absence of functional p53, indicating a p53-independent role for MDM2 in tumorigenesis [132]. Therefore, inhibition of the MDM2 p53-independent activity may be as important as the inactivation of its p53-dependent activity.

We have successfully designed anti-MDM2 antisense oligos that inhibit MDM2 expression in tumor cells *in vitro* and *in vivo*. We began the development of such oligos with the successful identification of one that effectively inhibits MDM2 expression in tumor cells containing MDM2 gene amplifications [133, 134]. These PS oligos were initially screened in two cell lines, JAR (choriocarcinoma) and SJSA (osteosarcoma), which contain wild-type p53, amplified MDM2 genes, and overexpressed the MDM2 oncoprotein. Out of the nine PS oligos screened, oligo AS5 (5′-GATCACTCCCACCTTCAAGG-3′), which hybridizes to a position ~360 bp downstream of the translation start codon, reproducibly decreased MDM2 protein levels in both cell lines by 3–5-fold at concentrations of 100–400 nM [133]. The mismatch control oligo M4 (5′-GATGACTCACACCATCAAGG-3′) had no effect on MDM2 expression. In this study, oligo AS5 induced RNase H cleavage of the target MDM2 mRNA, resulting in truncation and degradation of the target. Following Northern blot hybridization, AS5 caused a slight decrease in the molecular weight of MDM2 mRNA. This is consistent with RNase H cleavage at the target of AS5 (~700 nucleotides from the 5 end), which would reduce the molecular weight of the mRNA (~5500 nucleotides) by ~12%. Further studies demonstrated that, following AS5 treatment, the p53 protein level was elevated and its activity was increased. A dose-dependent induction of p21 expression up to 6.6-fold by AS5 was observed at the optimal concentration of 200 nM, suggesting that p53 transcriptional activity may be increased following inhibition of MDM2 expression. JAR cells treated with AS5 showed an increase in the levels of apoptosis.

A different antisense oligo, AS5–2, which was effective in 26 cell lines (16 types of human cancers), enhanced the p53 activity in all cells, even those with low levels of wild-type p53 and in those with only low levels of MDM2 expression [19]. This oligo was subsequently modified to be a MBO to be used for further *in vitro* and *in vivo* studies [135–139].

In vitro, the novel anti-MDM2 AS MBO specifically inhibited MDM2 expression in tested cells in a dose-dependent manner, regardless of the p53 status [135–139]. The mismatch control oligo had little or no effect. The *in vivo* antitumor effects of the test MBO on tumor growth were first evaluated using a nude mouse SJSA tumor xenograft model [135]. The mismatch control oligo had no appreciable effect on tumor growth, but a dose-dependent growth inhibition on SJSA tumor xenografts was found following treatment with the anti-MDM2 AS MBO [135]. Notably, in SJSA xenograft mice, the test MBO increased the therapeutic effects of the cancer chemotherapeutic agents, 10-hydroxycamptothecin and adriamycin, in a dose-dependent manner [135]. The mismatch control showed no effect on the therapeutic effectiveness of these agents. The synergistic effects between MDM2 inhibition and cancer cytotoxic agents were further demonstrated in the JAR xenograft model [135].

The novel MBO targeting the MDM2 oncogene has now been further evaluated in other types of human cancers, including colon, lung, breast and prostate carcinoma as well as glioma [135–139]. The selected antisense MBO was evaluated for its *in vitro* and *in vivo* antitumor activity in human cancer models, both those expressing wild-type p53 and those with mutant p53. In cancer cells with wild-type p53, the p53 and p21 levels were elevated, resulting from specific inhibition of MDM2 expression by the antisense MBO [135–139]. In cancer cells with mutant p53, p21 levels were elevated following inhibition of MDM2 expression, although the p53 levels remained unchanged [135–139]. In both models (p53 wild-type or mutant), the inhibition of MDM2 resulted in *in vivo* synergistic or additive therapeutic effects with the cancer chemotherapeutic agents irinotecan, 5-fluorouracil, and taxol [135–139].

These results suggest that MDM2 has a role in tumor growth and progression through both the p53-dependent and -independent pathways, including the response to therapy.

The anti-MDM2 MBO has also been examined for radiosensitization effects in several *in vitro* and *in vivo* human cancer models [137, 138]. It was evaluated for its *in vitro* radiosensitization activity in cell lines of human lung cancer (A549), prostate cancer (LNCaP and PC-3) and glioma (U87MG and A172), and for its *in vivo* activity in xenograft models of human prostate (LNCaP and PC-3), breast (MCF-7 and MDA-MB-468) and pancreatic cancer (PANC-1). In cells containing at least one functional p53 allele (A549, LNCaP, U87MG and A172), p53 and p21 levels were elevated following specific inhibition of MDM2 expression by the antisense oligo.

Over the years, there have been concerns that have limited the enthusiasm for the development of antisense oligos as therapeutic agents. Nevertheless, we have demonstrated that the specific anti-human-MDM2 MBO has antitumor activity in both *in vitro* and *in vivo* human cancer models, regardless of p53 status, suggesting that MDM2 has a role in the development and progression of various cancers through both p53-dependent and p53-independent mechanisms. The MDM2 antisense oligo thus stands as a proof-of-principle for the rational development of drugs, and demonstrates the utility of antisense oligo drugs.

6 Conclusion

In the last decade, progress has been made in the development of antisense oligos as therapeutic agents. Perhaps the most important aspects of therapeutic oligos that have been recently improved are the identification and validation of new gene targets, and the improvements made in the targeting effectiveness of the antisense drugs. Many antisense antitumor oligos are being evaluated in humans, and are showing promise used either alone or in combination with other therapeutic agents. Future studies are needed not only to confirm the efficiency and specificity of their antisense effects, but also to meet the requirements for antisense therapy to be a widely accepted therapeutic approach. The underlying mechanisms of action (antisense, sequence-dependent non-antisense, and non-sequence-specific) responsible for the observed biological effects, including therapeutic effects and unwanted side effects, must be investigated to understand all of the effects of the antisense drugs. More rational selection of targets and drugs, especially more well-designed clinical studies and new approaches to resolve regulatory issues related to antisense drugs are needed. The new generations of antisense drugs being created are expected to be more effective, more specific, and to have better safety profiles than drugs tested previously. Thus, based on the results from previous and current clinical trials, and the improvements being made, antisense oligos are likely to become more widely utilized for therapy. It is likely that other antisense drugs will soon join Vitravene for the treatment of human disease.

No discussion of gene silencing strategies is complete without mentioning a newly discovered method for preventing the expression of gene products. RNAi was first decribed in the early 1990s [140, 141], and has since been extensively investigated. RNAi, as mentioned in an earlier section of this chapter, is similar to antisense in that RNAi molecules also activate an enzyme complex, and result in the degradation of a targeted mRNA. RNAi molecules will theoretically silence any gene for which the sequence is known, permitting a broad range of applications. The silencing targets include oncogenes, genes involved in the pathogenesis of disease, and mutated genes resulting in genetic disorders. RNAi has already proved to be a valuable tool in the laboratory, leading to the production of knockdown cell lines and animal models for easier analysis of gene function and interactions, as well as for the validation of target therapeutic molecules and detection of single nucleotide polymorphisms (SNPs).

Although impressive progress has been made in the last few years, the strategy is still in its infancy. Thus far, most published data are from *in vitro* studies, with remarkable variations in both specificity and efficacy [142, 143]. The major challenges are associated with *in vivo* stability, delivery, and silencing efficiency. As yet, no RNAi molecules have entered clinical trials. Nonspecific inhibition of related or unrelated genes is also a major concern [142, 143]. The potential of RNAi molecules as therapeutic agents depends on several factors, including their target specificity, *in vivo* silencing efficiency and stability, and their safety profiles. In particular, a novel design of these agents suitable for clinical use is needed before the ultimate utility of this approach for therapy can be demonstrated. Thus, while RNAi may eventually prove to be a therapeutic modality, its development is likely to take several years. The information gathered during preclinical and clinical trials with antisense oligos will aid in the development of RNAi, and as new information is found using RNAi, antisense strategies will likely benefit as well. Thus, research using both types of gene silencing strategies will advance the treatment of human diseases.

Acknowledgements

This project was supported by grants from National Institutes of Health/ National Cancer Institute (R01 CA 80698 and R01 CA112029). Dr. H. Wang was supported in part by funds from the Comprehensive Cancer Center, University of Alabama at Birmingham. Members of the Zhang Laboratory contributed substantially to studies cited in this article.

References

1 Hanahan D, Weinberg R (2000) The hallmarks of cancer. *Cell* 100: 57–70
2 Zamecnik P, Stephenson M (1978) Inhibition of Rous sarcoma virus replication and cell transformation by a specific oligodeoxynucleotide. *Proc Natl Acad Sci USA* 75: 280–284
3 Simons R (1988) Naturally occurring antisense RNA control, a brief review. *Gene* 72: 35–44
4 Dean N, Bennett C (2003) Antisense oligonucleotide-based therapeutics for cancer. *Oncogene* 22: 9087–9096
5 Agrawal S, Kandimalla E (2000) Antisense therapeutics: Is it simple as complementary base recognition? *Mol Med Today* 6: 72–81
6 Wang H, Prasad G, Buolamwini J, Zhang R (2001) Antisense anticancer oligonucleotide therapeutics. *Curr Cancer Drug Targets* 1: 177–196
7 Crooke, S (2001) *Antisense drug technology. Principles, strategies, and applications.* Marcel Dekker: New York
8 Cho-Chung Y (2003) Antisense DNAs as targeted genetic medicine to treat cancer. *Arch Pharm Res* 6:183–191
9 Crooke S (2004) Antisense strategies. *Curr Mol Med* 4: 465–487
10 Crooke S (1998) Vitravene – Another piece in the mosaic. *Antisense Nucleic Acid Drug Dev* 8: vii–viii
11 Agrawal S (1996) Antisense oligonucleotides: Towards clinical trials. *Trends Biotechnol* 14: 376–387
12 Rayburn E, Wang H, He J and Zhang R (2005) RNA silencing technologies in drug discovery and target validation. *Lett Drug Dis Dev* 5: 173–190
13 Gewirtz A (2000) Oligonucleotide therapeutics: A step forward. *J Clin Oncol* 18: 1809–1811
14 Crooke S (2000) Potential roles of antisense technology in cancer chemotherapy. *Oncogene* 19: 6651–6659

15 Agrawal S (1999) Importance of nucleotide sequence and chemical modifications of antisense oligocnucleotides. *Biochim Biophys Acta* 1489: 53–68
16 Lebedeva I, Stein C (2001) Antisense oligonucleotides: Promise and reality. *Annu Rev Pharm Toxicol* 41: 403–419
17 Crooke S (1999) Molecular mechanisms of action of antisense drugs. *Biochim Biophys Acta* 1489: 31–44
18 Crooke S (2000) Comments on evaluation of antisense drugs in the clinic. *Antisense Nucleic Acid Drug Dev* 10: 225–227
19 Diasio R, Zhang R (1997) Pharmacology of therapeutic oligonucleotides. *Antisense Nucleic Acid Drug Dev* 7: 239–243
20 Wu H, Lima W, Zhang H, Fan A, Sun H, Crooke S (2004) Determination of the role of the human RNase H1 in the pharmacology of DNA-like antisense drugs. *J Biol Chem* 279: 17181–17189
21 Urban E, Noe C (2003) Structural modifications of antisense oligonucleotides. *Farmaco* 58: 243–258
22 Zellweger T, Miyake H, July L, Akbari M, Kiyama S, Gleave M (2001) Chemosensitization of human renal cell cancer using antisense oligonucleotides targeting the antiapoptotic gene clusterin. *Neoplasia* 3: 360–367
23 Bartel F, Harris L, Wurl P, Taubert H (2004) MDM2 and its splice variant messenger RNAs: expression in tumors and down-regulation using antisense oligonucleotides. *Mol Cancer Res* 2: 29–35
24 Kurreck J (2003) Antisense technologies. Improvement through novel chemical modifications. *Eur J Biochem* 270: 1628–1644
25 Agrawal S, Iyer R (1997) Perspectives in antisense therapeutics. *Pharmacol Ther* 76: 151–160
26 Zhang Z, Li M, Wang H, Agrawal S, Zhang R (2003) Antisense therapy targeting MDM2 oncogene in prostate cancer: Effects on proliferation, apoptosis, multiple gene expression, and chemotherapy. *Proc Natl Acad Sci USA* 100: 11636–11641
27 Prasad G, Wang H, Agrawal S, Zhang R (2002) Antisense anti-MDM2 oligonucleotides as a novel approach to the treatment of glioblastoma multiforme. *Anticancer Res* 22:107–116
28 Knight S, Bass B (2001) A role for the RNase III enzyme DCR-1 in RNA interference and germ line development in Caenorhabditis elegans. *Science* 293: 2269–2271
29 Dean N (2001) Functional genomics and target validation approaches using antisense oligonucleotide technology. *Curr Opin Biotechnol* 12: 622–625
30 Garcia-Chaumont C, Seksek O, Grzybowska J, Borowski E, Bolard J (2000) Delivery systems for antisense oligonucleotides. *Pharmacol Ther* 87: 255–277
31 Lysik M, Wu-Pong S (2003) Innovations in oligonucleotide drug delivery. *J Pharm Sci* 92: 1559–1573
32 Astriab-Fisher A, Fisher M, Juliano R, Herdewijn P (2004) Increased uptake of antisense oligonucleotides by delivery as double stranded complexes. *Biochem Pharmacol* 68: 403–407
33 Roth C, Sundaram S (2004) Engineering synthetic vectors for improved DNA delivery: insights from intracellular pathways. *Annu Rev Biomed Eng* 6: 397–426
34 Agrawal S, Kandimalla E, Yu D, Hollister B, Chen S, Dexter D, Alford T, Hill B, Bailey K, Bono C et al (2001) Potentiation of antitumor activity of irinotecan by chemically modified oligonucleotides. *Int J Oncol* 18: 1061–1069

35 Wang H, Nan L, Yu D, Agrawal S, Zhang R (2001) Antisense anti-MDM2 oligonucleotides as a novel therapeutic approach to human breast cancer: *in vitro* and *in vivo* activities and mechanisms. *Clin Cancer Res* 7: 3613–3624

36 Wang H, Wang S, Nan L, Yu D, Agrawal S, Zhang R (2002) Antisense anti-MDM2 mixed backbone oligonucleotides enhance therapeutic efficacy of topoisomerase I inhibitor irinotecan in nude mice bearing human cancer xenografts: *In vivo* activity and mechanisms. *Int J Oncol* 20: 745–752

37 Webb M, Tortora N, Cremese M, Kozlowska H, Blaquiere M, Devine D, Kornbrust D (2001) Toxicity and toxicokinetics of a phosphorothioate oligonucleotide against the c-myc oncogene in cynomolgus monkeys. *Antisense Nucleic Acid Drug Dev* 11: 155–163

38 Raoof A, Chiu P, Ramtoola Z, Cumming I, Teng C, Weinbach S, Hardee G, Levin A, Geary R (2004) Oral bioavailability and multiple dose tolerability of an antisense oligonucleotide tablet formulated with sodium caprate. *J Pharm Sci* 93: 1431–1439

39 Tanaka M, Nyce J (2001) Respirable antisense oligonucleotides: a new drug class for respiratory disease. *Respir Res* 2: 5–9

40 Templin M, Levin A, Graham M, Aberg P, Axelsson B, Butler M, Geary R, Bennett C (2000) Pharmacokinetic and toxicity profile of a phosphorothioate oligonucleotide following inhalation delivery to lung in mice. *Antisense Nucleic Acid Drug Dev* 10: 359–368

41 Geary R, Yu R, Watanabe T, Henry S, Hardee G, Chappell A, Matson J, Sasmor H, Cummins L, Levin A (2003) Pharmacokinetics of a tumor necrosis factor-alpha phosphorothioate 2 -*O*-(2-methoxyethyl) modified antisense oligonucleotide: comparison across species. *Drug Metab Dispos* 31: 1419–1428

42 Jansen B, Wacheck V, Heere-Ress E, Schlagbauer-Wadl H, Hoeller C, Lucas T, Hoermann M, Hollenstein U, Wolff K, Pehamberger H (2000) Chemosensitisation of malignant melanoma by BCL2 antisense therapy. *Lancet* 356: 1728–1733

43 Zhang R, Yan J, Shahinian H, Amin G, Lu Z, Liu T, Saag MS, Jiang Z, Temsamani J et al (1995) Pharmacokinetics of an oligodeoxynucleotide phosphorothioate (GEM 91) in HIV-infected subjects. *Clin Pharmacol Ther* 58: 44–53

44 Agrawal S, Zhao Q, Jiang Z, Oliver C, Giles H, Heath J, Serota D (1997) Toxicologic effects of an oligodeoxynucleotide phosphorothioate and its analogs following intravenous administration in rats. *Antisense Nucleic Acid Drug Dev* 7: 575–584

45 Henry S, Zuckerman J, Rojko J, Hall W, Harman R, Kitchen D, Crooke S (1997) Toxicological properties of several novel oligonucleotide analogs in mice. *Anticancer Drug Des* 12: 1–14

46 Agrawal S, Zhao Q (1998) Mixed backbone oligonucleotides: Improvement in oligonucleotide-induced toxicity *in vivo*. *Antisense Nucleic Acid Drug Dev* 8: 135–139

47 Agrawal S, Iadarola P, Temsamani J, Zhao Q, Shaw D (1996) Effect of G-rich sequences on the synthesis, purification, binding, cell uptake, and hemolytic activity of oligonucleotides. *Bioorg Med Chem Lett* 6: 2219–2224

48 Ahn C, DeGeorge J (1998) Preclinical development of antisense oligonucleotide therapeutics for cancer: Regulatory aspects. In: E Wickstrom (ed): *Clinical trials of genetic therapy with antisense DNA and DNA vectors*. Marcel Dekker, New York, 39–52

49 Chanan-Khan A, Czuczman M (2004) Bcl-2 antisense therapy in B-cell malignant proliferative disorders. *Curr Treat Options Oncol* 5: 261–267

50 Nahta R, Esteva F (2003) Bcl-2 antisense oligonucleotides: a potential novel strategy for the treatment of breast cancer. *Semin Oncol* 30: 143–149
51 Klasa R, Gillum A, Klem R, Frankel S (2002) Oblimersen Bcl-2 antisense: facilitating apoptosis in anticancer treatment. *Antisense Nucleic Acid Drug Dev* 12: 193–213
52 van de Donk N, Kamphuis M, van Dijk M, Borst H, Bloem A, Lokhorst H (2003) Chemosensitization of myeloma plasma cells by an antisense-mediated downregulation of Bcl-2 protein. *Leukemia* 17: 211–219
53 Liu Q, Gazitt Y (2003) Potentiation of dexamethasone-, paclitaxel-, and Ad-p53-induced apoptosis by Bcl-2 antisense oligodeoxynucleotides in drug-resistant multiple myeloma cells. *Blood* 101: 4105–4114
54 Herbst R, Frankel S (2004) Oblimersen sodium (Genasense bcl-2 antisense oligonucleotide): a rational therapeutic to enhance apoptosis in therapy of lung cancer. *Clin Cancer Res* 10: 4245s–4248s
55 Dean N, McKay R, Condon T, Bennett C (1994) Inhibition of protein kinase C-alpha expression in human A549 cells by antisense oligonucleotides inhibits induction of intercellular adhesion molecule 1 (ICAM-1) mRNA by phorbol esters. *J Biol Chem* 269: 16416–16424
56 Dean N, McKay R (1994) Inhibition of protein kinase C-alpha expression in mice after systemic administration of phosphorothioate antisense oligodeoxynucleotides. *Proc Natl Acad Sci USA* 91: 11762–11766
57 Geiger T, Muller M, Dean N, Fabbro D (1998) Antitumor activity of a PKC-alpha antisense oligonucleotide in combination with standard chemotherapeutic agents against various human tumors transplanted into nude mice. *Anticancer Drug Des* 13: 35–45
58 Tortora G, Ciardiello F (2003) Antisense strategies targeting protein kinase C: preclinical and clinical development. *Semin Oncol* 30: 26–31
59 Lahn M, Sundell K, Moore S (2003) Targeting protein kinase C-alpha (PKC-alpha) in cancer with the phosphorothioate antisense oligonucleotide aprinocarsen. *Ann N Y Acad Sci* 1002: 263–270
60 Adjei A (2001) Blocking oncogenic Ras signaling for cancer therapy. *J Natl Cancer Inst* 93: 1062–1074
61 Wickstrom E (2001) Oligonucleotide treatment of ras-induced tumors in nude mice. *Mol Biotechnol* 18: 35–55
62 Cunningham C, Holmlund J, Geary R, Kwoh T, Dorr A, Johnston J, Monia B, Nemunaitis J (2001) A phase I trial of H-ras antisense oligonucleotide ISIS 2503 administered as a continuous intravenous infusion in patients with advanced carcinoma. *Cancer* 92: 1265–1271
63 Adjei A, Rowinsky E (2003) Novel anticancer agents in clinical development. *Cancer Biol Ther* 2: S5–15
64 Cho-Chung Y, Pepe S, Clair T, Budillon A, Nesterova M (1995) cAMP-dependent protein kinase: role in normal and malignant growth. *Crit Rev Oncol Hematol* 21: 33–61
65 Cho-Chung Y, Clair T (1993) The regulatory subunit of cAMP-dependent protein kinase as a target for chemotherapy of cancer and other cellular dysfunctional related diseases. *Pharmacol Ther* 60: 265–288
66 Young M, Montpetit M, Lozano Y, Djordjevic A, Devata S, Matthews J, Yedavalli S Chejfec G (1995) Regulation of Lewis lung carcinoma invasion and metastasis by protein kinase A. *Int J Cancer* 61: 104–109

67 Miller W, Hulme M, Bartlett J, MacCallum J, Dixon J (1997) Changes in messenger RNA expression of protein kinase A regulatory subunit Iα in breast cancer patients treated with tamoxifen. *Clin Cancer Res* 3: 2399–2404

68 McDaid H, Cairns M, Atkinson R, McAleer S, Harkin D, Gilmore P, Johnston P (1999) Increased expression of the RIα subunit of the cAMP-dependent protein kinase A is associated with advanced stage ovarian cancer. *Br J Cancer* 79: 933–939

69 Bradbury A, Carter D, Miller W, Cho-Chung Y, Clair T (1994) Protein kinase A (PK-A) regulatory subunit expression in colorectal cancer and related mucosa. *Br J Cancer* 69: 738–742

70 Cho Y, Park Y, Lee Y, Kim M, Bates S, Tan L, Cho-Chung Y (2000) Extracellular protein kinase A as a cancer biomarker: its expression by tumor cells and reversal by a myristate-lacking Cα and RIIβ subunit overexpression. *Proc Natl Acad Sci USA* 97: 835–840

71 Abraham I, Chin K, Gottesman M, Mayo J, Sampson K (1990) Transfection of a mutant regulatory subunit gene of cAMP-dependent protein kinase causes increased drug sensitivity and decreased expression of P-glycoprotein. *Exp Cell Res* 189: 133–141

72 Rohlff C, Glazer R (1995) Regulation of multidrug resistance through the cAMP and EGF signalling pathways. *Cell Signal* 7: 431–434

73 Cvijic M, Chin K (1998) Effects of RIα overexpression on cisplatin sensitivity in human ovarian carcinoma cells. *Biochem Biophys Res Commun* 249: 723–727

74 Ramage A, Langdon S, Ritchie A, Urns D, Miller W (1995) Growth inhibition by 8-chloro-cyclic AMP of human HT29 colorectal and ZR-75–1 breast carcinoma xenografts is associated with selective modulation of protein kinase A isoenzymes. *Eur J Cancer* 31A: 969–973

75 Cho-Chung Y, Nesterova M, Pepe S, Lee GR, Noguchi K, Srivastava R, Srivastava A, Alper O, Park Y, Lee Y (1999) Antisense DNA-targeting protein kinase A-RIα subunit: a novel approach to cancer treatment. *Front Biosci* 4: d859–868

76 Wang H, Cai Q, Zeng X, Yu D, Agrawal S, Zhang R (1999) Anti-tumor activity and pharmacokinetics of a mixed-backbone antisense oligonucleotide targeted to RIα subunit of protein kinase A after oral administration. *Proc Natl Acad Sci USA* 96: 13989–13994

77 Tortora G, Bianco R, Damiano V, Fontanini G, De Placido S, Bianco A, Ciardiello F (2000) oral antisense that targets protein kinase A cooperates with taxol and inhibits tumor growth, angiogenesis, and growth factor production. *Clin Cancer Res* 6: 2506–2512

78 Chen H, Marchall J, Ness E, Martin R, Dvorchik B, Rizi N, Marquis J, McKinlay M, Dahur W, Hawkins M (2000) A safety and pharmackinetic study of a mixed-backbone oligonucleotide (GEM231) targeting the type I protein kinase A by two-hour infusion in patients with refractory solid tumors. *Clin Cancer Res* 6: 1259–1266

79 Agrawal S, Zhang X, Zhao H, Lu Z, Yan J, Cai H, Diasio R, Habus I, Jiang Z, Iyer R et al (1995) Absorption, tissue distribution and *in vivo* stability in rats of a hybrid antisense oligonucleotide following oral administration. *Biochem Pharm* 50: 571–576

80 Yang L, Mashima T, Sato S, Mochizuki M, Sakamoto H, Yamori T, Oh-Hara T, Tsuruo T (2003) Predominant suppression of apoptosome by inhibitor of apoptosis protein in non-small cell lung cancer H460 cells: therapeutic effect of a novel polyarginine-conjugated Smac peptide. *Cancer Res* 63: 831–837

81 Rajcan-Separovic E, Liston P, Lefebvre C, Korneluk R (1996) Assignment of human inhibitor of apoptosis protein (IAP) genes xiap, hiap-1, and hiap-2 to chromosomes Xq25 and 11q22-q23 by fluorescence in situ hybridization. *Genomics* 37: 404–406
82 Bratton S, Cohen G (2003) Death receptors leave a caspase footprint that Smacs of XIAP. *Cell Death Differ* 10: 4–6
83 Deveraux Q, Leo E, Stennicke H, Welsh K, Salvesen G, Reed J (1999) Cleavage of human inhibitor of apoptosis protein XIAP results in fragments with distinct specificities for caspases. *EMBO J* 18: 5242–5251
84 Suzuki Y, Nakabayashi Y, Takahashi R (2001) Ubiquitin-protein ligase activity of X-linked inhibitor of apoptosis protein promotes proteasomal degradation of caspase-3 and enhances its anti-apoptotic effect in Fas-induced cell death. *Proc Natl Acad Sci USA* 98: 8662–8667
85 Hu Y, Cherton-Horvat G, Dragowska V, Baird S, Korneluk R, Durkin J, Mayer L, LaCasse E (2003) Antisense oligonucleotides targeting XIAP induce apoptosis and enhance chemotherapeutic activity against human lung cancer cells *in vitro* and *in vivo*. *Clin Cancer Res* 9: 2826–2836
86 Yang L, Cao Z, Yan H, Wood W (2003) Coexistence of high levels of apoptotic signaling and inhibitor of apoptosis proteins in human tumor cells: implication for cancer specific therapy. *Cancer Res* 63: 6815–6824
87 Tamm I, Kornblau S, Segall H, Krajewski S, Welsh K, Kitada S, Scudiero D, Tudor G, Qui Y, Monks A et al (2000) Expression and prognostic significance of IAP-family genes in human cancers and myeloid leukemias. *Clin Cancer Res* 6: 1796–1803
88 Yan Y, Mahotka C, Heikaus S, Shibata T, Wethkamp N, Liebmann J, Suschek C, Guo Y, Gabbert H, Gerharz C et al (2004) Disturbed balance of expression between XIAP and Smac/DIABLO during tumour progression in renal cell carcinomas. *Br J Cancer* 91: 1349–1357
89 Ramp U, Krieg T, Caliskan E, Mahotka C, Ebert T, Willers R, Gabbert H, Gerharz C (2004) XIAP expression is an independent prognostic marker in clear-cell renal carcinomas. *Hum Pathol* 35: 1022–1028
90 Cummins J, Kohli M, Rago C, Kinzler K, Vogelstein B, Bunz F (2004) X-linked inhibitor of apoptosis protein (XIAP) is a nonredundant modulator of tumor necrosis factor-related apoptosis-inducing ligand (TRAIL)-mediated apoptosis in human cancer cells. *Cancer Res* 64: 3006–3008
91 Bilim V, Kasahara T, Hara N, Takahashi K, Tomita Y (2003) Role of XIAP in the malignant phenotype of transitional cell cancer (TCC) and therapeutic activity of XIAP antisense oligonucleotides against multidrug-resistant TCC *in vitro*. *Int J Cancer* 103: 29–37
92 McManus D, Lefebvre C, Cherton-Horvat G, St-Jean M, Kandimalla E, Agrawal S, Morris S, Durkin J, Lacasse E (2004) Loss of XIAP protein expression by RNAi and antisense approaches sensitizes cancer cells to functionally diverse chemotherapeutics. *Oncogene* 23: 8105–8117
93 Chawla-Sarkar M, Bae S, Reu F, Jacobs B, Lindner D, Borden E (2004) Downregulation of Bcl-2, FLIP or IAPs (XIAP and survivin) by siRNAs sensitizes resistant melanoma cells to Apo2L/TRAIL-induced apoptosis. *Cell Death Differ* 11: 915–923
94 Shi W, Siemann D (2002) Inhibition of renal cell carcinoma angiogenesis and growth by antisense oligonucleotides targeting vascular endothelial growth factor. *Br J Cancer* 87: 119–126

95 Riedel F, Gotte K, Li M, Hormann K, Grandis J (2003) Abrogation of VEGF expression in human head and neck squamous cell carcinoma decreases angiogenic activity *in vitro* and *in vivo*. *Int J Oncol* 23: 577–583
96 Lacombe J, Viazovkina E, Bernatchez P, Galarneau A, Damha M, Sirois M (2002) Antisense inhibition of Flk-1 by oligonucleotides composed of 2′ -deoxy-2′-fluoro-beta-D-arabino- and 2′-deoxy-nucleosides. *Can J Physiol Pharmacol* 80: 951–961
97 Chesire D, Isaacs W (2003) Beta-catenin signaling in prostate cancer: an early perspective. *Endocr Relat Cancer* 10: 537–560
98 Luu H, Zhang R, Haydon R, Rayburn E, Kang Q, Si W, Park J, Wang H, Peng Y, Jiang W et al (2005) Wnt/β-catenin signaling pathway as novel cancer drug targets. *Curr Cancer Drug Targets* 4: 653–671
99 Roh H, Green D, Boswell C, Pippin J, Drebin J (2001) Suppression of beta-catenin inhibits the neoplastic growth of APC-mutant colon cancer cells. *Cancer Res* 61: 6563–6568
100 Green D, Roh H, Pippin J, Drebin J (2001) Beta-catenin antisense treatment decreases beta-catenin expression and tumor growth rate in colon carcinoma xenografts. *J Surg Res* 101: 16–20
101 Veeramachaneni N, Kubokura H, Lin L, Pippin J, Patterson G, Drebin J, Battafarano R (2004) Down-regulation of beta catenin inhibits the growth of esophageal carcinoma cells. *J Thorac Cardiovasc Surg* 127: 92–98
102 Chung E, Hwang S, Nguyen P, Lee S, Kim J, Kim J, Henkart P, Bottaro D, Soon L, Bonvini P et al (2002) Regulation of leukemic cell adhesion, proliferation, and survival by beta-catenin. *Blood* 100: 982–990
103 Easwaran V, Lee S, Inge L, Guo L, Goldbeck C, Garrett E, Wiesmann M, Garcia P, Fuller J, Chan V et al (2003) beta-Catenin regulates vascular endothelial growth factor expression in colon cancer. *Cancer Res* 63: 3145–3153
104 Ambrosini G, Adida C, Altieri D (1997) A novel anti-apoptosis gene, survivin, expressed in cancer and lymphoma. *Nat Med* 3: 917–921
105 Altieri D (2003) Survivin, versatile modulation of cell division and apoptosis in cancer. *Oncogene* 22: 8581–8589
106 Grossman D, Kim P, Blanc-Brude O, Brash D, Tognin S, Marchisio P, Altieri D (2001) Transgenic expression of survivin in keratinocytes counteracts UVB-induced apoptosis and cooperates with loss of p53. *J Clin Invest* 108: 991–996
107 Fukuda S, Mantel C, Pelus L (2004) Survivin regulates hematopoietic progenitor cell proliferation through p21WAF1/Cip1-dependent and -independent pathways. *Blood* 103: 120–127
108 Schimmer A (2004) Inhibitor of apoptosis proteins: translating basic knowledge into clinical practice. *Cancer Res* 64: 7183–7190
109 Liu T, Brouha B, Grossman D (2004) Rapid induction of mitochondrial events and caspase-independent apoptosis in Survivin-targeted melanoma cells. *Oncogene* 23: 39–48
110 Dohi T, Beltrami E, Wall N, Plescia J, Altieri D (2004) Mitochondrial survivin inhibits apoptosis and promotes tumorigenesis. *J Clin Invest* 114: 1117–1127
111 Carter B, Wang R, Schober W, Milella M, Chism D, Andreeff M (2003) Targeting Survivin expression induces cell proliferation defect and subsequent cell death involving mitochondrial pathway in myeloid leukemic cells. *Cell Cycle* 2: 488–493

112 Tu S, Jiang X, Lin M, Cui J, Yang Y, Lum C, Zou B, Zhu Y, Jiang S, Wong W et al (2003) Suppression of survivin expression inhibits *in vivo* tumorigenicity and angiogenesis in gastric cancer. *Cancer Res* 63: 7724–7732

113 Ansell S, Arendt B, Grote D, Jelinek D, Novak A, Wellik L, Remstein E, Bennett C, Fielding A (2004) Inhibition of survivin expression suppresses the growth of aggressive non-Hodgkin's lymphoma. *Leukemia* 18: 616–623

114 Kanwar J, Shen W, Kanwar R, Berg R, Krissansen G (2001) Effects of survivin antagonists on growth of established tumors and B7–1 immunogene therapy. *J Natl Cancer Inst* 93: 1541–1552

115 Cao C, Mu Y, Hallahan D, Lu B (2004) XIAP and survivin as therapeutic targets for radiation sensitization in preclinical models of lung cancer. *Oncogene* 23: 7047–7052

116 Adamzik I, Kabelitz D, Dreger P, Schmitz N, Heiser A (2003) Generation of cytotoxic responses in mice and human individuals against hematological malignancies using survivin-RNA-transfected dendritic cells. *J Immunol* 170: 5391–5397

117 Fakharzadeh S, Trusko S, George D (1991) Tumorigenic potential associated with enhanced expression of a gene that is amplified in a mouse tumor cell line. *EMBO J* 10: 1565–1569

118 Prives C, Hall P (1999) The p53 pathway. *J Pathol* 187: 112–126

119 Freedman D, Levine A (1999) Regulation of the p53 protein by the MDM2 oncoprotein—Thirty-eighth G.H.A. Clowes Memorial Award lecture. *Cancer Res* 59: 1–7

120 Hupp T, Lane D, Ball K (2000) Strategies for manipulating the p53 pathway in the treatment of human cancer. *Biochem J* 352: 1–17

121 Lane D, Lain S (2002) Therapeutic exploitation of the p53 pathway. *Trends Mol Med* 8: S38-S42

122 Michael D, Oren M (2002) The p53 and mdm2 families in cancer. *Curr Opin Genet Dev* 12: 53–59

123 Silvestrini R, Daidone M, Benini E, Faranda A, Tomasic G, Boracchi P, Salvadori B, Veronesi U (1996) Validation of p53 accumulation as a predictor of distant metastasis at 10 years of follow-up in 1400 node-negative breast cancers. *Clin Cancer Res* 2: 2007–2013

124 Slaton J, Benedict W, Dinney C (2001) P53 in bladder cancer: mechanism of action, prognostic value, and target for therapy. *Urology* 57: 852–859

125 Weller M (1998) Predicting response to cancer chemotherapy: the role of p53. *Cell Tissue Res* 292: 435–445

126 Lang F, Yung W, Raju U, Libunao F, Terry N, Tofilon P (1998) Enhancement of radiosensitivity of wild-type p53 human glioma cells by adenovirus-mediated delivery of the p53 gene. *J Neurosurg* 89: 125–132

127 Muschel R, Soto D, McKenna W, Bernhard E (1998) Radiosensitization and apoptosis. *Oncogene* 17: 3359–3363

128 Momand J, Wu H, Dasgupta G (2000) MDM2 – master regulator of the p53 tumor suppressor protein. *Gene* 242: 15–29

129 Zhang R, Wang H (2000) MDM2 oncogene as a novel target for human cancer therapy. *Curr Pharm Design* 6: 393–416

130 Momand J, Jung D, Wilczynski S, Niland J (1998) The MDM2 gene amplification database. *Nucleic Acids Res* 26: 3453–3459

131 Zhang Z, Wang H, Li M, Agrawal S, Chen X, Zhang R (2004) MDM2 is a negative regulator of $p21^{WAF1/CIP1}$, independent of p53. *J Biol Chem* 279: 16000–16006

132 Jones S, Hancock A, Vogel H, Donehower L, Bradley A (1998) Overexpression of Mdm2 in mice reveals a p53-independent role for Mdm2 in tumorigenesis. *Proc Natl Acad Sci USA* 95: 1508–1512
133 Chen L, Agrawal S, Zhou W, Zhang R, Chen J (1998) Synergistic activation of p53 by inhibition of MDM2 expression and DNA damage. *Proc Natl Acad Sci USA* 95: 195–200
134 Chen L, Lu W, Agrawal S, Zhou W, Zhang R, Chen J (1999) Ubiquitous induction of p53 in tumor cells by antisense inhibition of MDM2 expression. *Mol Med* 5: 21–34
135 Wang H, Zeng X, Oliver P, Le L, Chen J, Chen L, Zhou W, Agrawal S, Zhang R (1999) MDM2 oncogene as a target for cancer therapy: An antisense approach. *Int J Oncol* 15: 653–660
136 Wang H, Nan L, Yu D, Lindsey J, Agrawal S, Zhang R (2002) Anti-tumor efficacy of a novel antisense anti-mdm2 mixed-backbone oligonucleotide in human colon cancer models: p53-dependent and p53-independent mechanisms. *Mol Med* 8: 185–199
137 Wang H, Yu D, Agrawal S, Zhang R (2003) Experimental therapy of human prostate cancer by inhibiting MDM2 expression with novel mixed-backbone antisense oligonucleotides: *In vitro* and *In vivo* activities and mechanisms. *Prostate* 54: 194–205
138 Wang H, Oliver P, Zhang Z, Agrawal S, Zhang R (2003) Chemosensitization and radiosensitization of human cancer by antisense anti-MDM2 oligonucleotides: *In vitro* and *In vivo* activities and mechanisms. *Ann New York Acad Sci* 1002: 217–235
139 Zhang Z, Wang H, Prasad G, Li M, Yu D, Bonner J, Agrawal S, Zhang R (2004) Radiosensitization by antisense anti-MDM2 mixed-backbone oligonucleotide in *in vitro* and *in vivo* human cancer models. *Clin Cancer Res* 10: 1263–1273
140 Jorgensen R (1990) Altered gene expression in plants due to trans interactions between homologous genes. *Trends Biotechnol* 8: 340–344
141 Fire A, Xu S, Montgomery M, Kostas S, Driver S, Mello C (1998) Potent and specific genetic interference by double-stranded RNA in *Caenorhabditis elegans*. *Nature* 391: 806–811
142 Jackson A, Bartz S, Schelter J, Kobayashi S, Burchard J, Mao M, Li B, Cavet G, Linsley P (2003) Expression profiling reveals off-target gene regulation by RNAi. *Nat Biotechnol* 21: 635–637
143 Jackson A, Linsley P (2004) Noise amidst the silence: off-target effects of siRNAs? *Trends Genet* 20: 521–524
144 Orr RM (2001) GTI-2040. Lorus Therapeutics. *Curr Opin Investig Drugs* 2: 1462–1466
145 Tu G, Tu X (2001) GTI-2501. Lorus Therapeutics. *Curr Opin Investig Drugs* 2001 2: 1467–1470
146 Mani S, Goel S, Nesterova M, Martin R, Grindel J, Rothenberg M, Zhang R, Tortora G, Cho-Chung Y (2003) Clinical studies in patients with solid tumors using a second-generation antisense oligonucleotide (GEM 231) targeted against protein kinase A type I. *Ann N Y Acad Sci* 1002: 252–262
147 Davis A, Gelmon K, Siu L, Moore M, Britten C, Mistry N, Klamut H, D'Aloisio S, MacLean M, Wainman N et al (2003) Phase I and pharmacologic study of the human DNA methyltransferase antisense oligodeoxynucleotide MG98 given as a 21-day continuous infusion every 4 weeks. *Invest New Drugs* 21: 85–97
148 Iversen P, Arora V, Acker A, Mason D, Devi G (2003) Efficacy of antisense morpholino oligomer targeted to c-myc in prostate cancer xenograft murine model and a Phase I safety study in humans. *Clin Cancer Res* 9: 2510–2519

149 Stephens A (2004) Technology evaluation: AVI-4126, AVI BioPharma. *Curr Opin Mol Ther* 6: 551–558

150 Arora V, Cate M, Ghosh C, Iversen P (2002) Phosphorodiamidate morpholino antisense oligomers inhibit expression of human cytochrome P450 3A4 and alter selected drug metabolism. *Drug Metab Dispos* 30: 757–762

151 Antisense Pharma (2005) Antisense Pharma completes patient recruitment for AP 12009 phase II trial, April 28, 2005: *http://www.antisensepharma.com/news/pressrelease/f_pressrelease.htm* (Accessed May 2005)

152 Oza A, Elit L, Swenerton K, Faught W, Ghatage P, Carey M, McIntosh L, Dorr A, Holmlund J, Eisenhauer E (2003) NCIC Clinical Trials Group Study. Phase II study of CGP 69846A (ISIS 5132) in recurrent epithelial ovarian cancer: an NCIC clinical trials group study (NCIC IND.116). *Gynecol Oncol* 89: 129–133

153 Moreira J, Simoes S (2003) Technology evaluation: LErafAON, NeoPharm. *Curr Opin Mol Ther* 5: 547–552

154 Rudin C, Marshall J, Huang C, Kindler H, Zhang C, Kumar D, Gokhale P, Steinberg J, Wanaski S, Kasid U et al (2004) Delivery of a liposomal c-raf-1 antisense oligonucleotide by weekly bolus dosing in patients with advanced solid tumors: a phase I study. *Clin Cancer Res* 10: 7244–7251

155 Gleave M, Nelson C, Chi K (2003) Antisense targets to enhance hormone and cytotoxic therapies in advanced prostate cancer. *Curr Drug Targets* 4: 209–221

156 Orr R (1999) Technology evaluation: leukemia therapy, University of Pennsylvania. *Curr Opin Mol Ther* 1: 399–403

157 Bishop M, Iversen P, Bayever E, Sharp J, Greiner T, Copple B, Ruddon R, Zon G, Spinolo J, Arneson M et al (1996) Phase I trial of an antisense oligonucleotide OL(1)p53 in hematologic malignancies. *J Clin Oncol* 14: 1320–1326

158 Yuen A, Sikic B (2000) Clinical studies of antisense therapy in cancer. *Front Biosci* 5: D588–593

159 Cummings J, Ward TH, LaCass E, Lefebvre C, St-Jean M, Durkin J, Ranson M, Dive C (2005) Validation of pharmacodynamic assays to evaluate the clinical efficacy of an antisense compound (AEG 35156) targeted to the X-linked inhibitor of apoptosis protein XIAP. *Br J Cancer* 92: 532–538

160 Holmlung JT (2003) Applying antisense technology: Affinitak and other antisense oligonucleotides in clinical development. *Ann N Y Acad Sci* 1002: 244–251

161 Ko Y, Devi G, London C, Kayas A, Reddy M, Iversen P, Bubley G, Balk S (2004) Androgen receptor down-regulation in prostate cancer with phosphorodiamidate morpholino antisense oligomers. *J Urol* 172: 1140–1144

162 Ying H, Yu Y, Xu Y (2000) Antisense of ATP synthase subunit e inhibits the growth of human hepatocellular carcinoma cells. *Oncol Res* 12: 485–490

163 Hayward R, Macpherson J, Cummings J, Monia B, Smyth J, Jodrell D (2004) Enhanced oxaliplatin-induced apoptosis following antisense Bcl-xl down-regulation is p53 and Bax dependent: Genetic evidence for specificity of the antisense effect. *Mol Cancer Ther* 3: 169–178

164 Zangemeister-Wittke U (2003) Antisense to apoptosis inhibitors facilitates chemotherapy and TRAIL-induced death signaling. *Ann N Y Acad Sci* 1002: 90–94

165 Hyer M, Sudarshan S, Kim Y, Reed J, Dong J, Schwartz D, Norris J (2002) Down-regulation of c-FLIP sensitizes DU145 prostate cancer cells to Fas-mediated apoptosis. *Cancer Biol Ther* 1: 401–406

166 Aharinejad S, Paulus P, Sioud M, Hofmann M, Zins K, Schafer R, Stanley ER, Abraham D (2004) Colony-stimulating factor-1 blockade by antisense oligonucleotides and small interfering RNAs suppresses growth of human mammary tumor xenografts in mice. *Cancer Res* 64: 5378–5384

167 Sak A, Stuschke M, Wurm R, Schroeder G, Sinn B, Wolf G, Budach V (2002) Selective inactivation of DNA-dependent protein kinase with antisense oligodeoxynucleotides: consequences for the rejoining of radiation-induced DNA double-strand breaks and radiosensitivity of human cancer cell lines. *Cancer Res* 62: 6621–6624

168 Niwa H, Wentzel A, Li M, Gooding W, Lui V, Grandis J (2003) Antitumor effects of epidermal growth factor receptor antisense oligonucleotides in combination with docetaxel in squamous cell carcinoma of the head and neck. *Clin Cancer Res* 9: 5028–5035

169 Washio K, Aoe M, Toyooka S, Mushiake H, Tsukuda K, Shimizu N (2003) The effect of epidermal growth factor receptor antisense morpholino oligomer on non-small cell lung cancer cell line. *Oncol Rep* 10: 1967–1971

170 Baron V, Duss S, Rhim J, Mercola D (2003) Antisense to the early growth response-1 gene (Egr-1) inhibits prostate tumor development in TRAMP mice. *Ann N Y Acad Sci* 1002: 197–216

171 Chan K, Chan J, Chung K, Fung K (2004) Inhibition of cell proliferation in human breast tumor cells by antisense oligonucleotides against facilitative glucose transporter 5. *J Cell Biochem* 93: 1134–1142

172 Yang D, Jiang X, Elliott R, Head J (2002) Antisense ferritin oligonucleotides inhibit growth and induce apoptosis in human breast carcinoma cells. *Anticancer Res* 22: 1513–1524

173 Hirai K, Sasaki H, Sakamoto H, Takeshita F, Asano K, Kubota Y, Ochiya T, Terada M (2003) Antisense oligodeoxynucleotide against HST-1/FGF-4 suppresses tumorigenicity of an orthotopic model for human germ cell tumor in nude mice. *J Gene Med* 5: 951–957

174 Liu Y, Han T, Yu J, Bitterman A, Le A, Giuliano A, Cabot M (2004) Oligonucleotides blocking glucosylceramide synthase expression selectively reverse drug resistance in cancer cells. *J Lipid Res* 45: 933–940

175 Deng W, Li R, Guerrera M, Liu Y, Ladisch S (2002) Transfection of glucosylceramide synthase antisense inhibits mouse melanoma formation. *Glycobiology* 12: 145–152

176 Zheng G, Zhang J, Liu F, Wang X, Zhang X (2002) Molecular mechanism of antisense glycosyltransferase oligonucleotide inhibiting human gliomas cell line SWO-38. *Ai Zheng* 21: 1095–1099

177 Rait A, Pirollo K, Ulick D, Cullen K, Chang E (2003) HER-2-targeted antisense oligonucleotide results in sensitization of head and neck cancer cells to chemotherapeutic agents. *Ann N Y Acad Sci* 1002: 78–89

178 Rait A, Pirollo K, Xiang L, Ulick D, Chang EH (2002) Tumor-targeting, systemically delivered antisense HER-2 chemosensitizes human breast cancer xenografts irrespective of HER-2 levels. *Mol Med* 8: 475–486

179 Dai S, Huang M, Hsu C, Chao K (2003) Inhibition of hypoxia inducible factor 1alpha causes oxygen-independent cytotoxicity and induces p53 independent apoptosis in glioblastoma cells. *Int J Radiat Oncol Biol Phys* 55: 1027–1036

180 Liu S, Sun W, Cao Y, Ma C, Han L, Zhang L, Wang Z, Zhu F (2004) Antisense oligonucleotide targeting at the initiator of hTERT arrests growth of hepatoma cells. *World J Gastroenterol* 10: 366–370

181 Kinzel B, Hall J, Natt F, Weiler J, Cohen D (2002) Downregulation of Hus1 by antisense oligonucleotides enhances the sensitivity of human lung carcinoma cells to cisplatin. *Cancer* 94: 1808–1814
182 Zang X, Lerner M, Dunn S, Brackett D, Pento J (2003) Antisense KGFR oligonucleotide inhibition of KGF-induced motility in breast cancer cells. *Anticancer Res* 23: 4913–4919
183 Kausch I, Jiang H, Brocks C, Bruderek K, Kruger S, Sczakiel G, Jocham D, Bohle A (2004) Ki-67-directed antisense therapy in an orthotopic renal cell carcinoma model. *Eur Urol* 46: 118–124
184 Nakada Y, Saito S, Ohzawa K, Morioka CY, Kita K, Minemura M, Takahara T, Watanabe A (2001) Antisense oligonucleotides specific to mutated K-ras genes inhibit invasiveness of human pancreatic cancer cell lines. *Pancreatology* 1: 314–319
185 Aoki K, Ohnami S, Yoshida T (2004) Suppression of pancreatic and colon cancer cells by antisense K-ras RNA expression vectors. *Methods Mol Med* 106: 193–204
186 Rashmi R, Kumar S, Karunagaran D (2004) Ectopic expression of Bcl-XL or Ku70 protects human colon cancer cells (SW480) against curcumin-induced apoptosis while their down-regulation potentiates it. *Carcinogenesis* 25: 1867–1877
187 Belenkov A, Paiement J, Panasci L, Monia B, Chow T (2002) An antisense oligonucleotide targeted to human Ku86 messenger RNA sensitizes M059K malignant glioma cells to ionizing radiation, bleomycin, and etoposide but not DNA cross-linking agents. *Cancer Res* 62: 5888–5896
188 Khazenzon N, Ljubimov A, Lakhter A, Fujita M, Fujiwara H, Sekiguchi K, Sorokin L, Petajaniemi N, Virtanen I, Black K et al (2003) Antisense inhibition of laminin-8 expression reduces invasion of human gliomas *in vitro*. *Mol Cancer Ther* 2: 985–994
189 Thallinger C, Wolschek M, Wacheck V, Maierhofer H, Gunsberg P, Polterauer P, Pehamberger H, Monia B, Selzer E, Wolff K et al (2003) Mcl-1 antisense therapy chemosensitizes human melanoma in a SCID mouse xenotransplantation model. *J Invest Dermatol* 120: 1081–1086
190 Rittierodt M, Tschernig T, Harada K (2004) Modulation of multidrug-resistance-associated P-glycoprotein in human U-87 MG and HUV-ECC cells with antisense oligodeoxynucleotides to MDR1 mRNA. *Pathobiology* 71: 123–128
191 London C, Sekhon H, Arora V, Stein D, Iversen P, Devi G (2003) A novel antisense inhibitor of MMP-9 attenuates angiogenesis, human prostate cancer cell invasion and tumorigenicity. *Cancer Gene Ther* 10: 823–832
192 Matsumoto Y, Miyake K, Kunishio K, Tamiya T, Seigo N (2004) Reduction of expression of the multidrug resistance protein (MRP)1 in glioma cells by antisense phosphorothioate oligonucleotides. *J Med Invest* 51: 194–201
193 Pession A, Tonelli R, Fronza R, Sciamanna E, Corradini R, Sforza S, Tedeschi T, Marchelli R, Montanaro L, Camerin C et al (2004) Targeted inhibition of NMYC by peptide nucleic acid in N-myc amplified human neuroblastoma cells: cell-cycle inhibition with induction of neuronal cell differentiation and apoptosis. *Int J Oncol* 24: 265–272
194 Fan Y, Borowsky A, Weiss R (2003) An antisense oligodeoxynucleotide to p21(Waf1/Cip1) causes apoptosis in human breast cancer cells. *Mol Cancer Ther* 2: 773–782
195 Sonnemann J, Gekeler V, Ahlbrecht K, Brischwein K, Liu C, Bader P, Muller C, Niethammer D, Beck J (2004) Down-regulation of protein kinase Ceta by antisense

oligonucleotides sensitises A549 lung cancer cells to vincristine and paclitaxel. *Cancer Lett* 209: 177–185
196 Wang C, Hu F, Lu Y, Wang S, Ma D (2002) Effects of RelA antisense oligonucleotide on apoptosis of ovarian cancer cells COC1. *Zhonghua Fu Chan Ke Za Zhi* 37: 202–204
197 Gardner-Thorpe J, Ito H, Ashley S, Whang E (2003) Ribosomal protein P2: a potential molecular target for antisense therapy of human malignancies. *Anticancer Res* 23: 4549–4560
198 Fluiter K, ten Asbroek A, van Groenigen M, Nooij M, Aalders M, Baas F (2002) Tumor genotype-specific growth inhibition *in vivo* by antisense oligonucleotides against a polymorphic site of the large subunit of human RNA polymerase II. *Cancer Res* 62: 2024–2028
199 Fluiter K, ten Asbroek A, de Wissel M, Jakobs M, Wissenbach M, Olsson H, Olsen O, Oerum H, Baas F (2003) *In vivo* tumor growth inhibition and biodistribution studies of locked nucleic acid (LNA) antisense oligonucleotides. *Nucleic Acids Res* 31: 953–962
200 Rubenstein M, Slobodskoy L, Mirochnik Y, Guinan P (2003) Inhibition of PC-3 prostate cancer cell growth *in vitro* using both antisense oligonucleotides and taxol. *Med Oncol* 20: 29–35
201 Fujiwara M, Jin E, Ghazizadeh M, Kawanami O (2002) Antisense oligodeoxynucleotides against thrombomodulin suppress the cell growth of lung adenocarcinoma cell line A549. *Pathol Int* 52: 204–213
202 Berg R, Ferguson P, Vincent M, Koropatnick D (2003) A "combination oligonucleotide" antisense strategy to downregulate thymidylate synthase and decrease tumor cell growth and drug resistance. *Cancer Gene Ther* 10: 278–286
203 Salatino M, Schillaci R, Proietti C, Carnevale R, Frahm I, Molinolo A, Iribarren A, Charreau E, Elizalde P (2004) Inhibition of *in vivo* breast cancer growth by antisense oligodeoxynucleotides to type I insulin-like growth factor receptor mRNA involves inactivation of ErbBs, PI-3K/Akt and p42/p44 MAPK signaling pathways but not modulation of progesterone receptor activity. *Oncogene* 23: 5161–5174
204 Grzmil M, Hemmerlein B, Thelen P, Schweyer S, Burfeind P (2004) Blockade of the type I IGF receptor expression in human prostate cancer cells inhibits proliferation and invasion, up-regulates IGF binding protein-3, and suppresses MMP-2 expression. *J Pathol* 202: 50–59
205 D'Alessio S, Margheri F, Pucci M, Del Rosso A, Monia B, Bologna M, Leonetti C, Scarsella M, Zupi G, Fibbi G et al (2004) Antisense oligodeoxynucleotides for urokinase-plasminogen activator receptor have anti-invasive and anti-proliferative effects *in vitro* and inhibit spontaneous metastases of human melanoma in mice. *Int J Cancer* 110: 125–133

Progress in Drug Research, Vol. 63
(R. M. Schultz, Ed.)

Preclinical development of Alimta™ (Pemetrexed, LY231514), a multitargeted antifolate

Richard M. Schultz

Division of Cancer Research
Lilly Research Laboratories
Lilly Corporate Center
Indianapolis, IN 46285, USA
<Rick_1252@msn.com>

Glossary of abbreviations

AICARFT, aminoimidazole carboxamide ribonucleotide formyltransferase; BrdU, 5-bromodeoxyuridine; DHF, dihydrofolate; DHFR, dihydrofolate reductase; FPGS, folylpolyglutamate synthetase; FR, folate receptor; 5-FU, 5-fluorouracil; GARFT, glycinamide ribonucleotide formyltransferase; HGPRT, hypoxanthine phosphoribosyl transferase; LFD, low-folate diet; PCNA, proliferating cell nuclear antigen; RFC, reduced folate carrier; rh, recombinant human; rm, recombinant mouse; TK, thymidine kinase; TS, thymidylate synthase.

1 Introduction

Folate-requiring enzymes provide excellent targets for cancer chemotherapy due to the close relationship of folic acid metabolism to cell replication. Folate vitamins are a class of cofactors that serve as one-carbon donors in biochemical reactions that are needed for *de novo* synthesis of purines and pyrimidines. Antifolates act by interfering with the binding of natural folate cofactors to critical biosynthetic enzymes, thereby inhibiting growth or killing rapidly dividing cells, such as most cancer cells [1–3]. The folate-requiring enzymes include: thymidylate synthase (TS), which converts deoxyuridine monophosphate to deoxythymidine monophosphate for DNA synthesis; aminoimidazole carboxamide ribonucleotide formyltransferase (AICARFT) and glycinamide ribonucleotide formyltransferase (GARFT), which are key steps in the synthesis of purines for DNA and RNA; and dihydrofolate reductase (DHFR), which regenerates tetrahydrofolate. Inhibition of any of these enzymes will retard the synthesis of nucleotides and inhibit the synthesis of DNA and RNA.

N-[4-[2-(2-amino-3,4-dihydryo-4-oxo-7H-pyrrolo[2,3-d]pyrimidin-5-yl)-ethyl]-benzoyl]-L-glutamic acid (Alimta, Pemetrexed, LY231514) is a structurally novel antifolate that possesses a unique 6-5 fused pyrrolo[2,3-d]-pyrimidine nucleus instead of the more common 6-6 fused pteridine or quinazoline ring structure. Alimta was initially discovered through structure/activity relationship studies of the novel antipurine antifolate, lometrexol. Early studies demonstrated that the primary site of action of Alimta was thymidylate synthase [4, 5] rather than purine synthesis. It is interesting to note that complete protection of leukemia cells from Alimta cytotoxicity required both thymidine and hypoxanthine [5]. Further studies by the author using cell culture end-product reversal studies in multiple carcinoma cell lines have demonstrated that thymidine (5 µM) alone was not able to fully reverse the cytotoxic action of LY231514 [6–8] and only protected cells at low drug levels. Both thymidine (5 µM) and hypoxanthine (100 µM) were required to fully protect cells from the growth inhibitory action exerted by LY231514. This unique reversal pattern suggested that multiple targets were involved in Alimta-induced cytotoxicity.

Alimta is one of the best substrates that is known for the enzyme folyl-polyglutamate synthase (K_m = 1.6 µM and V_{max}/K_m = 621 [9]). Pemetrexed can be considered a pro-drug, because its pentaglutamate is a predominant intracellular form. Polyglutamation traps Alimta, thus enhancing its intracellular retention. Whereas Alimta only moderately inhibited TS (K_i = 340 nM, recombinant mouse), the pentaglutamate form was 100-fold more potent (K_i = 3.4 nM [5]), becoming one of the most potent folate-based TS inhibitors [10]. Studies have also shown that the polyglutamates of Alimta (e.g., the triglutamate glu_3 and pentaglutamate glu_5) potently inhibit several other key enzymes of the folate metabolism, including DHFR, GARFT, and AICARFT (Fig. 1) [8]. This chapter reviews the unique preclinical polypharmacology of Alimta.

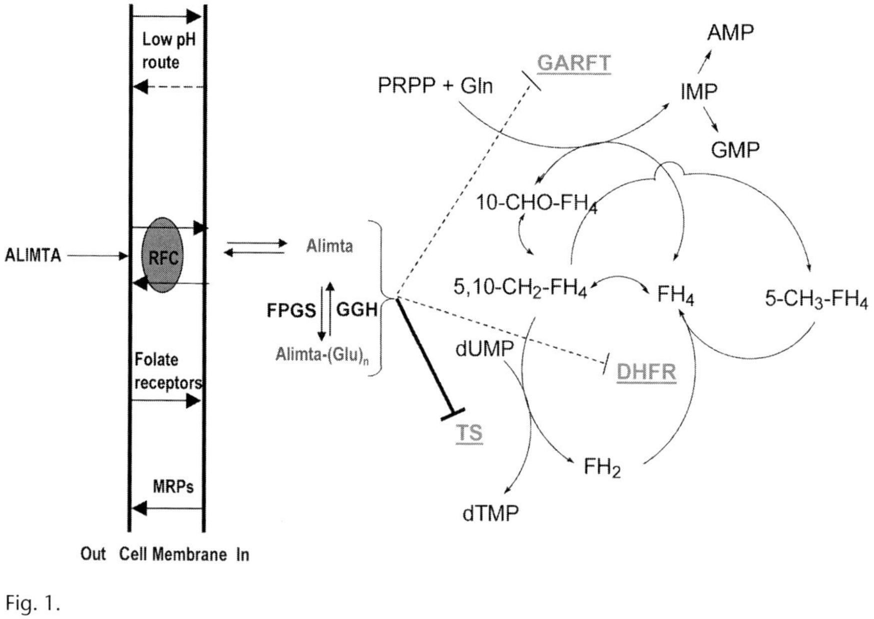

Fig. 1.
Mechanisms of action of Alimta. (Courtesy of Victor Chen).

2 End-product reversal studies and mechanism of action

Reversal conditions can help elucidate the mechanism of antitumor activity by antifolates. For example, inhibition of GARFT can be overcome by the salvage of exogenous hypoxanthine via hypoxanthine phosphoribosyl transferase (HGPRT), and GARFT inhibitors, such as lometrexol, do not inhibit cell growth in the presence of a plentiful supply of hypoxanthine. Similarly, thymidine supplementation can prevent growth inhibition by TS inhibitors because cells can salvage extracellular thymidine via thymidine kinase. Early studies indicated that the antiproliferative activity of Alimta was prevented by leucovorin, but incompletely reversed by thymidine in human CCRF-CEM and murine L1210 leukemia cells [4, 5]. Although thymidine could protect cells from Alimta at concentrations near the growth-inhibitory IC_{50}, higher concentrations of drug required both thymidine (5 µM) and hypoxanthine (100 µM) to fully protect cells. At higher drug concentrations, inhibition of DHFR and/or purine *de novo* biosynthetic enzymes appeared to be responsible for the secondary cytotoxic actions of Alimta. This reversal pattern was significantly different from other know antifolates such as methotrexate, Tomudex®, and lometrexol, and suggests that TS is only partially responsible for the antiproliferative action of this novel antifolate. It was for this reason that Alimta was referred to as the "multitargeted antifolate (MTA)" in early literature [6, 7]. In addition to leukemia cells, this reversal pattern was observed in various human carcinoma cell lines, including HCT-8 ileocecal carcinoma, GC3 colon carcinoma, and MCF-7 breast carcinoma ([8, 11]; Tab. 1). In contrast, the cytotoxic activity of the more selective TS inhibitor Tomudex was completely reversed by thymidine treatment (5 µM) alone.

The conditions for reversal of growth inhibitory activity were also used to characterize drug resistance. In resistant sublines with TS amplification, the reversal patterns were distinctly different from those observed in drug-naïve populations. Thymidine treatment did not significantly protect cells from Alimta cytotoxicity, whereas hypoxanthine alone completely protected these cells [11]. This suggested that selective inhibition of purine *de novo* biosynthesis was responsible for cytotoxic activity in cells containing elevated levels of TS. In contrast, a methotrexate-resistant CCRF-CEM leukemia line resulting from DHFR amplification demonstrated strong collateral resistance to

Table 1.
End-product reversal studies with Alimta in wild-type human cell lines.[a]

Cell line	IC_{50} (nM)[b]	Increase (fold) in IC_{50} with addition of:		
		5 µM dThd[c]	100 µM hypoxanthine	dThd + hypoxanthine
CCRF-CEM	25	5.5	1.3	>1600
GC3/cl1	34	18.7	1.0	>1176
HCT-8	220	14.1	4.9	>182

[a]Adapted from [8, 11].
[b]Cytotoxicity determined by MTT analysis after 72-h exposure to drug.
[c]dThd, thymidine; MTT, 3-[4,5-dimethylthiazol-2yl]-2,5 diphenyl-tetrazolium bromide.

Alimta, and Alimta cytotoxicity was largely prevented by thymidine treatment [12].

These studies using antifolate-resistant cell lines to characterize mechanisms of resistance [11, 12] demonstrated that Alimta was less dependent than methotrexate and Tomudex on DHFR and TS as targets, respectively. In TS-amplified lines resulting from resistance due to either Tomudex, Alimta, or 5-FU exposure, the cells were >160-fold less resistant to Alimta compared to the selective TS inhibitor, raltitrexed. DHFR-amplified leukemia cells with methotrexate resistance were 8-fold less resistant to Alimta than to methotrexate.

The cytotoxic potency of Alimta and the mechanism of action in tumor cells appear to be determined by several factors, including relative levels of target enzymes, purine/pyrimidine salvage, and intracellular concentrations of Alimta and its polyglutamates. The extremely high collateral resistance of the Alimta-resistant lines to raltitrexed (>3200-fold) [11] coupled with the loss of thymidine protection, suggest that modulation of TS inhibition is one of the early responses involved in Alimta resistance. The data clearly suggest that enzymatic targets for Alimta antitumor activity can shift during development of antifolate resistance.

3 Folate enzyme inhibition studies

The inhibition of recombinant human (rh)TS, rhDHFR, and recombinant mouse (rm)GARFT by Alimta and its polyglutamates (glu_3 and glu_5) [8] is

Table 2.
Inhibitory activity of Alimta, methotrexate, Tomudex, and their polyglutamates against rhTS, rhDHFR, and rmGARFT (K_i [mean ± SE, nM]).[a]

Compound	rhTS	rhDHFR	rmGARFT
Alimta	109 ± 9	7.0 ± 1.9	9300 ± 690
Alimta-glu_3	1.6 ± 0.1	7.1 ± 1.6	380 ± 92
Alimta-glu_5	1.3 ± 0.3	7.2 ± 0.4	65 ± 16
Methotrexate	13 000	0.004	80 000
Methotrexate-glu_5	47	0.004	2500
Tomudex	6.0 ± 0.9	45 ± 3	424 000
Tomudex-glu_5	1.4 ± 0.1	30 ± 3	132 000

[a]Adapted from [8, 13].

summarized in Table 2). The parent monoglutamate Alimta inhibited rhTS with a K_i of 109 nM. Mammalian TS shows a strong preference for polyglutamated folate substrates, and the addition of two extra γ-glutamyl residues (glu_3) to Alimta resulted in 68-fold reduction of the K_i value (K_i = 1.6 nM). Further extension of the polyglutamate tail (Alimta-glu_5) only slightly increased activity (K_i = 1.3 nM). Alimta and its polyglutamates inhibited rhTS in a competitive fashion with respect to the natural substrate [6R]-5,10-methylenetetrahydrofolate [8]. In comparison, another TS inhibitor, Tomudex was less dependent on polyglutamation. A 5-fold increase in affinity was observed for Tomudex polyglutamates toward rhTS. Chabner and coworkers [13] reported that the pentaglutamate (Glu_5) of methotrexate also demonstrated a significant increase in affinity toward rhTS (K_i = 47 nM) when compared with the parent monoglutamate.

Alimta was also found to be a potent inhibitor of human DHFR (K_i = 7.0 nM). Tight binding analysis showed that Alimta inhibited rhDHFR in a competitive fashion [8]. In contrast to rhTS, attachment of additional γ-glutamyl residues to Alimta had little effect on the inhibition of DHFR. Likewise, polyglutamation of Tomudex and methotrexate did not significant enhance affinity to DHFR. In our hands, Tomudex and its polyglutamates also inhibited rhDHFR but were 6-fold less potent than Alimta.

Drug inhibition against folate-requiring enzymes along the purine *de novo* biosynthetic pathway was also studied. Alimta only moderately inhibited rmGARFT (K_i = 9.3 μM). The triglutamate and pentaglutamate of Alimta significantly enhanced inhibitory activity against GARFT, with K_i values of

380 nM (24-fold) and 65 nM (144-fold), respectively. In comparison, Tomudex, methotrexate and their polyglutamates showed extremely weak inhibitory activity against GARFT. The second folate-requiring enzyme along the purine *de novo* biosynthetic pathway is AICARFT, which uses the same folate cofactor as GARFT, 10-formyl-tetrahydrofolate, as the one carbon donor in purine biosynthesis. Like GARFT inhibition, Alimta polyglutamates produced a similar trend of enhancement of affinity toward hAICARFT. The K_i values were 3.58 μM, 480 nM (7.5-fold), and 265 nM (13.5-fold) for the mono-, tri-, and pentaglutamyl derivatives of Alimta, respectively [8].

4 Transport and polyglutamation

Membrane transport can occur through normal active folate physiological pathways. At least two distinct carrier-mediated active transport systems are responsible for the cellular uptake of antifolates [14, 15]. Cells differentially regulate specific transport systems as a function of their metabolic requirements [16]. One transport mechanism, termed the reduced folate carrier (RFC), is a low-affinity transporter of both methotrexate and reduced folates with affinity constants in the micromolar range. This system also transports the naturally occurring reduced folates, including the rescue agent leucovorin. Alimta has an affinity for RFC about twice that of methotrexate in human and murine leukemia cells [17].

A second transport mechanism utilizes a high-affinity, membrane-associated folate-binding protein called the folate receptor (FR) system. The system has affinity constants for reduced folates and folic acid in the nanomolar range and is expressed in normal tissues and, at high levels, on the surface of some epithelial tumors such as ovarian cancer [18, 19]. Alimta has an affinity for FR-α that is comparable to that of folic acid, its preferred substrate, and at least two orders of magnitude greater than that for methotrexate [17]. It is presently unclear, however, as to the relative contributions of these two transport mechanisms to the delivery of Alimta to cells and the role that RFC and FR-α play as determinants of cytotoxicity.

We studied the roles of the RFC and FR-α in the cytotoxic activity of Alimta using ZR-75-1 human breast carcinoma sublines that differ in expression of RFC and FR-α [20]. Wild-type ZR-75-1 cells express RFC as the major transport route for natural reduced folate cofactors and antifolate compounds, and do not express detectable levels of FR-α. The predominant role of RFC in transport of Alimta is illustrated by the fact that wild-type ZR-75 cells with or without transfected FR-α were much more sensitive to drug cytotoxicity than sublines resistant to methotrexate through decreased RFC expression [8]. However, cells deficient in both transport routes were still sensitive to Alimta (growth inhibitory IC_{50} of 430 nM). Other mechanisms for antifolate membrane transport are a focus of continued research. For example, Zhao and coworkers [21] demonstrated the selective preservation of Alimta pharmacological activity in HeLa cells lacking the reduced folate carrier.

Alimta has previously been demonstrated to be an exceptionally efficient substrate for folylpolyglutamate synthetase (FPGS) (K_m = 1.9 µmol/L compared to 116 µmol/L for methotrexate) [5, 9]. Studies with recombinant human FPGS (RG Moran, personal communication) indicate that Alimta is one of the most efficient substrates for the enzyme FPGS tested to date. To evaluate the role of FPGS in the cytotoxic activity of Alimta, we used CR15 cells, a lometrexol-resistant CCRF-CEM human leukemia subline. This subline has previously been shown to have a markedly diminished capacity for accumulating lometrexol polyglutamates, and has approximately 10% of the FPGS activity of wild-type cells [22]. Impaired polyglutamation in CR15 cells was identified as the mechanism of resistance to the GARFT inhibitor, lometrexol. We observed that CR15 cells were markedly cross-resistant to Alimta [8], suggesting that polyglutamation is a major determinant of cytotoxicity. The addition of a polyglutamate tail to the folate or antifolate molecule by the enzyme FPGS serves three main purposes [23–25]: it facilitates the accumulation of intracellular reduced folates in excess of the monoglutamate pool that are freely transportable into and out of cells; it allows selective intracellular retention of these relatively large anionic molecules, and thus prolongs intracellular half-life; and it enhances folate cofactor affinity for several folate-dependent enzymes. As previously discussed, the pentaglutamate of Alimta is approximately 100-fold more potent than the parent compound for TS and GARFT (Tab. 2).

The sequence of events following the addition of Alimta to cells is (a) a rapid build-up of polyglutamates resulting in suppression of TS and cessation of the oxidation of 5,10-CH_2-tetrahydrofolate to DHF, so that DHF levels remain low; and (b) a continued build-up of Alimta polyglutamates in excess of the GARFT K_i resulting in suppression of GARFT and inhibition of purine synthesis [26, 27]. In this regard, cell culture experiments have demonstrated that the intracellular drug concentration of Alimta can reach levels of 50 µM in CCRF-CEM cells after 16-h exposure to 2 µM [^{14}C]Alimta (R. M. Schultz, unpublished observation). Similarly, treatment of CCRF-CEM cells for 24 h with 1 µM [^{3}H]Alimta produced an intracellular drug concentration of 41 µM. The penta- and hexaglutamated Alimta have been identified to be the major intracellular active forms [28]. These high intracellular drug concentrations of polyglutamated metabolites are sufficient to inhibit several folate-requiring enzymes, including potentially even C1 tetrahydrofolate synthase [8].

5 Resistance studies

Resistance to chemotherapeutic agents has proved to be a major barrier in the clinical management of neoplastic disease. The most common biochemical alterations associated with inherent and acquired resistance to classical antifolates are (a) elevated levels of the target enzymes (e.g., TS and DHFR), (b) decreased carrier-mediated membrane transport secondary to RFC and FR-α protein, (c) decreased binding affinity of the antifolate to its target enzyme from point mutations, and (d) decreased polyglutamation.

There have been several reports that induction of resistance to Alimta is associated with TS overexpression [11, 12, 29, 30]. It is interesting that resistant cells with TS overexpression had lower levels of resistance to Alimta than to the more selective TS inhibitor, Tomudex (Tab. 3) [11, 12]. This was the case whether resistance was induced by incremental exposure to Alimta, Tomudex, or 5-fluorouracil (FU) [11, 31, 32]. The lower resistance to Alimta was possibly due to Alimta's ability to inhibit several folate-dependent reactions. By analyzing end-product reversal patterns, Schultz hypothesized that Alimta has a unique ability to shift target enzymes through development of resistance [12]. In TS-amplified lines, hypoxanthine supplementation reversed Alimta-induced growth inhibition, but thymidine did not, indicating that GARFT inhibition is the mechanism underlying the cytotoxic effects [11, 12]. Freemantle and colleagues [33] demonstrated that small changes in TS levels may translate into clinically significant alterations in drug sensitivity. In a heterogeneous nonselected human colon carcinoma cell line panel of 13 lines, the best predictor for sensitivity to 5-FU was TS activity, but multiple sensitivity determinants were of importance for antifolate TS inhibitors, including FPGS activity and TS enzyme kinetics [34]. Sensitivity to Alimta did not correlate with TS, FPGS or reduced folate carrier activity, or methotrexate

Table 3.
Cytotoxic activity of Alimta, methotrexate (MTX), and Tomudex (TDX) against resistant human cell lines.[a]

Cell line[b]	Mechanism	Resistance factor[c]		
		Alimta	Tomudex	Methotrexate
MCF-7_{TDX}	↑ TS	89	16 917	NT[d]
H630R$10_{5\text{-}FU}$	↑ TS	5	6434	NT
GC3_{Alimta}	↑ TS	140	23 503	31
CCRF-CEM-R_{MTX}	↑ DHFR	53	3	437
CCRF-CEM_{Alimta}	↓ accumulation	729	7252	1
HCT-8_{Alimta}	↓ accumulation	117	3571	1
CCRF-CEM-T_{MTX}	↓ RFC transport	90	315	690
ZR-75-1_{MTX}	↓ RFC transport	4	64	NT

[a]Adapted from [11, 12].
[b]Subscript denotes agent that resistance was developed against.
[c]Resistance factor is calculated as IC_{50} resistance cells/IC_{50} sensitive cells (where IC_{50} is the concentration of drug required to inhibit cell growth by 50%).
[d]NT, not tested.

accumulation. It is likely that a combination of many factors, rather than a single factor, determines sensitivity to Alimta. Pestalozzi and coworkers [35] demonstrated that increased TS protein levels are principally associated with proliferation but not cell cycle phase in asynchronous human cancer cells.

Several investigators have demonstrated that loss of FPGS activity can be a dominant mechanism of resistance to polyglutamylation-dependent antifolates, including Alimta in several human tumor cell lines [36–39]. As previously discussed, the inhibitory activity of Alimta for TS and GARFT is increased approximately 100-fold by polyglutamation. We observed that CR15, a lometrexol-resistant CCRF-CEM subline with approximately 10% of the FPGS activity of wild-type cells [22], were markedly cross-resistant to Alimta (growth inhibitory IC_{50} >200 μM *versus* 25 nM in wild-type cells) [8].

Decreased drug accumulation in cells is another important acquired resistance mechanism for Alimta. In CCRF-CEM and HCT-8 cells, which were Alimta resistant owing to a decrease of more than 90% in drug accumulation, the cells were much more resistant to Tomudex than Alimta, and only thymidine and hypoxanthine supplementation together could modulate the cytotoxicity of Alimta [11]. This end-product reversal pattern is reminiscent of that seen with DHFR inhibitors. Biochemically, reduced drug accumulation could result from an alteration in the membrane-associated drug carrier, reduced cellular polyglutamation or both. Among the three major, potential enzyme targets of Alimta, both TS and GARFT show preference for the higher polyglutamate forms of the drug. However, DHFR is insensitive to the extent of polyglutamation. Thus, reduced polyglutamation might have led to poor drug retention in the cells and low drug accumulation. However, the concentration of drug that accumulated appeared to be high enough to inhibit DHFR, but not sufficiently polyglutamated to inhibit TS and GARFT, leading to a shift in the metabolic protection profile. Tomudex-resistant L1210 murine leukemia and 41M human ovarian carcinoma cells that have decreased drug accumulation due to reduced FPGS and/or reduced folate carrier expression were also less resistant to Alimta than to Tomudex [31]. This suggests that Alimta is less sensitive than Tomudex to decreased drug accumulation. It is noteworthy that in most resistant lines (either secondary to effects on target enzyme or drug accumulation), the degree of resistance is less for Alimta than for other antifolate compounds such as methotrexate and especially Tomudex.

In addition to downregulation of FPGS, the accumulation of polyglutamated antifolates can be limited by overexpression of glutamyl hydrolase, the enzyme that removes glutamate residues from polyglutamated metabolites. Alimta poly-γ-glutamates are effective substrates for glutamyl hydrolase and their pharmacological effectiveness bears an inverse relationship to cellular glutamyl hydrolase activity [40]. In the H35D rat hepatoma cell line with increased glutamyl hydrolase activity due to acquired drug resistance, the cells had an 80–90% reduction in Alimta polyglutamate accumulation and were 55-fold more resistant to Alimta than antifolate-naive cells.

We also tested the cytotoxic activity of Alimta in a methotrexate-resistant CCRF-CEM leukemia line with 18-fold DHFR amplification [12]. This line demonstrated collateral (54-fold) resistance to Alimta, but was 8-fold less resistant to Alimta than methotrexate. Alimta cytotoxicity was largely overcome by thymidine addition. The cytotoxic potency of Alimta and the mechanism of action in tumor cells appear to be determined by several factors, including relative levels of target enzymes, purine/pyrimidine salvage, and intracellular concentrations of Alimta and its polyglutamates.

In general, the Alimta IC_{50} values of the resistant cells studied were <10 μM, which is much less than the plasma C_{max} (about 160 μM) attainable in patients receiving Alimta at the proposed clinical dose of 500 mg/m^2.

Thus, Alimta may be useful in tumors resistant to other antifolates. This lower resistance to Alimta compared to other antifolates supports the hypothesis that Alimta can inhibit multiple folate-dependent reactions.

6 Antithymine *versus* antipurine effects

The cell cycle is a tightly controlled progression through the four phases of cell division: G_1, S (DNA synthesis), G_2, and M (mitosis) phases. Various stresses, such as DNA damage, can initiate a signal transduction pathway involving the tumor-suppressor genes P53 and RB, which arrests the cells at the G_1/S phase boundary. Using DNA flow cytometric techniques, Tonkinson and coworkers [41] demonstrated that relatively pure inhibitors of TS and inhibitors of GARFT produce distinct cell cycle alterations. They examined cell cycle-related events in CCRF-CEM leukemia cells subsequent to inhibition of TS with Tomudex or to inhibition of GARFT with 6R-5,10-dideazatetrahydrofolate (lometrexol). Cell populations treated for up to 96 h with lometrexol did not replicate, and maintained a cell cycle distribution with distinct G_1, S and G_2/M regions. The number of S-phase cells in treated populations was slightly elevated relative to controls, as measured by DNA content and proliferating cell nuclear antigen (PCNA). However, these cells were unable to incorporate 5-bromodeoxyuridine (BrdU). Throughout treatment, cells incubated with GARFT inhibitors maintained intact membranes and respired at a level comparable to untreated cells. In contrast, cells treated with the TS inhibitor, Tomudex as well as Alimta, induced synchronization of the treated population at the G_1/S interface within 12 h of drug addition. This was followed by synchronous entry of the population into S phase. After 24 h of treatment, more than 90% of the cells were capable of incorporating BrdU and stained positive for PCNA. DNA fragmentation and cell death occurred in cells treated with Tomudex or Alimta after 36 h of exposure, indicative of apoptosis, but not in those treated with GARFT inhibitors.

Smith and coworkers [42] compared the cytotoxicity of lometrexol and Tomudex in human WiDr colonic carcinoma cells. Tomudex was highly cytotoxic (>3 logs of cell kill) after a 4-h exposure to 1 μM drug, or a 24-h exposure to very low concentrations (40 nM). On the other hand, the cytotoxicity of lometrexol was substantially lower, with 2 logs of cell kill requiring >100 μM for 4 h or 40 μM for 72 h of drug exposure. Maximal cell kill induced by Tomudex was 5–6 logs, consistent with elimination of all viable cells except preexisting mutants. A maximum of 2–3 logs of cell death was observed with lometrexol. The morphologies of the cells treated with the two drugs were markedly different. Tomudex-treated cells detached from the dish within 1–2 days, whereas lometrexol-treated cells remained adherent to the dishes for at least 10 days of treatment. The addition of thymidine to Tomudex-treated cultures or hypoxanthine to lometrexol-treated cells after up to 20 h of drug exposure completely prevented cytotoxicity of either drug. However, the cytotoxicity of both drugs progressively increased with longer exposures in spite of such rescue. These results indicate that the rate of commitment to cell death and the extent of cell kill was greater with a pure inhibitor of TS. The cells could withstand inhibition of the supply of thymidylate or of newly synthesized purines for 20–24 h without effect, but longer periods of interruption of either pathway commits cells to death.

VanTriest and coworkers [43] studied the downstream molecular determinants of response to 5-FU and antifolate TS inhibitors. The precise mechanism by which TS inhibition leads to cell death is still not completely resolved. TS inhibition results in depletion of 2′-deoxythymidine-5′-triphosphate (dTTP), an essential precursor for DNA, and an increase in 2′-deoxyuridine-5′-triphosphate (dUTP). This leads to the so-called "thymine-less death" due to misincorporation of dUTP into DNA: its excision, catalyzed by uracil-DNA glycosylase, results in DNA damage. Both this imbalance in dTTP/dUTP and DNA damage can result in induction of downstream events, leading to apoptosis. On the other hand, a specific interaction exists between oncogenes and TS, by binding of TS protein to p53 and c-myc RNA, while wild-type p53 can also inhibit TS promoter activity. TS inhibition by either 5-FU or antifolates can also result in a depression of TS protein-mediated inhibition of TS mRNA translation, leading to induction of more TS protein synthesis, and p53 protein may further deregulate this process. These authors further postulated a combined prognostic role for TS and p53 in the clinical response to TS inhibitors.

The action of Alimta against both purine and thymidylate synthesis pathways has complicated interpretation of the contribution of each pathway to the cytotoxicity of Alimta. In this regard, there have been suggestions that inhibition of purine synthesis by methotrexate may limit the cytotoxicity caused by its inhibition of TS [44, 45]. The classic studies by Borsa and Whitmore [44] led to the conclusion that the cytotoxicity of methotrexate to L-cells resulted from inhibition of TS, and that the concurrent inhibition of purine synthesis tended to prevent efficient cell killing. Conceptually, this effect has been attributed to accumulation of cells in G_1 as a result of inhibition of RNA synthesis. As a result of such inhibition of cell cycle progression, the entry of methotrexate-treated cells into S phase is thought to be limited by inhibition of RNA synthesis, with a resultant decrease in the efficiency of "thymine-less death" [44, 46]. A source of purines increased cell kill by methotrexate in these studies. Houghton and coworkers [47] proposed that wild-type p53 caused cell cycle arrest in thymine-less conditions, and thus protected cells. Fisher et al. [48] examined the relation of apoptosis, triggered by treatment with TS inhibitors, to expression of bcl-2, and found that bcl-2 expression protected cells from cytotoxicity induced by TS inhibitors.

Other investigators have demonstrated synergistic cytotoxicity when an inhibitor of DHFR is combined with an antifolate inhibitor of TS or with an antifolate inhibitor of GARFT [49, 50]. Kisliuk and coworkers [49] demonstrated that these synergistic interactions are dependent on medium folic acid concentration, and are greatly enhanced by increasing folic acid levels. Synergism was seen only when the TS or GARFT inhibitor is polyglutamylable. Faessel et al. [50] presented evidence that the ideal requirement for folic acid-enhanced synergy is that a nonpolgluamylatable DHFR inhibitor be combined with a polyglutamylatable inhibitor of another folate-requiring enzyme. It is not known whether this effect can be utilized for enhanced antitumor efficacy *in vivo*. However, a favorable interaction has been observed between methotrexate and lometrexol on survival of mice bearing L1210 tumors [51].

7 *In vivo* antitumor action

Thymidine can reverse the activity of TS inhibitors *in vitro* and *in vivo* [8, 52–55]. Although thymidine levels in the plasma compartment in humans are quite low, and thus not likely to attenuate TS inhibition, substantial levels of thymidine are found in mouse plasma (approximately 1 µM [56]), which are high enough for *in vitro* reversal of the growth-inhibitory effects of TS inhibitors. High circulating thymidine levels in rodents complicate the assessment of both antitumor activity and toxicity associated with TS inhibitors. Thymidine salvage involves the enzyme thymidine kinase (TK), which phosphorylates the nucleoside to produce thymidine monophosphate, which is then further phosphorylated to the triphosphate for incorporation into DNA. A high TK activity may provide enough thymidine nucleotides to bypass DNA synthesis inhibition resulting from TS inhibition.

To overcome the salvage problem that complicates antitumor efficacy studies in mice, a TK-deficient mutant of the human GC3 colon carcinoma (provided by Janet Houghton [57]) was used to evaluate *in vivo* antitumor activity [58]. Thymidine at physiological levels in mouse plasma (approximately 1 µM) produced only a 2.6-fold shift in the IC_{50} for Alimta-mediated cytotoxicity in TK-proficient GC3/c11 cellscompared to a 128-fold shift for Tomudex. Alimta treatment (i.p., q.d. × 10) significantly delayed tumor growth in the GC3 carcinoma xenograft model. However, the TK-deficient mutant of this same tumor line demonstrated heightened sensitivity to the *in vivo* antitumor activity of Alimta with complete regression of established tumors and a large number of tumor-free survivors after one course of treatment. These data demonstrate that inhibition of TS is a prominent mechanism for antitumor activity by Alimta, but important secondary sites of action exist for this multitargeted molecule. Another TK-deficient tumor, L5178Y/TK-/HX- murine lymphoma, in contrast to wild-type L5178Y-S cells, was also exquisitely sensitive to the antitumor activity of Alimta [59]. The role of thymidine salvage in this antitumor activity was complicated by the additional deficiency in hypoxanthine phosphoribosyl transferase, which makes this tumor incapable of salvage of the purines hypoxanthine and guanine. We also noted a 2.6-fold increase in the growth inhibitory IC_{50} for Alimta at 1 µM thymidine with TK-proficient L5178Y/S cells. It is interesting that such a modest 2.6-fold difference in the IC_{50}s of Alimta under physiological mouse thymidine plasma conditions translates into such a major difference in the *in vivo* antitumor activity between TK-proficient and TK-deficient tumors.

Alimta administered as a single course [i.p. daily for 10 days at maximally tolerated doses (300 and 100 mg/kg/dose, respectively)] in two TK-competent models (GC3 colon carcinoma xenograft and L5178Y/S murine lymphoma) showed significant inhibition of tumor growth at the initial tumor measurement taken shortly after completion of therapy, but after a few days delay, the tumors resumed growth [58, 59]. Significant antitumor activity was also observed in VRC5 human colon carcinoma, BXPC3 human pancreatic carcinoma, LX-1 human lung carcinoma and MX-1 human breast carcinoma (60–78% tumor inhibition). The requirement for prolonged treatment protocols for TS inhibitors in the mouse may be related to the requirement for plasma thymidine levels to fall to a level that does not compromise inhibition of TS [53]. However, it is pertinent to point out that plasma thymidine levels in man are lower (approximately 0.1–0.2 μM) and are not likely to limit the efficacy of Alimta in humans [60].

8 Combination effects

Alimta has been investigated with a variety of other conventional anticancer agents for tumor cytotoxicity in human cancer cell lines. Scheduling of drugs in combination studies appears to be very important, since many of these studies have demonstrated sequence dependency for optimal antitumor activity. For example, Schultz and coworkers [61] combined Alimta with doxorubicin in ZR-75-1 human breast carcinoma cells. Preincubation with Alimta for 24 h followed by exposure to doxorubicin for 72 h resulted in highly synergistic activity, whereas the opposite sequence or simultaneous exposure produced mainly an additive response. DNA flow cytometry studies indicated that Alimta causes a build-up of cells near the G_1/S interface after 24 h of incubation in ZR-75-1 cells. A similar sequence dependency has been demonstrated with combinations of Alimta with taxol or taxotere. When Alimta preceded taxane treatment by 24 h, marked synergy was observed in NCI-H23 and NCI-H460 non-small cell lung cancer cells [62].

Several investigators have tested combinations of Alimta with Gemcitabine. Tonkinson and associates [63] provided *in vitro* and *in vivo* data that the cytotoxicity of gemcitabine for HT29 human colon carcinoma cells was increased by 2- to 7-fold when Alimta was administered 24 h before gemcitabine. No increase in potency or cell kill was observed when the two compounds were added simultaneously. These investigators hypothesized that pretreatment of cells with Alimta would increase the potency of gemcitabine by synchronizing the population for DNA synthesis. The sequence dependency was also evaluated *in vivo* in HT29 colon carcinoma xenografts. Again, the tumor growth delay was greatest when Alimta was administered before gemcitabine, compared with simultaneous drug administration or the reverse sequence. However, another report demonstrated synergistic cytotoxicity for the opposite sequence of drug exposure in HCT-8 human colon carcinoma [64, 65]. We have recently evaluated combinations of Alimta and gemcitabine in GC3 TK- and HCT-116 human colon carcinoma cells. In these cell lines, the simultaneous addition of both drugs produced profound antagonism (R. M. Schultz, unpublished observations). However, when Alimta was administered 24 h prior to gemcitabine (or the reverse order), the response ranged from modest antagonism to additivity. Tesei and coworkers [66] also demonstrated that the concurrent addition of both drugs gave antagonistic results in LRWZ and WiDr, but additive effects in LOVO colon carcinoma cells. However, sequential treatment gave additive-to-synergistic effects in the three cell lines, with the sequence of gemcitabine preceding Alimta being preferred.

Combinations of Alimta and platinum analogs have also been evaluated. Interactions of Alimta with cisplatin in MSTO-211H human mesothelioma cells have been demonstrated to be synergistic and sequence independent, although there was a slight preference for simultaneous treatment [67]. DNA flow cytometry studies indicated that Alimta induces a build-up of cells starting at the G_1/S interface preceding into S-phase at 24 h of incubation and apoptosis within 48 h. Synergistic growth inhibitory activity was observed with low concentrations of cisplatin in cultures that were devoid of cell cycle and apoptotic activity. Carboplatin and cisplatin were also evaluated with Alimta in NCI-H460 non-small cell lung carcinoma, SKOV-3 ovarian carcinoma and HT29 colon carcinoma cells [62, 68]. The interaction was additive in these cell lines regardless of the sequence of drug administration.

The triple combination of Alimta, oxaliplatin, and gemcitabine was studied in three colorectal cell lines, LOVO, HT290, and COLO 320DM [69]. The drug effects were evaluated with respect to the rate of drug-induced apoptosis as determined by spectrophotometry. In this study, the activity of oxaliplatin alone was found to greatly exceed that of Alimta or gemcitabine alone. The disparity in activity between the compounds made it impossible to obtain meaningful results in the combinations when oxaliplatin was added prior to the other compounds. Of the remaining combinations, the highest apoptotic responses were observed with the sequence in which Alimta and gemcitabine were administered either individually or concurrently for either 6 or 24 h prior to oxaliplatin.

Van der Wilt and associates [70] tested the effects of combining Alimta and 5-FU in colorectal carcinoma cells. They reported that this combination is additive regardless of the sequence of drug addition in LS174T cells, but antagonistic in WiDr cells.

9 Role of folic acid in modulating toxicity

Folate depletion has been demonstrated to increase the sensitivity of solid tumor cell lines to antifolates [15, 71]. The mechanism by which natural folates protect cells *in vitro* from the toxic effects of antifolates is generally believed to be the result of competition at the levels of transport into the cell, polyglutamation, or target inhibition, either independently or in combination [72]. The very complexity of the processes involved suggests ways in which the antifolates could be tuned to have a selective advantage against tumors compared with normal tissues [73]. Protection from toxicities without impairment of drug efficacy suggests a differential response to the folate/drug combination between tumor cells and normal cells such that the outcome favors the survival of normal cells [74]. To evaluate the importance of dietary folate in modulating the toxicity of Alimta, LD_{50} values were determined in mice maintained on standard diet or on a special low-folate diet (LFD) [59, 75]. Alimta was administered i.p. daily for 10 days. It was estimated that mice on LFD consumed an average of 0.003 mg/kg/day of folic acid *versus* 0.75–1.5 mg/kg/day for mice on standard diet. Thus, mice on standard diet had a daily intake of approximately 250–500 times more folic acid than mice on LFD. Alimta was much more toxic in several strains of mice maintained on LFD, with the LD_{50} values being 30- to 250-fold lower than mice on standard diet. The therapeutic index of Alimta against the L5178Y/TK-/HX- tumor was greatly diminished when the mice were placed on LFD for 2 weeks prior to tumor implantation with no folate supplementation. For these mice on LFD, Alimta at 0.3 and 1 mg/kg (q.d. x 10, i.p.) produced 100% inhibition of L5178Y/TK-/HX- lymphoma growth, and significant lethality occurred at =3 mg/kg. For mice on standard diet, Alimta produced >95% inhibition of lymphoma growth over a broader dose range (30–300 mg/kg), but all mice died when given 800 mg/kg. In the L5178Y/TK-/HX- model, folic acid supplementation was demonstrated to preserve the antitumor activity of Alimta in mice on LFD, while reducing toxicity. Since circulating folate levels in humans closely resemble those of mice on LFD [76, 77], it was suggested that folate supplementation could increase the antitumor effects of Alimta in patients and reduce the risk of toxic side effects.

10 Conclusion

The early clinical development of Alimta has been the subject of several reviews over the last few years [74, 78–88]. In this chapter, I have attempted to review the preclinical data that led to the clinical development of this novel antifolate. Although it primarily acts against TS, several lines of evidence demonstrate that Alimta may act as a multitargeted antifolate with additional targets, including GARFT, DHFR and AICARFT. These include: (a) the cytotoxicity reversal pattern for Alimta in a variety of human cancer cell lines, including colon carcinoma, breast carcinoma, and leukemia, which demonstrates that, although TS may be a major site of action for Alimta at concentrations near the IC_{50}, higher concentrations can lead to inhibition of DHFR and/or other enzymes along the purine pathway [6-8, 11]; (b) Alimta being an excellent substrate for FPGS, with K_i values for the pentaglutamate of Alimta of 1.3, 7.2, 65 and 265 nM for inhibition of TS, DHFR, GARFT, and AICARFT, respectively [8]; (c) that intracellular concentrations of Alimta and its polyglutamates can reach 50 µM in leukemia cells; (d) that Alimta produces distinctive effects on intracellular nucleotide levels that are different from those of Tomudex, methotrexate, and a selective GARFT inhibitor, LY309887 [89]; and (e) that the profile of metabolic protection against the growth inhibitory effects of Alimta changed in resistant populations [11, 12].

These changes in conditions for end-product reversal of cytotoxicity were quite dramatic [11]. In cells that were deficient in drug accumulation, thymidine alone became ineffective at reducing cytotoxicity. Instead, the prevention of Alimta-induced cytotoxicity was only accomplished by the combination of thymidine and hypoxanthine. This observation suggested that the biochemical changes in resistant cells resulted in Alimta shifting its main target from TS to DHFR. In cell lines with TS amplification, hypoxanthine alone was observed to protect cells from Alimta cytotoxicity, suggesting that GARFT inhibition had become the primary cytotoxic locus. In cells with DHFR amplification, Alimta cytotoxicity was generally prevented by thymidine alone without any need for hypoxanthine [12]. These secondary targets that emerge during development of Alimta resistance may have very important clinical implications.

High circulating thymidine levels in rodents complicate the assessment of both antitumor activity and toxicity associated with TS inhibitors. Alimta demonstrated good *in vivo* antitumor activity in various preclinical tumor models and potent activity in TK-deficient models. These models suggest that TS is probably the first rate-limiting step in the initial exposure of tumor cells to Alimta. This is exemplified by the ability of thymidine to completely protect cells at drug concentrations near the IC_{50}, and by the large difference in antitumor activity between TK-proficient and -deficient models [58]. Other studies have suggested the potential to reduce toxic effects and increase the therapeutic index of Alimta by folate supplementation [75]. Based on these observations and clinical toxicities, folic acid and vitamin B_{12} dietary supplementation have been introduced into Alimta clinical trials [90]. Further biochemical and mechanistic studies are needed to better characterize the multi-targeted nature of Alimta action.

References

1 Jackson RC (1984) Biological effects of folic acid antagonists with antineoplastic activity. *Pharmacol Ther* 25: 61–82

2 Allegra CJ (1990) Antifolates. In: BA Chabner, JM Collins (eds): Cancer chemotherapy: principles and practice. JB Lippincott, New York, 110

3 Schultz RM (1995) Newer antifolates in cancer therapy. In: E Jucker (ed): *Progress in Drug Research, Vol. 44*. Birkhauser Verlag, Basel, 129–157

4 Grindey GB, Shih C, Barnett CJ, Pearce HL, Engelhardt JA, Todd GC, Rinzel SM, Worzalla JF, Gossett LS, Everson TP et al (1992) LY231514, a novel pyrrolopyrimidine antifolate that inhibits thymidylate synthase (TS). *Proc Am Assoc Cancer Res* 33: 411

5 Taylor EC, Kuhnt D, Shih C, Rinzel SM, Grindey GB, Barredo J, Jannatipour M, Moran RG (1992) A dideazatetrahydrofolate analogue lacking a chiral center at C-6, N-[4-[2-(2-amino-3,4-dihydryo-4-oxo-7H-pyrrolo[2,3-d]pyrimidin-5-yl)ethyl]-benzoyl]-L-glutamic acid, is an inhibitor of thymidylate synthase. *J Med Chem* 35: 4450–4454

6 Schultz RM, Andis SL, Bewley JR, Chen VJ, Habeck LL, Mendelsohn LG, Patel VF, Rutherford PG, Self TD, Shih C et al (1996) Antitumor activity of the multitargeted antifolate LY231514. *Proc Am Assoc Cancer Res* 37: 380

7 Schultz RM, Andis S, Chen V, Mendelsohn L, Patel V, Shih C, Houghton J (1996) Comparative antitumor activity of the multitargeted antifolate LY231514 and the thymidylate synthase (TS) inhibitor ZD1694. *NCI EORTC Symp New Drugs Cancer Ther,* abstr 290

8 Shih C, Chen VJ, Gossett LS, Gates SB, MacKellar WC, Habeck LL, Shackelford KA, Mendelsohn LG, Soose DJ, Patel VF et al (1997) LY231514, a pyrrolo [2,3-d]pyrimidine-based antifolate that inhibits multiple folate-requiring enzymes. *Cancer Res* 57: 1116–1123

9 Habeck LL, Shih C, Gossett LS, Leitner TA, Schultz RM, Andis SL, Moran RG, Mendelsohn LG (1995) Substrate specificity of mammalian folylpolyglutamate synthetase for 5,10-dideazatetrahydrofolate analogs. *Mol Pharmacol* 48: 326–333

10 Touroutogolou N, Pazdur R (1996) Thymidylate synthase inhibitors. *Clin Cancer Res* 2: 227–243

11 Schultz RM, Chen VJ, Bewley JR, Roberts EF, Shih C, Dempsey JA (1999) Biological activity of the multitargeted antifolate, MTA (LY231514), in human cell lines with different resistance mechanisms to antifolate drugs. *Semin Oncol* 26, suppl 6: 68–73

12 Schultz RM, Chen VJ, Bertino JR (1999) The multitargeted antifolate: Shifting enzymatic targets during development of antifolate resistance. *Abstracts of the AACR-NCI-EORTC Internation Conference on Molecular Targets of Cancer Therapy* (November 16–19, Washington). Abst 654

13 Chabner BA, Allegra CJ, Curt GA, Clendeninn NJ, Baram J, Koizumi S, Drake JC, Jolivet J (1985) Polyglutamation of methotrexate: Is methotrexate a prodrug? *J Clin Invest* 76: 907–912

14 Matherly LH (2001) Molecular and cellular biology of the human reduced folate carrier. *Prog Nucleic Acid Res Mol Biol* 67: 131–162

15 Schultz RM, Andis SL, Shackelford KA, Gates SB, Ratnam M, Mendelsohn LG, Shih C, Grindey GB (1995) Role of membrane-associated folate binding protein in the cytotoxicity of antifolates in KB, IGROV1, and L1210A cells. *Oncol Res* 7: 97–102

16 Kamen BA, Capdevila A (1986) Receptor-mediated folate accumulation is regulated by the cellular folate content. *Proc Natl Acad Sci USA* 83: 5983–5987

17 Westerhof GR, Schornagel JH, Kathmann I, Jackman AL, Rosowsky A, Forsch RA, Hynes JB, Boyle FT, Peters GJ, Pinedo HM, Jansen G (1995) Carrier- and receptor-mediated transport of folae antagonists targeting folate-dependent enzymes: Correlates of molecular structure and biological activity. *Mol Pharmacol* 48: 459–471

18 Antony AC (1992) The biological chemistry of folate receptors. *Blood* 79: 2807–2820

19 Coney LR, Tomassetti A, Carayannopoulos L, Frasca V, Kamen BA, Colnaghi MI, Zurawski VR (1991) Cloning of a tumor-associated antigen: MOv8 and MOv19 antibodies recognize a folate-binding protein. *Cancer Res* 51: 6125–6132

20 Dixon KH, Mulligan T, Chung KN, Elwood PC, Cowan KH (1992) Effects of folate receptor expression following stable transfection into wild type and methotrexate transport-deficient ZR-75-1 human breast cancer cells. *J Biol Chem* 26: 24140–24147

21 Zhao R, Hanscom M, Chattopadhyay S, Goldman ID (2004) Selective preservation of pemetrexed pharmacological activity in HeLa cells lacking the reduced folate carrier: Association with the presence of a secondary transport pathway. *Cancer Res* 64: 3313–3319

22 Pizzorno G, Moroson BA, Cashmore AR, Russelo O, Mayer JR. Galivan J, Bunni MA, Priest DG, Beardsley GP (1995) Multifactorial resistance to 5,10-dideazatetrahydrofolic acid in cell lines derived from human lymphoblastic leukemia CCRF-CEM. *Cancer Res* 55: 566–573

23 Shane B (1989) Folylpolyglutamate synthesis and role in the regulation of one-carbon metabolism. *Vitam Horm* 45: 263–335

24 Sun X, Cross JA, Bognar AL (2001) Folate-binding triggers the activation of folylpolyglutamate synthetase. *J Mol Biol* 310: 1067–1078

25 Purcell WT, Ettinger DS (2003) Novel antifolate drugs. *Curr Oncol Rep* 5: 114–125

26 Goldman ID, Zhao R (2002) Molecular, biochemical, and cellular pharmacology of pemetrexed. *Semin Oncol* 29, suppl 18: 3–17

27 Chen VJ, Bewley JR, Smith PG, Andis SL, Schultz RM, Iversen PW, Tonkinson JL, Shih C (2000) An assessment of the antithymine and antipurine characteristics of MTA (LY231514) in CCRF-CEM cells. *Adv Enzyme Regul* 40: 143–154

28 Rhee MS, Ryan TJ, Gallivan J (1999) Glutamyl hydrolase and the multitargeted antifolate LY231514. *Cancer Chemother Pharmacol* 44: 427–432

29 Sigmond J, Backus, HHJ, Wouters D, Temmink OH, Jansen G, Peters GJ (2003) Induction of resistance to the multitargeted antifolate Pemetrexed (ALIMTA) in WiDr human colon cancer cells is associated with thymidylate synthase overexpression. *Biochem Pharmacol* 66: 431–438

30 Schultz RM, Bewley JR, Dempsey JA, Roberts EF, Shih C, Chen VJ (1998) Mechanisms of acquired resistance to the multitargeted antifolate (MTA, LY231514) in human leukemia and colon carcinoma cell lines continuously exposed to stepwise increasing drug concentrations. *Ann Oncol* 9, suppl 2: 587

31 Jackman AL, Kelland LR, Kimbell R, Brown M, Gibson W, Aherne GW, Hardcastle A, Boyle FT (1995) Mechanisms of acquired resistance to the quinazoline thymidylate synthase inhibitor ZD1694 (Tomudex) in one mouse and three human cell lines. *Br J Cancer* 71: 914–924

32 Curtin NJ, Hughes AN (2001) Pemetrexed disodium, a novel antifolate with multiple targets. *Lancet Oncol* 2: 298–306

33 Freemantle SJ, Jackman AL, Kelland LR, Calvert AH, Lunec J (1995) Molecular characterization of two cell lines selected for resistance to the folate-based thymidylate synthase inhibitor, ZD1694. *Br J Cancer* 71: 925–930

34 van Triest B, Pinedo HM, van Hensbergen Y, Smid K, Telleman F, Schoenmakers PS, van der Wilt CL, van Laar JAM, Noordhuis P, Jansen G et al (1999) Thymidylate synthase level as the main predictive parameter for sensitivity to 5-fluorouracil, but not for folate-based thymidylate synthase inhibitors, in 13 nonselected colon cancer cell lines. *Clin Cancer Res* 5: 643–654

35 Pestalozzi BC, McGinn CJ, Kinsella TJ, Drake JC, Glennon MC, Allegra CJ , Johnston PG (1995) Increase thymidylate synthase protein levels are principally associated with proliferation but not cell cycle phase in asynchronous human cancer cells. *Br J Cancer* 71: 1151–1157

36 Liani E, Rothem L, Bunni MA, Smith CA, Jansen G, Assaraf YG (2003) Loss of folylopoly-γ-glutamate synthetase activity is a dominant mechanism of resistance to polyglutamylation-dependent novel antifolates in multiple human leukemia sublines. *Int J Cancer* 103: 487–599

37 Lu K, Yin M-B, McGuire JJ, Bonmassar E, Rustum YM (1995) Mechanisms of resistance to N-[5-[n-(3,4-dihydro-2-methyl-4-oxoquinazolin-6-ylmethyl)-N-methylamino]-2-thenoyl]-L-glutamic acid (ZD1694), a folate-based thymidylate synthase inhibitor, in the HCT-8 human ileocecal adenocarcinoma cell line. *Biochem Pharmacol* 50: 391–398

38 Wang Y, Zhao R, Goldman ID (2003) Decreased expression of the reduced folate carrier and folylpolyglutamate synthetase is the basis for acquired resistance to the pemetrexed antifolate (LY231514) in an L1210 murine leukemia cell line. *Biochem Pharmacol* 65: 1163–1170

39 Takemura Y, Kobayashi H, Gibson W, Kimbell R, Miyachi H, Jackman AL (1996) The influence of drug-exposure conditions on the development of resistance to methotrexate or ZD1694 in cultured human leukaemia cells. *Int J Cancer* 66: 29–36

40 Rhee MS, Ryan TJ, Gallivan J (1999) Glutamy hydrolase and the multitargeted antifolate LY231514. *Cancer Chemother Pharmacol* 44: 427–432
41 Tonkinson JL, Marder P, Andis SL, Schultz RM, Gossett LS, Shih C, Mendelsohn LG (1997) Cell cycle effects of antifolate antimetabolites: implications for cytotoxicity and cytostasis. *Cancer Chemother Pharmacol* 39: 521–531
42 Smith SG, Lehman NL, Moran RG (1993) Cytotoxicity of antifolate inhibitors of thymidylate and purine synthesis to WiDr colonic carcinoma cells. *Cancer Res* 53: 5697–5706
43 Van Triest B, Pinedo HM, Giaccone G, Peters GJ (2000) Downstream molecular determinants of response to 5-fluorouracil and antifolate thymidylate synthase inhibitors. *Ann Oncol* 11: 385–391
44 Borsa J, Whitmore GF (1969) Cell killing studies on the mode of action of methotrexate on L-cells *in vitro*. *Cancer Res* 29: 737–744
45 Kwok JBJ, Tattersall MHN (1991) Inhibition of 2-desamino-2-methyl-10-propargyl-5,8-dideazafolic acid cytotoxicity by 5,10-dideazatetrahydrofolate in L1210 cells with decrease in DNA fragmentation and deoxyadenosine triphosphate pools. *Biochem Pharmacol* 42: 507–513
46 Taylor W, Slowiaczek P, Francis PR, Tattersall MHN (1982) Biochemical and cell cycle perburbations in methotrexate-treated cells. *Mol Pharmacol* 21: 204–210
47 Houghton JA, Harwood FG, Houghton PJ (1994) Commitment to thymineless death is influenced by cell cycle control processes. *Proc Am Assoc Cancer Res* 35: 316
48 Fisher TC, Milner AE, Gregory CD, Jackman Al, Aherme GW (1993) bcl-2 modulation of apoptosis induced by anticancer drugs: resistance to thymidylate stress is independent of classical resistance pathways. *Cancer Res* 53: 3321–3328
49 Kisliuk RL (2000) Synergistic interactions among antifolates. *Pharmacol Ther* 85: 183–190
50 Faessel HM, Slocum HK, Jackson RC, Boritzki TJ, Rustum YM, Nair MG, Greco WR (1998) Super *in vitro* synergy between inhibitors of dihydrofolate reductase and inhibitors of other folate-requiring enzymes: the critical role of polyglutamylation. *Cancer Res* 58: 3036–3050
51 Ferguson K, Boschelli D, Hoffman P, Oronsky A, Whitely J, Webber S, Gallivan J, Freisheim J, Hynes J, Kerwar SS (1990) Synergy between 5,10-dideaza-5,6,7,8-tetrahydrofolic acid and methotrexate in mice bearing L1210 tumors. *Cancer Chemother Pharmacol* 25: 173–176
52 Takemura Y, Jackman AL (1997) Folate-based thymidylate synthase inhibitors in cancer chemotherapy. *Anticancer Drugs* 8: 3–16
53 Jackman AL, Taylor GA, Calvert AH, Harrap KR (1984) Modulation of the anti-metabolite effects. Effects of thymidine on the efficacy of the quinazoline-based thymidylate synthase inhibitor, CB3717. *Biochem Pharmacol* 33: 3269–3275
54 Jackman AL, Taylor GA, Gibson W, Kimbell R, Brown M, Calvert AH, Judson IR, Hughes LR (1991) ICI D1694, a quinazoline antifolate thymidylate synthase inhibitor that is a potent inhibitor of L1210 cell growth *in vitro* and *in vivo*, a new agent for clinical study. *Cancer Res* 51: 5579–5586
55 Banks SD, Waters KA, Barrett LL, Dickerson S, Pendergast W, Smith GK (1994) Destruction of WiDr multicellular tumor spheroids with the novel thymidylate synthase inhibitor 1843U89 at physiological thymidine concentrations. *Cancer Chemother Pharmacol* 33: 455–459

56 Nottebrock H, Then R (1977) Thymidine concentrations in serum and urine of different animal species and man. *Biochem Pharmacol* 26: 2175–2179

57 Houghton PJ, Houghton JA, Germain G, Torrance PM (1987) Development and characterization of a human colon adenocarcinoma xenograft deficient in thymidine salvage. *Cancer Res* 47: 2117–2122

58 Schultz RM, Patel VF, Worzalla JF, Shih C (1999) Role of thymidylate synthase in the antitumor activity of the multitargeted antifolate, LY231514. *Anticancer Res* 19: 437–444

59 Worzalla JF, Shih C, Schultz RM (1998) Role of folic acid in modulating the toxicity and efficacy of the multitargeted antifolate, LY231514. *Anticancer Res* 18: 3235–3240

60 Houghton PJ, Houghton JA, Hazelton BJ, Radparvar S (1989) Biochemical mechanisms in colon xenografts: thymidylate synthase as a target for therapy. *Invest New Drugs* 7: 59–69

61 Schultz RM, Dempsey JA (2001) Sequence dependence of Alimta (LY231514, MTA) combined with doxorubicin in ZR-75-1 human breast carcinoma cells. *Anticancer Res* 21: 3209–3214

62 Schultz RM, Dempsey JA, Kraus LA, Schmid SM, Calvete JA, Laws AL (1999) *In vitro* sequence dependence for the multitargeted antifolate (MTA, LY231514) combined with other anticancer agents. *Eur J Cancer* 35, suppl 4: S194

63 Tomkinson JL, Worzalla JF, Teng C-H, Mendelsohn LG (1999) Cell cycle modulation by a multitargeted antifolate, LY231514, increases the cytotoxicity and antitumor activity of gemcitabine in HT29 colon carcinoma. *Cancer Res* 59: 3671–3676

64 Adjei AA, Erlichman C, Thornton D (1998) Synergistic cytotoxicity of MTA (LY231514) and gemcitabine *in vitro* and *in vivo*. *Ann Oncol* 9, suppl 2: 168

65 Adjei AA, Erlichman C, Sloan JA (2000) Phase 1 and pharmacologic study of sequences of gemcitabine and the multitargeted antifolate agent in patients with advanced solid tumors. *J Clin Oncol* 8: 1748–1757

66 Tesei A, Ricotti L, dePaola F, Amadori D, Frassinet GL, Zoli W (2002) *In vitro* schedule-dependent interactions between the multitargeted antifolate LY231514 and gemcitabine in human colon adenocarcinoma cell lines. *Clin Cancer Res* 8: 233–239

67 Dempsey JA, Laigle DK, Schultz RM (2000) Effect of the multitargeted antifolate (MTA, Alimta) on human mesothelioma cell lines. *Proc Am Assoc Cancer Res* 41: 127

68 Schultz RM, Dempsey JA, Teicher BA, Harrison DS, Shih C, Kraus LA, Schmid SM (1998) Interactions between the multitargeted antifolate (MTA, LY231514) and cisplatin in non-small cell lung cancer (NSCLC) cell lines. *Proc Am Assoc Cancer Res* 39: 308

69 Schultz R, Rothenberg M, Kourny M, Hankins WD, Kravtsov V (2000) Sequence dependence using combinations of ALIMTA (pemetrexed disodium, LY231514, MTA), gemcitabine and oxaliplatin in human colorectal carcinoma cell lines. *Clin Cancer Res* 6: 1078

70 van der Wilt CL, Kuiper CM, Peters GJ (1999) Combination studies with antifolates and 5-fluorouracil in colon cancer cell lines. *Oncol Res* 11: 383–391

71 Backus HHJ, Pinedo HM, Wouters D, Padron JM, Molders N, van der Wilt CL, van Groeningen CJ, Jansen G, Peters GJ (2000) Folate depletion increases sensitivity of solid tumor cell lines to 5-fluorouracil and antifolates. *Int J Cancer* 87: 771–778

72 Jackson RD, Fry DW, Boritz K (1984) Biochemical pharmacology of the lipophilic antifolate, trimetrexate. *Adv Enzyme Regul* 22: 187–206

73 Calvert H (1999) An overview of folate metabolism: features relevant to the action and toxicities of antifolate anticancer agents. *Semin Oncol* 26, suppl 6: 3–10

74 Hanauske A-R, Chen V, Paoletti P, Niyikiza C (2001) Pemetrexed disodium: a novel antifolate clinically active against multiple solid tumors. *Oncologist* 6: 363–373

75 Worzalla JF, Self TD, Theobald KS, Schultz RM, Mendelsohn LG, Shih C (1997) Effects of folic acid on toxicity and antitumor activity of LY231514 multitargeted antifolate (MTA). *Proc Am Assoc Cancer Res* 38: 478

76 Alati T, Warzalla JF, Shih C, Bewley JR, Lewis S, Moran RG, Grindey GB (1996) Augmentation of the therapeutic activity of lometrexol [(6-R)5,10-dideazatetrahydrofolate] by oral folic acid. *Cancer Res* 56: 2331–2335

77 Schmitz JC, Grindey GB, Schultz RM, Priest DG (1992) Impact of dietary folic acid on reduced folates in mouse plasma and tissues: relationship to dideazatetrahydrofolate sensitivity. *Biochem Pharmacol* 48: 319–325

78 Graul A, Tracy M, Castaner J (1998) Pemetrexed disodium. *Drug Fut* 23: 498–507

79 Norman P (2001) Pemetrexed disodium. *Curr Opin Invest Drugs* 2: 1611–1622

80 Calvert H, Bunn PA (2002) Future directions in the development of pemetrexed. *Semin Oncol* 29, suppl 5: 54–61

81 Hanauske AR (2002) Pemetrexed: translational research in breast cancer. *Semin Oncol* 29, suppl 9: 40–42

82 Anonymous (2000) Pemetrexed disodium (alimta). *Drugs Fut* 25: 527–534

83 Adjei AA (2004) Pemetrexed (alimta), a novel multitargeted antineoplastic agent. *Clin Cancer Res* 10: 4276s–4280s

84 Adjei AA (2003) Pemetrexed (alimta): a novel multitargeted antifolate agent. *Expert Rev Anticancer Ther* 3: 145–156

85 Manegold C (2003) Pemetrexed (alimta, MTA, multitargeted antifolate, LY231514) for malignant pleural mesothelioma. *Semin Oncol* 30, suppl 10: 32–36

86 Manegold C, Aisner J (2002) Pemetrexed for diffuse malignant pleural mesothelioma. *Semin Oncol* 20, suppl 5: 30–35

87 Shepherd FA (2002) Pemetrexed in the treatment of non-small cell lung cancer. *Semin Oncol* 29, suppl 18: 43–48

88 O'Shaughnessy JA (2002) Pemetrexed: an acive new agent for breast cancer. *Semin Oncol* 29, suppl 18: 57–62

89 Chen VJ, Bewley JR, Andis SL, Schultz RM, Iversen PW, Shih C, Mendelsohn LG, Seitz DE, Tonkinson JL (1999) Cellular pharmacology of MTA: a correlation of MTA-induced cellular toxicity and *in vitro* enzyme inhibition with its effects on intracellular folate and nucleoside triphosphate pools in CCRF-CEM cells. *Semin Oncol* 26, Suppl 6: 48–54

90 Niyikiza C, Baker SD, Seitz DE, Walling JM, Nelson K, Rusthoven JJ, Stabler SP, Paoleti P, Calvert AH, Allen RH (2002) Homocysteine and methylmalonic acid: markers to predict and avoid toxicity from pemetrexed therapy. *Mol Cancer Ther* 1: 545–552

Index

The PDR-Series
Progress in Drug Research

Progress in Drug Research is a prestigious book series which provides extensive expert-written reviews on highly topical areas in current pharmaceutical and pharmacological research.

Founded in 1959 by Ernst Jucker, the series moved from its initial focus on medicinal chemistry to a much wider scope. Today it encompasses all fields concerned with the development of new therapeutic drugs and the elucidation of their mechanisms of action, reflecting the increasingly complex nature of modern drug research. Invited authors present their biological, chemical, biochemical, physiological, immunological, pharmaceutical, toxicological, pharmacological and clinical expertise in carefully written reviews and provide the newcomer and the specialist alike with an up-to-date list of prime references.

Starting with volume 61, *Progress in Drug Research* is continued as a series of monographs.

Forthcoming titles:

Imaging in Drug Discovery and Early Clinical Trials (PDR 62), M. Rudin (Editor), 2005
Unbiased Approaches to Drug Target Finding and Validation (PDR 64), D. Jeffery (Editor), 2006
Systems Biological Approaches in Infectious Diseases (PDR 65), H.I. Boshoff (Editor), 2006

Available volumes:

Peptide Transport and Delivery into the Central Nervous System (PDR 61), L. Prokai, K. Prokai-Tatrai (Editors), 2003
Progress in Drug Research, volumes 1–60, E. Jucker (Editor), 1959–2003